INTERVENTIONS FOLLOWING
MASS VIOLENCE AND DISASTERS

Interventions Following Mass Violence and Disasters

Strategies for Mental Health Practice

edited by

ELSPETH CAMERON RITCHIE
PATRICIA J. WATSON
MATTHEW J. FRIEDMAN

THE GUILFORD PRESS
New York   London

© 2006 The Guilford Press
A Division of Guilford Publications, Inc.
72 Spring Street, New York, NY 10012
www.guilford.com

Printed in the United States of America

This book is printed on acid-free paper.

Last digit is print number: 9   8   7   6   5   4   3   2   1

Library of Congress Cataloging-in-Publication Data

Interventions following mass violence and disasters: strategies for mental
health practice / edited by Elspeth Cameron Ritchie, Patricia J. Watson,
Matthew J. Friedman.
    p. cm.
  Includes bibliographical references and index.
  ISBN 1-59385-256-8 (hardcover)
  1. Post-traumatic stress disorder—Treatment. 2. Psychic trauma—
Treatment. 3. Psychotherapy. I. Ritchie, Elspeth Cameron. II. Watson,
Patricia J. III. Friedman, Matthew J.
  RC552.P67I68 2006
  616.85'21—dc22

                                                    2005019698

About the Editors

Elspeth Cameron Ritchie, MD, MPH, is Psychiatry Consultant to the U.S. Army Surgeon General. Her assignments and other missions have taken her to Korea, Somalia, Iraq, Israel, and Vietnam. An internationally recognized expert, Dr. Ritchie brings a unique public health approach to the management of disaster and combat mental health issues. She has published numerous articles on forensic, disaster, and military operational psychiatry.

Patricia J. Watson, PhD, is an Educational Specialist for the National Center for Post-Traumatic Stress Disorder (PTSD) and Assistant Professor in the Department of Psychiatry at Dartmouth Medical School. At the National Center for PTSD, she collaborates with the Substance Abuse and Mental Health Services Administration, the Centers for Disease Control and Prevention, and subject-matter experts to create publications for public and mental health interventions following large-scale terrorism, disasters, and pandemic flu. Dr. Watson is also a project coordinator for the interagency agreement with the Emergency Disaster Branch of the Center for Mental Health Services. Special areas of professional interest include science-to-service interventions in disaster/terrorism events, early intervention treatments for trauma, the effects of childhood trauma on adult coping and development, trauma in children and adolescents, the interface between disability/injury and quality of life, and growth aspects of trauma.

Matthew J. Friedman, MD, PhD, is Executive Director of the U.S. Department of Veterans Affairs National Center for PTSD and Professor of Psychiatry and Pharmacology at Dartmouth Medical School. He has worked with patients with PTSD as a clinician and researcher for 30 years and has published extensively on stress and PTSD, biological psychiatry, psychopharmacology, and clinical outcome studies on depression, anxiety, schizo-phrenia, and chemical dependency. Dr. Friedman has written or coedited 15 books and monographs, 52 book chapters, and 93 peer-reviewed articles in scientific journals. Listed in *The Best Doctors in America*, he is a Distin-guished Fellow of the American Psychiatric Association, past president of the International Society for Traumatic Stress Studies (ISTSS), and Chair of the scientific advisory board of the Anxiety Disorders Association of Amer-ica. He has received many honors, including the ISTSS Lifetime Achieve-ment Award in 1999.

Contributors

Margarita Alegría, PhD, Multicultural Mental Health Research Center, Cambridge Health Alliance, Somerville, Massachusetts; Department of Psychiatry, Cambridge Hospital, Harvard Medical School, Cambridge, Massachusetts

Paul Bartone, PhD, Industrial College of the Armed Forces, National Defense University, Fort McNair, Washington, DC

Richard A. Bryant, PhD, School of Psychology, University of New South Wales, Sydney, Australia

Melissa J. Brymer, PsyD, National Child Traumatic Stress Network, Los Angeles, California

Judith A. Cohen, MD, Center for Traumatic Stress in Children and Adolescents, Department of Psychiatry, Allegheny General Hospital, Pittsburgh, Pennsylvania; Department of Psychiatry, Drexel University College of Medicine, Philadelphia, Pennsylvania

Stephen J. Cozza, MD, Department of Psychiatry, Walter Reed Army Medical Center, Washington, DC

Catherine M. DeBoer, BS, Psychiatry Consultation Liaison Services, Walter Reed Army Medical Center, Washington, DC

James Demer, MD, 10th Mountain Division, U.S. Army, Fort Drum, New York

Matthew J. Friedman, MD, PhD, National Center for PTSD, Veterans Affairs Medical Center, White River Junction, Vermont; Department of Psychiatry, Dartmouth Medical School, Hanover, New Hampshire

Laura E. Gibson, PhD, Behavior Therapy and Psychotherapy Center, University of Vermont, Burlington, Vermont

Geoffrey G. Grammer, MD, Medical Corps, U.S. Army; Psychiatry Consultation Liaison Services, Walter Reed Army Medical Center, Washington, DC

Fred D. Gusman, MSW, National Center for PTSD, Veterans Affairs Palo Alto Health Care System, Menlo Park, California

Jessica L. Hamblen, PhD, National Center for PTSD, Veterans Affairs Medical Center, White River Junction, Vermont; Department of Psychiatry, Dartmouth Medical School, Hanover, New Hampshire

Jack Herrmann, MEd, Center for Disaster Medicine and Emergency Preparedness and Department of Psychiatry, University of Rochester Medical Center, Rochester, New York

William J. Huleatt, LCSW, Walter Reed Army Medical Center, North Atlantic Regional Medical Command, Washington, DC

Adrian T. Kent, JD, PhD, Department of Psychiatry and Behavioral Sciences, University of Oklahoma Health Sciences Center, Tulsa, Oklahoma

Lisa R. LaDue, MSW, National Mass Fatalities Institute, Kirkwood Community College, Cedar Rapids, Iowa

Gregory A. Leskin, PhD, National Center for PTSD, Veterans Affairs Palo Alto Health Care System, Menlo Park, California

Brett T. Litz, PhD, National Center for PTSD, Boston Department of Veterans Affairs Health Care System, Boston, Massachusetts; Department of Psychology, Boston University, Boston, Massachusetts

Anthony P. Mannarino, PhD, Department of Psychiatry, Allegheny General Hospital, Pittsburgh, Pennsylvania; Department of Psychiatry, Drexel University College of Medicine, Philadelphia, Pennsylvania

James E. McCarroll, PhD, Center for the Study of Traumatic Stress, Department of Psychiatry, Uniformed Services University of the Health Sciences, Bethesda, Maryland

Laura Murray, PhD, Department of International Health, Boston University School of Public Health, Boston University, Boston, Massachusetts

April J. Naturale, MSW, Disaster Mental Health Management and Training, Montclair, New Jersey

Fran H. Norris, PhD, National Center for PTSD, Veterans Affairs Medical Center, White River Junction, Vermont; Department of Psychiatry, Dartmouth Medical School, Hanover, New Hampshire

Roderick J. Ørner, PhD, Department of Psychological Services, Lincolnshire Partnership HHS Trust, Baverstock House, University of Lincoln, Lincoln, United Kingdom

Ross H. Pastel, PhD, Medical Service Corps, U.S. Army; Safety, Biosurety, Operations, Plans, and Security, U.S. Army Medical Research Institute of Infectious Diseases, Fort Detrick, Maryland

Betty J. Pfefferbaum, MD, JD, Department of Psychiatry and Behavioral Sciences, University of Oklahoma Health Sciences Center, Oklahoma City, Oklahoma

Jennifer L. Price, PhD, Department of Psychology, Georgetown College, Georgetown, Kentucky

Beverley Raphael, MD, Department of Mental Health, University of Western Sydney, Sydney, Australia

Elspeth Cameron Ritchie, MD, MPH, Department of Psychiatry, Uniformed Services University of the Health Sciences, Bethesda, Maryland

Craig S. Rosen, PhD, Department of Psychiatry and Behavioral Sciences, Stanford University School of Medicine, Stanford, California; National Center for PTSD, Veterans Affairs Palo Alto Health Care System, Menlo Park, California

Josef I. Ruzek, PhD, National Center for PTSD, Veterans Affairs Palo Alto Health Care System, Menlo Park, California

Mark S. Salzer, PhD, Department of Psychiatry, University of Pennsylvania, Philadelphia, Pennsylvania

Arieh Y. Shalev, MD, Department of Psychiatry, Hadassah Medical Center, Jerusalem, Israel

Anthony H. Speier, PhD, Division of Program Development and Implementation, Louisiana Office of Mental Health, Baton Rouge, Louisiana

John Stasinos, MD, Department of Psychiatry, Tripler Army Medical Center, Honolulu, Hawaii

Susan P. Stevens, PsyD, National Center for PTSD, Veterans Affairs Medical

Center, White River Junction, Vermont; Department of Psychiatry, Dartmouth Medical School, Hanover, New Hampshire

Robert J. Ursano, MD, Center for the Study of Traumatic Stress, Department of Psychiatry, Uniformed Services University of the Health Sciences, Bethesda, Maryland

Harold J. Wain, PhD, Department of Psychiatry, Uniformed Services University of the Health Sciences, Bethesda, Maryland

Patricia J. Watson, PhD, National Center for PTSD, Veterans Affairs Medical Center, White River Junction, Vermont; Department of Psychiatry, Dartmouth Medical School, Hanover, New Hampshire

Marleen Wong, MSW, Los Angeles Unified School District, Los Angeles, California

Sally Wooding, PhD, Department of Mental Health, University of Western Sydney, Sydney, Australia

Bruce H. Young, MSW, National Center for PTSD, Veterans Affairs Palo Alto Health Care System, Menlo Park, California

Helena E. Young, PhD, National Center for PTSD, Veterans Affairs Palo Alto Health Care System, Menlo Park, California

Preface

In 2000 the editors of this book and other colleagues began planning an international conference on evidence-based early psychological intervention for victims and survivors of mass violence. The conference planning committee was led by psychiatrists and psychologists from the U.S. Departments of Defense, Veterans Affairs, Justice, and Health and Human Services and the American Red Cross, as well as by numerous international experts. The goal of the conference was to attempt to reach consensus on best practices for early intervention following mass violence.

The focus of the conference was practical. The intent was to provide disaster mental health workers in the field with useful guidance on how to proceed in the wake of mass violence. (Proceedings of this meeting are currently available on the Internet at www.nimh.nih.gov/publicat/massviolence.pdf.) Ironically, the conference had been scheduled, months in advance, for October 29–November 1, 2001, only 6 weeks after the September 11 attacks. As a result, the aftermath of that terrible event provided an immediate context for the discussion and recommendations that emerged. Although there was general agreement that empirical evidence supporting any early intervention was sparse, a surprisingly high level of agreement was achieved in several domains. These included key operating principles, effective early interventions, timing, screening, surveillance, research, and ethical issues.

The events of September 11, 2001, heightened the urgency behind the work of the consensus conference. This book represents a continuation of the process initiated by that conference. It documents clinical and scientific advances that have occurred since September 11 and outlines an agenda for the future. The contributors to this volume represent some of the leaders in this effort, who have participated in empirical research and working meetings with the goal of specifying best practices for mental health disaster response. Though research is ongoing, this volume presents the current state of the art in this area. In addition, the current military mental health experience at the frontlines or with returnees from Iraq and Afghanistan has informed several chapters. There are also chapters that deal in depth with topical issues, such as the aftermath of chemical, biological, or radiological attacks; the care of the wounded; and setting up a family assistance center.

The book consists of five parts containing 21 chapters. The chapters in Part I provide a brief historical overview and a critical review of the core theoretical assumptions and various models for early intervention. Part II covers individual and community preparation, training issues, and needs assessment.

Part III focuses on specific mental health interventions that have been employed in the wake of disasters. Chapters in this section review specific approaches designed for different phases of intervention (corresponding to periods of time) following the disaster. This section also includes chapters on consultation and program evaluation.

Part IV comprises chapters on unique populations and specific intervention approaches. Populations addressed include children and adolescents, ethnocultural minorities, and war zone veterans requiring medical or surgical hospitalization. Intervention scenarios include family assistance centers; large-scale outreach initiatives; psychological management following chemical, biological, radiological, or nuclear attack; and lessons learned from New York City after the 9/11 attacks.

The book finishes with two chapters oriented to scholarly, academic, and policy-minded readers. Chapter 20 delves into the challenges of conducting good research on disaster interventions. Chapter 21 offers general conclusions and proposes an agenda for future research, practice, and policy.

To summarize, this book attempts to specify what is known about early and later interventions following mass casualties and how such knowledge can be used across different settings, contexts, events, and populations. It covers the complete spectrum of current information on such interventions from public mental health approaches for resilient individuals to acute treatment for individuals with significant psychiatric problems. This book has been designed as an accessible, comprehensive, and useful guide for disaster planners and mental health clinicians that will serve as a handbook on contemporary advances in the field. It will provide both a benchmark against which to gauge future accomplishments as well as an impetus toward the achievement of such progress.

ELSPETH CAMERON RITCHIE, MD, MPH
PATRICIA J. WATSON, PhD
MATTHEW J. FRIEDMAN, MD

Acknowledgments

Elspeth Cameron Ritchie would like to thank the members of her family, including Elisavietta and Lyell E. Ritchie, and her husband and children, James, Jessie, and Lyell Curtis. Special thanks as well to Elisavietta for her technical editing.

Patricia J. Watson would like to thank her family and friends, including Jim, Judy, Marsella, Paige, and Jim Watson; Randy Parker; Sharon Thomas; Hemo Tortora; Karen Widerstrom; and Eleanor and David Winters. Special thanks to colleagues Jim Benedict, Matt Friedman, Paula Schnurr, Fran Norris, Joe Ruzek, Jessica Hamblen, Laura Gibson, Seth Hassett, Cecilia Casale, April Naturale, Shauna Spencer, Cam Ritchie, and Dori Reisman.

Matthew J. Friedman would like to thank his family, especially his wife, Gayle Smith, and his children, Abigail, Ezra, Jessica, and Rebecca. He also dedicates this book to the memory of his brother, Dick, and to his parents, Dr. Harry Friedman and Gertrude Friedman Tumarkin.

We, the editors, acknowledge Jan Clark and Peggy Willoughby for providing key support for the project at the National Center for Post-Traumatic Stress Disorder. We also thank all the members of the original October 2001 Mass Violence Consensus Conference and all others who have been involved in related conferences and collaborations since then.

Finally, special thanks to all first responders, public and mental health providers, and military and civilian survivors of mass trauma who have taught all of us what interventions are needed and how they should be provided.

Contents

III. MENTAL HEALTH INTERVENTIONS

IV. SPECIFIC SITUATIONS AND POPULATIONS

V. CREATING AN AGENDA FOR THE FUTURE

PART I

INTRODUCTION

CHAPTER 1

Overview

MATTHEW J. FRIEDMAN, ELSPETH CAMERON RITCHIE,
and PATRICIA J. WATSON

To set this volume in context, it is useful to consider the historical background. The current field of disaster mental health originated in military psychiatry. Frontline treatment (or forward psychiatry), first developed during World War I, has been extensively used, especially by Israel, Norway, Sweden, Australia, and the United States. As developed during World War II by the U.S. military psychiatrist Thomas W. Salmon, frontline treatment emphasizes the importance of administering psychological interventions as close to the front as possible. This process has been modified over time (Artiss, 1963; Kardiner & Spiegel, 1947; Neria & Solomon, 1999; Solomon & Benbenishty, 1986) but has retained the following three major principles:

1. *Proximity*—providing intervention as close to the active (combat) zone as possible.
2. *Immediacy*—providing intervention as soon as possible after an acute combat stress reaction.
3. *Expectancy*—emphasizing that acute stress reaction is a normal response to an overwhelming event, and that rapid recovery and resumption of normal duties are expected.

Many publications on frontline treatment attest to its effectiveness in returning soldiers to duty and in minimizing later morbidity, although little

3

solid empirical evidence supports these claims. The best recent data were obtained in a quasi-experimental study concerning Israeli Defense Force (IDF) personnel during the 1982 War in Lebanon. IDF troops with combat stress reactions (CSRs) either received frontline treatment in a forward-echelon medical unit, close to the battlefield, or were evacuated to rear-echelon units in Israel. Among those who received frontline treatment, 60% returned to active duty and 40% developed posttraumatic stress disorder (PTSD) at 1-year follow-up. In contrast, among those who received rear-echelon treatment, only 22% returned to active duty while 71% met diagnostic criteria for PTSD at 1-year follow-up (Milgram, 1986; Neria & Solomon, 1999; Solomon, Shklar, & Mikulincer, 1987). A recent 20-year follow-up study (Solomon, & Mikulincer, 2004) shows that soldiers who received frontline treatment have lower rates of posttraumatic and other psychiatric symptoms, experience less loneliness, and report better interpersonal functioning compared to similarly traumatized soldiers treated in rear-echelon facilities. Thus, frontline treatment seemed effective for ameliorating the immediate distress of CSR and for preventing later PTSD.

Frontline treatment is a flexible, individualized approach whereby the soldier remains in uniform, stays active with useful (but simple) chores, has the structure and order of a safe environment, has the opportunity to talk at his or her own pace if and when ready, is provided nurturance and peer support by comrades when possible, and is not forced to participate in psychological treatment. In contrast, psychological debriefing (see below) is often mandatory, follows a rigid format, is time limited, is not individualized, and might not be provided by colleagues.

Important early articles and books on frontline treatment from the United States and the United Kingdom include Ahrenfeldt (1958), Salmon (1919), Kardiner (1941), Kardiner and Speigel (1947), Glass (1954), and Artiss (1963).

DISASTER MENTAL HEALTH

Whereas frontline treatment has been focused on combat and the military, disaster mental health focuses on unpredictable events that happen to a civilian population.

Defusing

Defusing is designed as a brief (10–30 minutes) conversational intervention that can occur informally (e.g., during a meal or while standing in line for services). Defusings are designed to give survivors support, reassurance, and information. They may be used when an individual appears preoccupied with thoughts about a stressful event and indicates willingness to discuss them. A typical defusing progresses through four phases: fact finding, inquiring about thoughts, inquiring about feelings, and support and reassurance (Young, Ford, Ruzek, Friedman, & Gusman, 1998).

A report on 510 Swedish peacekeepers deployed to Bosnia showed that peer support followed by defusing led by the platoon commander had a positive effect on both the immediate and the postservice mental health of participants in contrast to other interventions or to no intervention. Defusing had significantly better outcomes than psychological debriefing (Larsson, Per-Olof, & Lundin, 2000). Frontline treatment or its key components have supported earlier conclusions by military psychiatrists that this approach effectively reduces acute combat stress reactions and prevents PTSD (Kardiner & Speigel, 1947; Neria & Solomon, 1999; Solomon & Benbenishty, 1986).

Psychological Debriefing

Psychological debriefing (PD) was initially an application of frontline psychiatry—proximity, immediacy, expectancy—principles to civilian disaster situations. Critical incident stress debriefing (CISD), one type of PD (Mitchell, 1983; Raphael, 1986), is a one-time approach whereby groups of 10–20 trauma-exposed individuals participate in 2- to 3-hour procedures. PD is a group-oriented onsite intervention that occurs shortly after the traumatic event. Although there are variations, a typical debriefing includes seven general components: introduction; review of facts; recounting thoughts and impressions; sharing emotional reactions; normalization of feelings/reactions; future planning/coping/psychoeducation; and disengagement (Bisson, McFarlane, & Rose, 2000; Bryant & Litz, Chapter 9, this volume; Dyregov, 1997).

There is little empirical evidence supporting the efficacy of PD or showing that it prevents PTSD. Some research suggests that PD may even exacerbate posttraumatic distress under certain conditions (by exacerbating intrusive recollections or producing secondary traumatization) thereby increasing the incidence of PTSD (Bisson et al., 2000; Neria & Solomon, 1999).

At the National Institute of Mental Health consensus conference the following recommendation was approved:

> Early intervention in the form of a single one-on-one recital of events and expression of emotions evoked by a traumatic event (as advocated in some forms of psychological debriefing) does not consistently reduce risks of later developing PTSD or related adjustment difficulties. Some survivors (e.g., those with high arousal) may be put at heightened risk for

adverse outcomes as a result of such early interventions. (National Institute of Mental Health, 2002, p. 8)

PUBLISHED LITERATURE

Another way to assess the growth of disaster mental health and PSTD fields is to review the relevant literature. The most authoritative source is the National Center for PTSD's (www.ncptsd.va.gov) PILOTS database (Published Literature on Traumatic Stress), the largest and most comprehensive database (currently over 28,000 citations) on stress, trauma, acute posttraumatic distress, PTSD, and related topics.

Before 1980, the English language literature on PTSD included 207 published articles; most (175) were devoted to combat stress reactions/war neurosis or military-related PTSD. Seminal publications by then included studies of World War I veterans (Kardiner, 1941; Rivers, 1918) and World War II veterans (Archibald & Tuddenham, 1966; Artiss, 1963; Bourne, 1970; Futterman & Pumpion-Mindlin, 1951; Glass, 1954, 1955; Grinker & Speigel, 1945; Salmon, 1919). There was also an outpouring of major articles concerning war neurosis/PTSD, depression, alcoholism, and substance abuse among American veterans of the Vietnam War (Borus, 1973, 1974; DeFazio, 1975; Figley, 1978; Haley, 1974; Helzer, Robins, & Davis, 1976; Howard, 1976; Lifton, 1973; Nace, Meyers, O'Brien, Ream, & Mintz, 1977; O'Neill & Fontaine, 1973; Shatan, 1973, 1978; Wilson, 1978).

The most important publication in 1980 was the American Psychiatric Association's (1980) DSM-III, which first proposed PTSD as an official psychiatric diagnosis and operationalized its diagnostic criteria. It is noteworthy that despite three subsequent revisions of the American Psychiatric Association's canon of diagnoses—DSM-III-R (1987), DSM-IV (1994), and DSM-IV-TR (2000)—the criteria for PTSD have held up quite well.

The trauma, acute stress, and PTSD literature has grown remarkably since 1980. Among the 28,000 publications in the current PILOTS database, over 800 are devoted entirely to the recognition and treatment of acute stress reactions and acute stress disorder.

A major new direction for the literature was the addition of a new diagnosis, acute stress disorder (ASD), in DSM-IV (American Psychiatric Association, 1994). ASD filled an important diagnostic niche between exposure to a traumatic event and potential onset of PTSD symptoms 1 month later. ASD also spurred important research on acute posttraumatic psychological reactions and clinical interventions. We address this in depth in subsequent chapters.

CONSENSUS CONFERENCE

In the Preface we discussed the 2001 Consensus Conference. Its major recommendations focused on key operating principles of early intervention, guidance to evidence-based practice, optimal timing of early interventions, screening for survivors, follow-up guidelines, expertise and training, research and evaluation, and ethical issues. Crucial gaps in knowledge were also identified. The full report is available elsewhere (National Institute of Mental Health, 2002; www.nimh.nih-gov/research/massviolence.pdf).

ACTIVITIES SINCE THE CONSENSUS CONFERENCE

Two major developments among those of the past 3 years that moved the disaster mental health field forward at an accelerating pace are most significant: first, our collective experience with the aftermath of September 11, and second, the current military mental health experience at the frontlines or with returnees from Iraq and Afghanistan.

A major player in learning and disseminating information has been the Center for Mental Health Services (CMHS), a division of the U.S. Department of Health and Human Services' Substance Abuse and Mental Health Services Administration (SAMHSA). This provides funding and assistance for mental health services and outreach following any national disaster through its crisis counseling program. Clinical experience and evaluation data obtained from the CMHS-supported post-9/11 crisis counseling program in New York, Project Liberty, has been a major addition to our understanding about the longitudinal course of acute posttraumatic distress and community-level approaches to alleviate it.

Numerous national surveys conducted within days of the September 11 attacks, some of which remain ongoing (Galea et al., 2002; Schuster et al., 2001; Silver, Holman, McIntosh, Poulin, & Gil-Rivas, 2002), have provided valuable information on the psychological impact of such events, on resilience and recovery among most affected survivors, and on vulnerability and psychiatric morbidity among a significant minority of victims. The bioterrorism program at the Uniformed Services University of the Health Sciences has made great strides in furthering our current understanding and in promoting policy and practice to help prepare for future episodes. The National Institute of Mental Health has published the aforesaid book on the consensus conference, promoted further research, and, in partnership with CMHS, convened several high-level roundtable discussions by national and international experts on methodologies for screening populations at risk and providing effective early interventions in the immediate aftermath of catastrophes. The Centers for Disease Control and Prevention in conjunction with the National Center for Child Traumatic Stress and National Center for PTSD took important steps to develop a public mental health strategy to alleviate the mental health consequences of future mass casualties. The Anxiety Disorders Association of America convened a conference in June 2002 to address key conceptual models and scientific findings pertinent to the phenomenology, psychology, psychobiology, and evidence-based early interventions for adults and children exposed to catastrophes (see Friedman, Foa, & Charney, 2003; Friedman, Hamblen, Foa, & Charney, 2004). Finally, CMHS has supported the National Center for PTSD's ongoing effort to develop evidence-based practice guidelines for early intervention. An important aspect of that initiative has been the development of case histories on Oklahoma City's mental health response following the terrorist bombing of the Murrah Federal Building and Project Liberty's efforts following the World Trade Center attacks (Norris, Watson, Hamblen, & Pfefferbaum, 2005; see also Norris et al., Chapter 18, this volume).

CURRENT STATUS OF THE FIELD

A Population Perspective

Although 95% of individuals exposed to some traumatic event reported some posttraumatic psychological distress, only 29% experienced reactions deemed serious from a clinical perspective. Most reactions were transient with symptom dissipation within a month for 42% and within a year for an additional 23%; only 30% experienced chronic symptoms lasting longer than a year (Norris, Murphy, Baker, & Perilla, 2003). Furthermore, a recent review of 160 studies on disaster survivors suggests that two-thirds will not develop clinically significant chronic psychiatric disorders that persists for months or years (Norris, Friedman, & Watson, 2002; Norris, Friedman, Watson, et al., 2002).

When considering the impact of terrorism, the prevalence of psychological distress appears to be considerably higher than for natural disasters. A random-digit dialing national survey of Americans completed within 3–5 days of September 11 indicated that 44% reported one or more substantial symptoms of severe distress, while 90% reported moderate distress (Schuster et al., 2001). Similar findings come from a Web-based survey of a national probability sample conducted 2 months after the World Trade Center attacks, indicating that 17% of the U.S. population outside New York reported symptoms of September 11-related posttraumatic stress (Silver et al., 2002). It is noteworthy that rates of posttraumatic distress in both studies are considerably higher than the prevalence of PTSD and depression, 7.5 and 9.7% respectively, among New Yorkers within weeks of the World Trade Center attacks (Galea et al., 2002).

Early Detection and Intervention

Although most people exposed to a terrorist attack exhibit psychological distress, we currently cannot distinguish vulnerable from resilient individuals immediately after a terrorist attack, mass casualty, or natural disaster. Whereas some survivors experience transient acute posttraumatic reactions that may be briefly incapacitating, others develop the initial stage of a severe, chronic, and potentially incapacitating psychiatric disorder. A number of prognostic candidates have been proposed as early indicators of future chronicity such as functional impairment (Norris et al., 2003), elevated heart rate (Shalev, Peri, Canetti, & Schreiber, 1996), and negative cognitions (Ehlers & Clark, 2003). Unfortunately, none of these has been tested sufficiently. In addition, the new DSM-IV diagnosis of ASD has had only limited usefulness as a screening criterion for the general population as the majority who develop PTSD will not have met ASD criteria beforehand (Bryant, 2003). Our current inability to develop reliable methods for differentiating resilient from vulnerable individuals immediately after a traumatic event is obviously a major concern for public mental health planners who, understandably, do not want to pathologize normal and transient posttraumatic distress and who do not want to use scarce and expensive clinical resources for individuals who will recover spontaneously or with minimal assistance.

As noted elsewhere (Friedman, 2005) early detection is important because different interventions may be indicated for people situated at different loci along the vulnerability to resilience spectrum. For example, very vulnerable survivors might be most susceptible to the potentially deleterious effects of psychological debriefing shortly after a terrorist attack (Rose & Bisson, 1998). They might do better if treatment is delayed at least several weeks, after which they should be offered a brief course of cognitive-behavioral treatment (Bryant, 2003). In contrast, the most resilient survivors might benefit most from not receiving any formal intervention during the acute posttraumatic phase so that natural recovery processes can run their course (Ehlers & Clark, 2003). They might benefit most from psychoeducational opportunities or family/peer group support.

To summarize, many differences apparently exist between individuals regarding posttraumatic vulnerability versus resilience, the likelihood of transient versus chronic posttraumatic reactions, and the best pretraumatic preparation and posttraumatic interventions.

EVIDENCE-BASED EARLY INTERVENTIONS

Data from both adults and children suggest that attending to basic needs (safety, security food, shelter, acute medical problems, etc.), psychological first aid, clinical assessment, screening, and surveillance may be the best intervention in the early phase of recovery (Friedman, 2005). Treatment at this time could be indirect, for example, focusing on sleep problems, providing educational information about normal reactions to traumatic stress, encouraging survivors to seek support from significant others, and helping parents with their anxiety so as not to frighten children. Focused cognitive-behavioral interventions may be best initiated at least several weeks and possibly several months after the trauma for those individuals still experiencing significant symptoms.

A more extensive discussion of evidence-based early intervention is beyond the scope of this overview. A thorough discussion of practical concerns and the current status of clinical evidence in this regard can be found in later chapters.

WHAT WE KNOW, WHAT WE DON'T KNOW, AND WHAT WE SHOULD DO[1]

We complete our summary with an adapted excerpt from an editorial titled "Toward Evidence-Based Early Intervention for Acutely Traumatized Adults and Children" (Friedman et al., 2003) that introduced a special issue of *Biological Psychiatry*.

Reproduced here are passages concerning phenomenology and early intervention (pp. 766–767).

Phenomenology

1. *We know* that the general response to trauma is one of immediate and significant distress; that most people recover spontaneously but a sizable minority progress to chronic incapacitating disorders such as PTSD or depression; that it is difficult to predict who will recover and who will develop trauma-related chronic disorders; that ASD has limited use as a screening criterion because most who develop PTSD never meet diagnostic criteria for PTSD; and that little current information pertains to children.

---

[1]Material in this section is adapted from Friedman et al. (2003). Copyright 2003, with permission from the Society of Biological Psychiatry.

2. *We don't know* the full range of psychological reactions in the acute phase regarding symptom profiles and functional impairment; how to weigh age, gender, and cultural differences; what measurable acute posttraumatic phenomenological, diagnostic, psychological, and biological factors will let us distinguish resilient survivors from those vulnerable to develop PTSD and other psychiatric problems; and the best methods and instruments to evaluate posttraumatic distress and monitor affected individuals over time.

3. *We can close the gaps in knowledge* by developing models that fully characterize acute phase reactions and predict chronicity; by conducting epidemiological research on the general population and longitudinal studies on specific vulnerable/resilient groups; by developing standard and reliable instrumentation and procedures for such research; and by promoting separate initiatives for children.

Early Intervention

1. *We know* that randomized clinical trials with cognitive-behavioral interventions successfully accelerated recovery and/or reduced PTSD incidence; that randomized trials on individual psychological debriefing indicate that such early intervention is either ineffective or may actually delay recovery; that acute pharmacotherapeutic interventions have been tested sparingly; and that no empirical studies exist on acute psychosocial interventions for children.

2. *We don't know* how knowledge of psychological and biological mechanisms can be translated to effective treatments; what treatments will help trauma survivors at what times; what acute psychotherapeutic and/or pharmacological interventions to recommend at present; and what societal interventions, such as education, preventive actions, community interventions, and risk communication strategies, should currently be recommended.

3. *We can close the gap* by investigating a wide spectrum of individual, group, and community interventions. Research on individual interventions should consider efficacy, effectiveness, timing, treatment setting, dosage, target population, cultural factors, and developmental level. Research on group interventions should rigorously test group debriefings, self-help initiatives, and other psychosocial approaches. Research on societal and community level interventions should systematically evaluate pretraumatic preparation as well as posttraumatic community/societal interventions, and a range of outcomes at both the individual and community level: adaptive functioning, mental/physical health, knowledge/attitudes concerning trauma, effective coping, and health-seeking behavior.

CONCLUSIONS

We have begun to make headway in filling some important gaps. Our growing understanding has enabled us to ask better questions, design more pertinent research, develop new tools for early intervention, and address major educational challenges such as training for professionals and education for the general population. We see this volume as the next step following the post–September 11 conferences and roundtables described in the beginning of this chapter. We hope it will spawn future policy, practice, and research to advance the field with vision, sophistication, humility, creativity, and a strong sense of urgency.

REFERENCES

Ahrenfeldt, R. H. (1958). *Psychiatry in the British Army in the Second World War.* New York: Columbia University Press.

Archibald, H. C., & Tuddenham, R. D. (1965). Persistent stress reaction after combat: A 20–year follow-up. *Archives of General Psychiatry, 12,* 475–481.

Artiss, K. L. (1963). Human behavior under stress: From combat to social psychiatry. *Military Medicine, 128,* 1011–1019.

American Psychiatric Association. (1980). *Diagnostic and statistical manual of mental disorders* (3rd ed.). Washington, DC: Author.

American Psychiatric Association. (1987). *Diagnostic and statistical manual of mental disorders* (3rd ed., rev.). Washington, DC: Author.

American Psychiatric Association. (1994). *Diagnostic and statistical manual of mental disorders* (4th ed.). Washington, DC: Author.

American Psychiatric Association. (2000). *Diagnostic and statistical manual of mental disorders* (4th ed., text rev.). Washington, DC: Author.

Bisson, J. I., McFarlane, A. C., & Rose, S. (2000). Psychological debriefing. In E. B. Foa, T. M. Keane, & M. J. Friedman (Eds.), *Effective treatments for PTSD: Practice guidelines from the International Society for Traumatic Stress Studies* (pp. 39–59). New York: Guilford Press.

Borus, J. F. (1973). Reentry: I. Adjustment issues facing Vietnam veterans. *Archives of General Psychiatry, 28,* 501–506.

Borus, J. F. (1974). Incidence of maladjustment in Vietnam returnees. *Archives of General Psychiatry, 30,* 554–557.

Bourne, P. G. (1970). *Men, stress and Vietnam.* Boston: Little, Brown.

Bryant, R. A. (2003). Early predictors of posttraumatic stress disorder. *Biological Psychiatry, 53,* 789–795.

DeFazio, V. J. (1975). The Vietnam era veteran: Psychological problems. *Journal of Contemporary Psychotherapy, 7,* 9–15.

Dyregrov, A. (1997). The process in psychological debriefings. *Journal of Traumatic Stress, 10,* 589–605.

Ehlers, A., & Clark, D. M. (2003). Early psychological interventions for adult survivors of trauma: A review. *Biological Psychiatry 53*, 817–826.

Figley, C. R. (1978). Symptoms of delayed combat stress among a college sample of Vietnam veterans. *Military Medicine, 143*, 107–110.

Friedman, M. J.(2005). Toward a public mental health approach for survivors of terrorism. *Journal of Aggression, Maltreatment, and Trauma, 10*, 527–539.

Friedman, M. J., Foa, E. B., & Charney, D. S. (2003). Toward evidence-based early interventions for acutely traumatized adults and children. *Biological Psychiatry, 53*, 765–768.

Friedman, M. J., Hamblen, J. L., Foa, E. B., & Charney, D. S. (2004). Fighting the psychological war on terrorism. *Psychiatry, 67*, 123–136.

Futterman, S., & Pumpian-Mindlin, E. (1951). Traumatic war neuroses five years later. *American Journal of Psychiatry, 108*, 401–408.

Galea, S., Ahern, J., Resnick, H. S., Kilpatrick, D. G., Bucuvalas, M. J., Gold, J., et al. (2002). Psychological sequelae of the September 11 terrorist attacks in New York City. *New England Journal of Medicine, 346*, 982–987.

Glass, A. J. (1954). Psychotherapy in the combat zone. *American Journal of Psychiatry, 110*, 725–731.

Glass, A. J. (1955). Principles of combat psychiatry. *Military Medicine, 117*, 27–33.

Grinker, R., & Spiegel, J. (1945). *Men under stress.* Philadelphia: Blakiston.

Haley, S. A. (1974). When the patient reports atrocities: Specific treatment considerations of the Vietnam veteran. *Archives of General Psychiatry, 30*, 191–196.

Helzer, J. E., Robins, L. N., & Davis, D. H. (1976). Depressive disorders in Vietnam veterans. *Journal of Nervous and Mental Disease, 163*, 526–529.

Howard, S. (1976). The Vietnam warrior his experience and implications for psychotherapy. *American Journal of Psychotherapy, 30*, 121–135.

Kardiner, A. (1941). *The traumatic neuroses of war.* Washington, DC: Hoeber.

Kardiner, A., & Spiegel, H. (1947). *War stress and neurotic illness.* New York: Hoeber.

Larsson, G., Per-Olof, M., & Lundin, T. (2000). Systematic assessment of mental health following various types of posttraumatic support. *Military Psychology, 12*, 121–135.

Lifton, R. J. (1973). *Home from the war: Vietnam veterans: Neither victims nor executioners.* New York: Simon & Schuster.

Milgram, N. (1986). *Stress and coping in time of war: Generalizations from the Israeli experience.* New York: Brunner/Mazel.

Mitchell, J. T. (1983). When disaster strikes: The Critical Incident Stress Debriefing. *Journal of Medical Emergency Services, 8*, 36–39.

Nace, E. P., Meyers, A., O'Brien, C. P., Ream, N., Mintz, J. (1977). Depression in veterans two years after Viet Nam. *American Journal of Psychiatry, 134*, 167–170.

National Institute of Mental Health Report. (2002). *Mental health and mass violence—Evidence-based early psychological intervention for victims/survivors of mass violence: A Workshop to Reach Consensus on Best Practices.* Washington, DC: U.S. Department of Defense; U.S. Department of Health and Human Services, the National Institute of Mental Health, the Substance Abuse and Mental Health Services Administration, Center for Mental Health Services; U.S. Department of Justice, Office for Victims of Crime; U.S. Department of Veterans Affairs, National Center for PTSD; and the American Red Cross.

Neria, Y., & Solomon, Z. (1999). Prevention of posttraumatic reactions: Debriefing and frontline treatment. In P. A. Saigh & J. D. Bremner (Eds.), *Posttraumatic stress disorder: A comprehensive test* (pp. 309–326). Boston: Allyn & Bacon.

Norris, F., Friedman, M., & Watson, P. (2002). 60,000 disaster victims speak: Part II. Summary and implications of the disaster mental health research. *Psychiatry, 65* 240—260.

Norris, F., Friedman, M., Watson, P., Byrne, C., Diaz, E., & Kaniasty, K. (2002). 60,000 disaster victims speak: Part I. An empirical review of the empirical literature, 1981–2001. *Psychiatry, 65,* 207–239.

Norris, F. H., Murphy, A. D., Baker, C. K., & Perilla, J. L. (2003). Severity, timing and duration of reactions to trauma in the population: An example from Mexico. *Biological Psychiatry, 53,* 769–778.

Norris, F., Watson, P., Hamblen, J., & Pfefferbaum, B. (2005). Provider perspectives on disaster mental health services in Oklahoma City. *Journal of Aggression, Maltreatment, and Trauma, 10,* 649–661.

O'Neill, D. J., & Fontaine, G. D. (1973). Counseling for the Vietnam veteran. *Journal of College Student Personnel, 14,* 153–155.

Raphael, B. (1986). *When disaster strikes: How individuals and communities cope with catastrophe.* New York: Basic Books.

Rivers, W. H. R. (1918). War neurosis and military training. *Mental Hygiene, 2,* 513–533.

Rose, S., & Bisson, J. I. (1998). Brief early psychological interventions following trauma: A systematic review of the literature. *Journal of Traumatic Stress, 11,* 697–710.

Salmon, T. W. (1919). The war neuroses and their lessons. *Journal of Medicine, 59,* 993–994.

Schuster, M., Bradley, D., Stein, M., Jaycox, L. H., Collins, R. L., Marshall, G. N., et al. (2001). A national survey of stress reactions after the September 11, 2001, terrorist attacks. *New England Journal of Medicine, 345,* 1507–1512.

Shalev, A. Y., Peri, T., Canetti, L., & Schreiber, S. (1996). Predictors of PTSD in injured trauma survivors: A prospective study. *American Journal of Psychiatry, 153,* 219–225.

Shatan, C. F. (1973). The grief of soldiers: Vietnam veterans self-help movement. *American Journal of Orthopsychiatry, 43,* 640–653.

Shatan, C. F. (1978). Stress disorders among Vietnam veterans: The emotional context of combat continues. In C. R. Figley (Ed.), *Stress disorders among Vietnam veterans: Theory, research and treatment* (pp. 43–52). New York: Brunner/Mazel.

Silver, R. C., Holman, E. A., McIntosh, D. N., Poulin, M., & Gil-Rivas, V. (2002). Nationwide longitudinal study of psychological responses to September 11. *Journal of the American Medical Association, 288,* 1235–1244.

Solomon, Z., & Benbenishty, R. (1986). The role of proximity, immediacy and expectancy in frontline treatment of combat stress reaction among Isreali CSR casualties. *American Journal of Psychiatry, 143,* 613–617.

Solomon, Z., & Mikulincer, M. (1987). Combat stress reactions, posttraumatic stress disorder, and social adjustment: A study of Israeli veterans. *Journal of Nervous and Mental Disease, 175,* 277–285.

Solomon, Z., Shklar, R., & Mikulincer, M. (2004, November). *A window of opportunity for psychological first aid: PIE revised 20 years after the Lebanon War.* Paper presented at the annual meeting of the International Society for Traumatic Stress Studies, New Orleans, LA.

Wilson, J. P. (1978). Conflict, stress and growth: The effects of the Vietnam war on psychosocial development among Vietnam veterans. In C. R. Figley & S. Levantman (Eds.), *Strangers at home: Vietnam veterans since the war* (pp. 123–166). New York: Praeger.

Young, B. H., Ford, J. D., Ruzek, J. I., Friedman, M. J., & Gusman, F. D. (1998). *Disaster mental health services: A guidebook for clinicians and administrators.* St. Louis, MO: National Center for PTSD, Department of Veterans Affairs Employee Education System.

CHAPTER 2

Models of Early Intervention Following Mass Violence and Other Trauma

JOSEF I. RUZEK

As trauma's negative effects on many victims of violent physical and sexual assault, disaster, mass violence, and war have become better recognized, there is increasing attention to the possibility that early intervention can reduce suffering and limit chronicity of problems. The evolving field of early intervention includes various practice domains and associated sets of interventions largely shaped by different pragmatic needs, historical experience, and theoretical orientations. These service models are each characterized by design features matched to the populations they serve and the goals they seek.

This chapter outlines three such models commonly applied in situations of mass violence—combat psychiatry, disaster mental health response, and high-risk occupation support—together with two additional models of early care—the rape crisis counseling model applied with numerous survivors of sexual violence, albeit on a sequential basis, and an evolving cognitive-behavioral model of early intervention with assault and accident survivors who receive hospital emergency medical care. Key issues in providing early intervention for survivors of mass violence are explored, in terms of the common assumptions of existing models of care, the nature and importance of "natural" recovery processes, range of potential targets of early intervention efforts, and ways of achieving target behavior change.

SERVICE DELIVERY MODELS

Empirical research into the impact of secondary prevention efforts with trauma survivors is only now beginning. But despite little being known about the effectiveness of such efforts, services intended to prevent or minimize trauma-related problems have routinely been delivered in many settings for years.

A first model of secondary prevention is *combat psychiatry*. War experiences are long recognized as potentially traumatic, and of crucial importance to military encounters, emotional casualties account for significant percentages of those unable to continue fighting. To keep personnel in the field, and to reduce psychiatric problems, armed forces developed principles of *frontline care*. Management of combat stress reactions in active-duty personnel has evolved to use frontline treatment as a way of increasing rate of return to military units and reducing psychological distress. The principles of frontline treatment are *proximity* (administer the intervention close to the traumatic event), *immediacy* (give treatment as soon as possible following onset of symptoms), *expectancy* (a crisis reaction is normal, and quick return to the unit is expected), and *simplicity* (keep interventions easy to deliver and understand). Although the effectiveness of frontline care in reducing the negative consequences of trauma (as opposed to enhancing return to combat) has to date received little empirical examination (Jones & Wessely, 2003), a recent follow-up of combat stress reaction casualties in the Lebanon War supports its use (Solomon, Shklar, & Mikulincer, 2004).

Disaster mental health services represent a second model. Immediate response to disaster is seldom concerned with specialist mental health care but with basic pragmatic assistance (e.g., safety, food, shelter, and communication with family, friends, and community) and psychological first aid (Young, Ford, Ruzek, Friedman, & Gusman, 1998). In the United States, disaster-affected communities may apply for grants for "crisis counseling" services: community education, brief individual and group counseling support, and active outreach programs. Counseling focuses on offering emotional support, "normalizing" expectable traumatic stress reactions, giving advice about coping, and referring to mental health counseling as warranted. Although many aspects of conventional disaster mental health services are consistent with current understanding of traumatic stress, their impact in preventing development of mental health problems is unclear.

A third model of care concerns *worker support in high-risk occupations*. Because response workers often face traumatic stimuli, groups such as police, firefighters, and emergency medical personnel evolved ways of staff support following work-related traumas. Programs can include thoughtful design of work roles, task rotation, peer support systems, involvement of chaplains and other support personnel, employee assistance program services, stress management training, and procedures for daily defusing. In group-administered stress debriefing, a single-session intervention is delivered to groups to promote disclosure of traumatic experiences, normalize reactions to trauma, educate participants about stress reactions, enhance coping, and identify those needing more intensive services. Despite widespread use, many recent reviewers question the approach (Bisson, McFarlane, & Rose, 2000; McNally, Bryant, & Ehlers, 2003), given that so far results of randomized controlled outcome trials indicate that psychological debriefing delivered to individual direct survivors does not prevent posttraumatic stress disorder (PTSD) or other psychopathology. Group debriefing may help group cohesion, morale, and other important outcomes, but we lack empirical proof.

Rape crisis counseling, provided by professional staff and trained volunteers, includes social support, assistance with challenges posttrauma, community education, and systems advocacy. Rape crisis hotlines offer easy-access support and information to survivors, who can seek support while remaining anonymous if preferred. Rape crisis counselors offer crisis counseling, encourage survivors to challenge rape myths, and draw attention to the larger societal environment, helping counteract environment features that may maintain or exacerbate problems. They provide referrals to various mental health, criminal justice system, and social services. Often, crisis counseling services are provided immediately following sexual assault, offering immediate help, 24 hours a day, to women receiving hospital medical care following rape. Sexual assault nurse examiner programs deliver care via hospital emergency departments and address the medical, emotional, and legal needs of women. Though more than 2,000 rape crisis advocacy programs operated across the last 20 years (Kilpatrick, Edmunds, & Seymour, 1992), relatively little is known about their efficacy.

Finally, *cognitive-behavioral early interventions* have recently been developed for use with many patients in hospital emergency services and trauma centers—important "capture sites" for survivors (Ruzek & Cordova, 2003) and also major response centers for survivors of mass violence, large-scale disaster, and toxic exposure (Ruzek, Young, Cordova, & Flynn, 2004). Several controlled trials suggest that brief (i.e., 4–5 sessions) cognitive-behavioral treatments, composed of education, breathing training/relaxation, imaginal and *in vivo* exposure, and cognitive restructuring, within weeks of the trauma, can prevent PTSD in many survivors who meet criteria for acute stress disorder (ASD) associated with nonsexual assault and motor vehicle and industrial accidents (Bryant, Harvey, Dang, Sackville, & Basten, 1998; Bryant, Sackville, Dang, Moulds, & Guthrie, 1999). We do not yet know if these findings also apply to survivors who do not meet criteria for ASD and to other traumatized populations, or whether cognitive-behavioral therapy (CBT) packages will be deliverable by nonspecialists in trauma. A similar (but more intensive) intervention, delivered from 1 to 34 months postbombing (median = 10 months) has been effective with mass violence survivors of a Northern Ireland car bombing (Gillespie, Duffy, Hackmann, & Clark, 2002). Efforts to treat 91 patients with PTSD produced a treatment effect size comparable to those found in CBT efficacy trials.

Some Assumptions of Service Delivery Models

The various models of early care clearly share many core assumptions and practices but differ in important ways.

• *Most people will recover.* The various models all validate the resilience of survivors, and emphasize that most will not develop PTSD or other chronic posttrauma problems. This is underlined by the "expectancy" construct of the combat stress model and underpins the reliance on one or two sessions of education and support on which most disaster mental health practice is based. Thus, CBT is offered only to those expected to fare poorly following trauma. Research on the longitudinal course of trauma symptoms broadly agrees with this view. While frequent, intense, acute stress reactions are common, most dissipate with time; that is, rape survivors report high levels of symptoms in week one but gradual diminishment across the following weeks (e.g., Rothbaum, Foa, Riggs, Murdock, & Walsh, 1992). For disaster survivors, symptoms usually peak in the first year and then diminish, leaving only a few individuals substantially impaired (Norris et al., 2002). However, research shows quite high percentages of survivors of mass violence with enduring problems. For example, a study of Oklahoma City bombing survivors showed that 45% of direct victims developed diagnosable mental health disorders, with extensive psychiatric comorbidity among PTSD cases (North et al., 1999). In such events, the assumption that most recover may restrict adequate planning for substantial numbers left chronically impaired.

• *It is important to intervene soon after trauma.* It is often assumed that interventions delivered in the first days or weeks following trauma are preferable to services delivered months afterward; this is reflected in the imperative of the PIES (proximity, immediacy, expectancy, simplicity) combat stress control model, and in the common early delivery of stress debriefing (e.g., within 72 hours of an event). Some theoreticians suggest that key processes leading to chronicity of problems may occur during month one after traumatization and therefore preventive activities should occur during this time. For example, Shalev (2003) hypothesized that the early weeks posttrauma might represent a critical period when progressive sensitization could create irreversible changes in the central nervous system. Pitman

(1989) hypothesized that increased levels of stress hormones posttrauma may lead to "overconsolidation" of traumatic memories, so early pharmacological intervention might limit this process. Bisson (2003) noted that, according to the logic of emotion processing theory, "the sooner individuals employ factors that promote emotional processing, the less opportunity there is for maladaptive and disruptive cognitive and behavioral patterns to become established" (p. 482). However, there is reason to question whether intervening sooner will result in better care. Ehlers and colleagues (2003) show that CBT delivered to survivors diagnosed with PTSD at approximately 4 months posttrauma could significantly reduce PTSD for most, and that there was no relationship between outcome and time since accident trauma. In their study of debriefing, Bisson, Jenkins, Alexander, and Bannister (1997) found that persons receiving debriefing closer to the time of their burn trauma fared worse. To date, only one study has set out to empirically compare alternative times of intervention. Campfield and Hills (2001) randomly assigned civilian robbery victims to immediate (less than 10 hours posttrauma) or delayed (more than 48 hours) critical incident stress debriefing. At postintervention and 2 weeks postrobbery, number and severity of PTSD symptoms fell in those receiving immediate debriefing. Consideration of when to intervene must depend on more empirical investigation.

   • *It is important to "normalize" acute stress reactions.* The approaches are united in stressing the importance of helping survivors understand that acute stress responses are normal, not dangerous or indicative of personal weakness or mental illness. This emphasis on normalization is consistent with some theory and research. For example, Ehlers and Clark's (2000) cognitive model of PTSD emphasizes appraisals of acute stress reactions as one determinant of subsequent symptoms; some early empirical evidence supports this component of the theory (Steil & Ehlers, 2000). The concept of "anxiety sensitivity" has been used as a summary term for a fear of anxiety-related symptoms that results from the belief that such symptoms have serious negative consequences; research shows that PTSD patients (combat veterans, rape victims, and accident victims) have high levels of anxiety sensitivity (e.g., Taylor, Koch, & McNally, 1992). The normalization construct has received little critical scrutiny, however. McFarlane (2003) notes the relative absence of research on normal distress itself following trauma exposure. Gersons (2003) suggests that describing all acute stress responses as normal is an incorrect public health education message for those who develop longer-term problems. Others note that setting a strong expectation that it is normal for reactions to subside over time may create negative consequences for those significant numbers of (especially, mass violence) survivors whose symptoms continue. To date, there are no studies evaluating the ability of early interventions to "normalize" early reactions, no studies demonstrating that such normalization is related to outcome, and no assessment tool specifically designed to measure normalization.

Just as normalization of responses is expected to set off processes to speed recovery, so pathologization of responses is feared to worsen reactions. Various actions, including use of diagnostic terms, screening for mental health problems, and involvement of mental health professionals in service delivery, are sometimes viewed as contributing to such pathologization. Therefore, diagnostic labels such as "acute stress disorder" and "posttraumatic stress disorder" are rarely used in the rape crisis, frontline psychiatry, disaster mental health, and workplace models. Only the CBT approach uses formal mental health terminology, perhaps because of its grounding in research on psychological treatment and psychopathology.

Concerns about pathologization extend beyond use of terms. Bryant (2003) suggested that identifying individuals needing services within days of trauma may communicate that they are responding in a maladaptive way. Early intervention itself might increase individual survivors' expectancies of developing psychological symptoms or increase awareness of psychological distress. Such concerns about pathologization have not yet been systematically formulated and researched.

• *Brief services will be adequate for most survivors.* In all early-intervention settings, and especially in situations of mass violence, services must be brief to be cost-effective. Brevity is also warranted given that immediate posttrauma distress will remit naturally for many, and may require only limited formal help. However, the preventive efficacy of very brief (i.e., 1–2 sessions) care has not been demonstrated (Bisson, 2003).

A corollary of brief services sufficing for most is that those who experience continuing problems will need more intensive services. Interventions presupposing resilience and effective functioning prior to trauma will be inadequate for many (Bisson, 2003). The need to create stepped-care approaches where levels of service are matched to levels of posttrauma problems is increasingly recognized.

• *It is important to focus on survivors' ongoing adaptive coping.* All service delivery models emphasize supporting adaptive functioning and enhancing coping. In the initial posttrauma period, most forms of intervention focus on pragmatic coping assistance. In disaster response, workers help individuals to reconnect with loved ones, apply for financial compensation, and generally negotiate the helping system. Rape crisis workers guide assault survivors through forensic gynecological exams, coping with stress reactions, and dealing with family members and friends and the legal system. The military understands the significance of homecoming and return to the family and tries to prepare those deployed for return to ordinary life. Support for adaptive coping sometimes involves efforts to return survivors to their functional roles. Frontline psychiatry emphasizes maintenance of work-related tasks during care.

All extant early intervention approaches provide information about useful ways of coping. Given this emphasis on existing care, unfortunately little is known about early coping. Whether existing practices successfully influence subsequent coping efforts, and whether any resulting changes in coping affect outcomes, is largely unknown. Few early interventions systematically teach coping skills. Stress inoculation training has been effective in treating chronic PTSD, and although it does not add to the effectiveness of combined exposure and cognitive restructuring for individuals with ASD (Bryant et al., 1999), it is not yet tested as a stand-alone early intervention.

• *It is important to offer social support.* Adaptive coping is universally understood to involve social support, an umbrella term describing various possible supportive activities, including practical help with problems, emotional understanding and acceptance, normalization of experiences, mutual instruction about coping, and informal cognitive therapy. Rape crisis work emphasizes mutual support among women; occupational stress support systems reinforce mutual support among workers; and combat stress control approaches focus on peer support. This emphasis on support is broadly backed by findings showing the importance of social support in trauma recovery. Lack of such support is a risk factor for PTSD (Brewin, Andrews, & Valentine, 2000). Greater received and perceived social support and higher levels of social embeddedness are associated with less distress among disaster survivors (Norris et al., 2002), and studies of military samples emphasize postdeployment family and community support (e.g., Bolton, Litz, Glenn, Orsillo, & Roemer, 2002). There is some suggestion that perceptions of inadequate social support or negative responses from others may be vital. Studies of sexual assault survivors show that negative responses from others are common and they predict PTSD symptoms better than positive social reactions (Ullman & Filipas, 2001). Zoellner, Foa, and Brigidi (1999), in a prospective study of women survivors of sexual and nonsexual assault, found that PTSD severity at 3 months posttrauma was predicted by degree of interpersonal friction shortly after the assault. While the impact of negative responses from others is evident for women, the importance of social reactions is also true for men. Studying male military peacekeepers, Bolton, Glenn, Orsillo, Roemer, and Litz (2003) found that those whose disclosures met with negative reactions reported more PTSD symptoms than those encountering positive responses.

The literature on disaster suggests that sustaining social support may be harder than mobilizing it (Kaniasty & Norris, 1993). With the departure of concerned media and supportive outsiders, social networks may succumb to fatigue, irritability, and scarcity of resources. Over time, PTSD symptoms may drive away sources of support. Generally, despite all the efforts to promote posttrauma social support across the models, little is known about how these efforts impact perceptions of support, actual support, or subsequent outcomes.

• *It is important to provide active outreach to survivors.* All approaches recognize that survivors must be actively located and engaged if they are to be educated and offered services, and various pragmatic strategies of outreach reflect this view. A central component of the disaster mental health approach is outreach via delivery of services where survivors congregate (e.g., shelters), through informal conversations with designated paraprofessional outreach workers. Rape crisis centers ensure easy access to services via hotlines and often offer services at a first possible point of contact, hospital emergency rooms. Recognizing the difficulty in engaging survivors is also reflected in the development of peer helping services in occupational stress management and military psychiatry. This emphasis on outreach is consistent with what is known about trauma survivor utilization of services—for example, in disasters, many closest to the event do not believe they need help and will not seek services, despite reporting significant emotional distress (Weisaeth, 2001). Following the 2001 attacks on the World Trade Center, Boscarino, Galea, Ahern, Resnick, and Vlahov (2002) found that 19.4% of Manhattan residents living in the most affected area saw a professional for mental health problems within 30 days, but this was little higher than they did in the 30 days *before* the disaster. Some 45% of current PTSD cases and 44% of current depression cases sought at least one mental health visit in the first month, suggesting that many who most needed mental health care ignored it. A study of children (grades 4–12) in 94 public schools 6 months after the attacks (Hoven et al., 2002) indicated that the parents of at least two-thirds of children with probable PTSD had not sought any mental health services for their children.

• *It is vital to identify high-risk survivors.* The models differ in the degree to which they emphasize identifying those at risk for continuing problems. Although all speak to the need to refer some individuals for mental health treatment, this is accomplished in nonsystematic ways in the various early-intervention environments. Mental health providers postdisaster make individual determinations of need for referral based on existing personal knowledge, but few disaster mental health training materials pay attention to evidence-based criteria for referral. Debriefing groups are partly intended to help identify those needing additional services, but their utility for this purpose has not been studied. The evolving CBT approaches emphasize using empirical criteria to select persons for participation in secondary prevention programs, and the studies conducted by Bryant and colleagues all were targeted at individuals at high risk for developing PTSD (i.e., those meeting criteria for a diagnosis of ASD). Although efforts to develop practical screening tools are underway, it is still unclear how best to identify those who may benefit from additional help. Early symptom levels are not necessarily indicative of risk, and predictors of PTSD may vary significantly across trauma populations (Brewin et al., 2000); moreover, the challenge is to predict other problems in addition to PTSD, including other anxiety, substance use, and mood disorders. Bryant (2003) suggests that it may be premature to identify individuals for intervention before 2 weeks posttrauma, that active CBT should not be offered before 2 weeks, and that delay in intervention may be recommended partly to allow survivors time to marshal resources and deal with practical problems.

In the case of biological or chemical attacks, the goal of identifying those needing more intensive care, physical and psychological, would be especially challenging. In particular, it would be hard for emergency medical practitioners to make accurate differential diagnoses, as exposure to various biological or chemical agents may mimic stress reactions or psychiatric problems (Ursano, Norwood, Fullerton, Holloway, & Hall, 2003). After the Aum Shinrikyo Cult sarin attacks in 15 Tokyo subway stations, approximately 5,000 people sought emergency care for exposure, although almost 75% of those seen in hospitals had not been exposed (Bowler, Murai, & True, 2001).

Commentary on Models

The models largely share common assumptions and each model has some notable strengths or emphases. Some are characterized by efficient ways to disseminate services (i.e., delivering debriefing and combat psychiatry via the workplace results in their widespread use). Of great relevance for incidents of mass violence are those approaches that give central importance to outreach systems and persuade survivors to access available services. Easy-access hotlines are routine in rape crisis centers and were recently intensively used by 9/11 survivors in New York. Several care systems focus on offering services at the immediate point of need: for rape and accident survivors in emergency rooms, for combat stress casualties in a war zone, and on-scene support in other disasters.

Several models attend to relatively overlooked processes or issues. Combat psychiatry is built around an awareness of incentives operating on the survivor. This model also shows most explicit efforts to maintain role functioning (e.g., military personnel withdrawn from the battlefront remain in uniform and continue to perform useful tasks). Rape crisis services include important consideration of the larger environments survivors face;

they draw attention to prominent societal "myths" about rape, try to raise community awareness, and advocate for women survivors in various community forums. With the exception of the rape crisis model, most models overlook gender issues, a glaring oversight given higher rates of PTSD in women and the possibility that women's and men's coping and recovery processes may differ. To date, the CBT approach focuses most explicitly on the delivery of evidence-based interventions, but emphasis on evidence is expected to grow in all models.

KEY QUESTIONS REGARDING NATURAL RECOVERY VERSUS FORMAL HELPING

Naturally Occuring Processes of Recovery

The processes of natural recovery from traumatic stress reactions are little understood. But the substantial rates of symptom reduction in the first days and weeks following trauma indicate that natural recovery is a powerful process. They also suggest that formal helping might usefully attempt to support, or promote, natural recovery. That some formal helping efforts might undermine naturally occurring processes of natural recovery has received increasing interest subsequent to studies suggesting that debriefing could worsen distress. A strong, related concern discussed earlier is that professional care may undermine more naturally occurring helping efforts (Bisson, 2003).

Discussion of the relative value of delivering versus withholding formal interventions must consider expected rates of natural recovery and the timing of intervention. While some individuals will likely recover within 1–2 months, others recover more gradually (e.g., after 6–12 months), and thus concerns about possible but not yet demonstrated negative effects of intervention must be balanced against possibilities of untreated survivors experiencing continuing distress. More centrally, any reliance on natural recovery is limited by its frequent failure, especially given mass violence. Research shows findings of high rates of ongoing problems, including PTSD, from these events. It must also be acknowledged that "natural processes" sometimes backfire. Significant others may disparage seeking social support, which may increase distress and inhibit recovery. Disclosure of traumatic experiences may not occur, or if it does, it may elicit various negative social reactions that exacerbate problems. For example, 14% of a sample of male Somalia peacekeepers reported a negative reaction to their disclosures, and 16% did not discuss their experiences with anyone (Bolton, Glenn, Orsillo, Roemer, & Litz, 2003). Others may constrain disclosure in various ways, with worse outcomes. In a study of rape survivors, specific negative social reactions of "treating the victim differently" (stigmatizing) and distraction (e.g., telling the victim to move on with her life) predicted PTSD symptom severity (Ullman & Filipas, 2001).

Formal Helping

If natural recovery processes account for some reduction in acute stress symptoms, then formal early-intervention efforts may benefit from strengthening these processes. Shalev and Ursano (2003) emphasized the role of trauma in eliciting powerful adaptive mechanisms, suggested that the helper's role may be to identify and manage obstacles to self-regulation on the survivor's part, and speculated that "ignorance of such adaptive forces and failure to engage them might have been the worst systematic error of early intervention programs devised so far" (p. 128). Therefore the aim of some forms of early intervention may be to encourage normal healing processes but to identify and intervene in individuals needing more help. For those at high risk for chronic PTSD, specialized formal helping efforts may possibly produce greater benefits than naturally occurring helping processes. Demonstrations of effective specialized helping interventions by trained mental health professionals in reducing chronic PTSD symptoms argue for early formal helping. Foa and Cahill (2002) argue that the same processes underlie change in both formal treatment and natural recovery: emotional engagement with feared stimuli; habituation, or the gradual reduction in fear from traumatic stimuli during successive psychological exposures; and modification of distressing trauma-related beliefs or cognitions. Social disclosure to nonprofessional support persons may organize memories and extinguish strong emotional responses (Bolton et al., 2003).

Nonetheless, formal help may provide a more systematic, sustained, or efficient approach to change (e.g., via multiple helping contacts between survivor and helpers) and better manipulate these change processes. Formal help may show a clearer "contract" between helper and survivor, more explicit goal setting, or the survivor's increased acceptance of responsibility for change. If theoretical accounts of recovery that emphasize emotion processing are correct, formal help may be necessary to increase the likelihood that survivors will process their experiences and emotions in ways that result in recovery. Perrin (2003) suggested that conditioning theory predicts that methods of bringing people into contact with the conditioned stimuli associated with traumatization—*in vivo* exposure, imaginal exposure, and writing or talking about the experience—will vary in effectiveness, and that by contrast with naturally occurring discussions of traumatic experiences, therapist-facilitated disclosure will seek to maximize recall of all stimuli encountered during the traumatic event (Perrin, 2003).

WHAT ARE APPROPRIATE TARGETS
OF EARLY INTERVENTION?

To date, evidence and theory are consistent with the targeting of a range of hypothetical behaviors and processes that may be expected to affect the trajectory of posttrauma reactions. Perhaps most important, they focus on the need to *increase therapeutic exposure* to the (internal and external) stimuli associated with the traumatic experience, variously construed as helping to extinguish conditioned emotional responses, accessing the fear network and incorporating new information, or constructing a narrative and better organizing the trauma memory. Whether individuals should be encouraged to talk in detail about their traumatic experiences soon after trauma occurs is complicated, and current opinion reflects a range of issues: that individuals should not be pushed to do so, that it may be contraindicated for some (e.g., recently traumatically bereaved individuals), that such exploration may in some cases have a negative impact, but that such a process may play a role in both natural recovery and therapist-facilitated treatments.

The cognitive-behavioral emotional processing approach also emphasizes the importance of *modifying negative trauma-related beliefs.* One goal of early intervention is to ensure that trauma survivors are making sense of their experience and its implications in adaptive and stress-containing or -reducing ways. In fact, much of existing practice in response to trauma survivors involves, in delivery contexts from rape crisis counseling to disaster mental health, the informal shaping of trauma-related beliefs, interpretations, and judgments. Education about trauma and its impact, the challenging of rape "myths," the normalization of acute stress reactions, and the instillation of hope for the future all involve the belief system of the survivor and its impact on recovery. A focus on posttrauma cognitive processes is in fact consistent with much current thinking about traumatic stress, and Bryant (2002) has found that cognitive therapy without exposure is an effective early intervention for those with ASD.

Because the research literature indicates that different forms of coping are associated with response to trauma, early interventions might (and do) seek to *improve coping efforts.* Indeed, in all models early helping efforts often include attention to *enhancing coping with posttrauma reactions* or "symptoms." Some include attempts to *reduce high arousal* during immediate posttrauma period, and most work to *decrease fear of acute stress reactions.* Important questions remain as to how central abilities to manage (or tolerate) acute anxiety levels are to recovery, and whether our efforts to help survivors with these are optimally effective. Most existing efforts involve simply providing information, and more sophisticated methods, including skills training, interoceptive exposure to anxiety sensations, and medications, require study. Evidence also suggests the potential importance of *preventing maladaptive coping* with acute stress reactions and trauma-related problems. Such problematic coping includes extreme avoidance, social isolation/withdrawal, and self-medication via alcohol and drugs. Early interventions may benefit from including systematic efforts to block maladaptive coping. In particular, existing evidence-based interventions aimed at reducing alcohol consumption should be investigated as posttrauma applications. Brief intervention with patients hospitalized for injury has reduced alcohol consumption in those with existing alcohol problems (Gentilello et al., 1999).

As noted previously, the consistent finding that perceived social support is associated with better outcomes posttrauma suggests that early helping efforts usefully attempt to *increase social support*. Although all the existing models emphasize the need to provide the survivor with social support, in most cases this is addressed in a relatively simple manner (e.g., pragmatic reconnection with loved ones, simple advice to seek and give support, and, for some, provision of professional-led or self-help support groups). Specific secondary prevention interventions attempting to shape social support are few, whether individual (Cordova, Ruzek, Benoit, & Brunet, 2003) or group based. Evidence to date suggests that such attempts should include efforts to reduce negative responses from others, especially partner/spouse and family (Bolton et al., 2003) and increase perceptions of support. Findings showing an association between degree of resource loss following disaster and depression suggest the importance of seeking to *prevent loss of resources and reduce continuing negative consequences* and of interventions designed to help survivors *maintain functioning* soon after the trauma.

HOW DO WE BEST FACILITATE BEHAVIOR CHANGE?

Education via Brief Information and Advice

All approaches considered in this chapter include significant efforts to educate survivors. Much of "early intervention" is really simple education giving survivors information intended to help them recover. Brief educational efforts are relatively nonstigmatizing, low-cost forms of care deliverable via public health media communication, informal conversations with a range of helpers, or structured formal presentations. While education is generally intended to achieve many of the goals delineated previously, probably only *some* objectives are routinely achieved by existing educational practices. Simple education is surely effective in informing survivors about sources of mental health counseling, and in sometimes effecting some change in targeted behaviors, such as reducing alcohol consumption or using formal counseling services. This may be particularly true when the required change is easily within the repertoire of the survivor, as in the seeking of counseling. When desired behaviors require more complex social performances (e.g., seeking social support), simple instruction may be less effective. Similarly, when they involve possible increases in negative emotion (e.g., talking about the experience of trauma) or other disincentives, education may have limited impact. For example, Ehlers and colleagues (2003) found that an educational self-help manual was ineffective in reducing PTSD symptoms, possibly because of difficulties in inducing self-managed exposure to feared situations. Currently, much of our posttrauma care involves simple survivor education, often via pamphlets, self-help materials, and informal discussions between trauma survivors and helpers. Little is currently known about the impact of such efforts, or of the more formal didactic educational presentations common in many posttrauma environments. Little is known about how well those receiving trauma-related information comprehend and retain that information. This is an important issue, given that acute stress reactions are likely to impair concentration and memory processes.

Education included in some early-intervention attempts failed to prevent or reduce PTSD (e.g., Bryant et al., 1999), although education has usually been delivered as part of a control (comparison) intervention. However, Resnick, Acierno, Holmes, Kilpatrick, and Jager (1999) demonstrated that simple education *can* produce some benefits for survivors. They showed a 17-minute educational videotape to recent rape victims, to prepare them for forensic rape examinations. Those who viewed the video, which presented information about and modeling of exam procedures, advice about ways of engaging in self-exposure to rape-related cues, information about cognitive and physiological reactions to rape, and ways of managing mood, demonstrated significant decreases in postexam distress ratings and anxiety symptoms.

Moderate-Intensity Interventions

In their International Society for Traumatic Stress Studies practice guideline for debriefing, Bisson and colleagues (2000) concluded that "more complex interventions for those individuals at highest risk may be the best way to prevent the development of PTSD following trauma" (p. 54). This conclusion agrees with current evidence and understanding of change processes. As noted, a primary limitation of any brief educational approach is that a single episode of advice and group discussion will likely be limited in impact on the more complex actions important to recovery. However, in moderate-intensity multisession interventions, key messages can be repeated; supportive relationships among members developed; skills instructed, practiced, and polished; recovery behaviors shaped and reinforced; and myriad group helping processes extended in duration. Multicontact interventions may enable applying some potentially powerful (and evidence-consistent) helping methods: skills training, therapeutic repetitive exposure, and cognitive restructuring (cognitive therapy). Skills-training technology (including skills instruction, practice, and coaching; demonstration or modeling of skills; self-monitoring of key behaviors; and use of task assignments in the real-world environment) remains to be more effectively harnessed as a potential early intervention. Teachable skills might include anxiety management, disclosure, social support seeking, support giving, and problem solving. Increased use of moderate-intensity interventions may also help ensure that the survivor's environment will facilitate recovery. Whereas many intervention approaches focus on intrapersonal processes and individual survivor behaviors, early intervention also needs to target the larger social environment, which can influence survivor behavior in various ways that negate or enhance the efforts of individual mental health providers. Interventions explicitly targeting social support processes require development, including efforts to build and maintain family support and to create support networks for those lacking it.

CONCLUSION

Early intervention services for survivors of mass violence and trauma are increasingly available and, in many contexts, have become part of routine service provision. Current models have evolved to fit the survivor populations they serve and the contexts of care in which they operate, include many innovative elements, and target processes of change that generally match current theories and research evidence. It remains unclear how effectively these systems accomplish the major tasks of early intervention: managing acute stress reactions, preventing and reducing the continuing negative trauma-related consequences, building recovery-supportive social environments, and, at the appropriate time, facilitating adaptive "emotional processing" of the trauma experience. As early interventions are increasingly based on systematic theory and subjected to empirical testing, surely some practices will be rejected, others maintained, and most modified to become more effective. Mental health workers and organizations must remain informed about ongoing developments and must find ways to combine experiential, theoretical, and research knowledge; remain flexible in selecting their methods and learning effective helping skills; and critically evaluate their early-intervention approaches.

REFERENCES

Bisson, J. I. (2003). Single-session early psychological interventions following traumatic events. *Clinical Psychology Review, 23,* 481–499.

Bisson, J., Jenkins, P., Alexander, J., & Bannister, C. (1997). A randomized controlled trial of psychological debriefing for victims of acute burn trauma. *British Journal of Psychiatry, 171,* 78–81.

Bisson, J. I., McFarlane, A. C., & Rose, S. (2000). Psychological debriefing. In E. B. Foa, T. M. Keane, & M. J. Friedman (Eds.), *Effective treatments for PTSD: Practice guidelines from the International Society for Traumatic Stress Studies* (pp. 39–59). New York: Guilford Press.

Bolton, E. E., Glenn, D. M., Orsillo, S., Roemer, L., & Litz, B. T. (2003). The relationship between self-disclosure and symptoms of posttraumatic stress disorder in peacekeepers deployed to Somalia. *Journal of Traumatic Stress, 16,* 203–210.

Bolton, E. E., Litz, B. T., Glenn, D. M., Orsillo, S., & Roemer, L. (2002). The impact of homecoming reception on the adaptation of peacekeepers following deployment. *Military Psychology, 14,* 241–251.

Boscarino, J. A., Galea, S., Ahern, J., Resnick, H., & Vlahov, D. (2002). Utilization of mental health services following the September 11th terrorist attacks in Manhattan, New York City. *International Journal of Emergency Mental Health, 4,* 143–155.

Bowler, R. M., Murai, K., & True, R. H. (2001). Update and long-term sequelae of the sarin attack in the Tokyo, Japan subway. *Chemical Health and Safety,* pp. 1–3.

Brewin, C. R., Andrews, B., & Valentine, J. D. (2000). Meta-analysis of risk factors for posttraumatic stress disorder in trauma-exposed adults. *Journal of Consulting and Clinical Psychology, 68,* 748–766.

Bryant. R. A. (2002, November 7–10). *Enhancing treatment effectiveness for acute stress disorder.* Paper presented at the annual meeting of the International Society for Traumatic Stress Studies, Baltimore.

Bryant, R. A. (2003). Cognitive behavior therapy of acute stress disorder. In R. Orner & U. Schnyder (Eds.), *Reconstructing early intervention after trauma: Innovations in the care of survivors* (pp. 159–168). Oxford, UK: Oxford University Press.

Bryant, R. A., Harvey, A. G., Dang, S. T., Sackville, T., & Basten, C. (1998). Treatment of acute stress disorder: A comparison of cognitive-behavioral therapy and supportive counseling. *Journal of Consulting and Clinical Psychology, 66,* 862–866.

Bryant, R. A., Sackville, T., Dang, S. T., Moulds, M., & Guthrie, R. (1999). Treating acute stress disorder: An evaluation of cognitive behavior therapy and supportive counseling techniques. *American Journal of Psychiatry, 156,* 1780–1786.

Campfield, K. M., & Hills, A. M. (2001). Effect of timing of critical incident stress debriefing (CISD) on posttraumatic symptoms. *Journal of Traumatic Stress, 14,* 327–340.

Cordova, M. J., Ruzek, J. I., Benoit, M., & Brunet, A. (2003). Promotion of emotional disclosure following illness and injury: A brief intervention for medical patients and their families. *Cognitive and Behavioral Practice, 10*, 359–372.

Ehlers, A., & Clark, D. M. (2000). A cognitive model of posttraumatic stress disorder. *Behaviour Research and Therapy, 38*, 319–345.

Ehlers, A., & Clark, D. M. (2003). Early psychological interventions for adult survivors of trauma: A review. *Biological Psychiatry, 53*, 817–826.

Ehlers, A., Clark, D. M., Hackmann, A., McManus, F., Fennell, M., Herbert, C., et al. (2003). A randomized controlled trial of cognitive therapy, self-help, and repeated assessment as early interventions for PTSD. *Archives of General Psychiatry, 60*, 1024–1032.

Foa, E. B., & Cahill, S. P. (2002). Specialized treatment for PTSD: Matching survivors to the appropriate modality. In R. Yehuda (Ed.), *Treating trauma survivors with PTSD* (pp. 43–62). Washington, DC: American Psychiatric Association Press.

Gentilello, L. M., Rivara, F. P., Donovan, D. M., Jurkovich, G. J., Daranciang, E., Dunn, C. W., et al. (1999). Alcohol interventions in a trauma center as a means of reducing the risk of injury recurrence. *Annals of Surgery, 230*, 473–483.

Gersons, B. P. R. (2003). Historical background: social psychiatry and crisis theory. In R. Orner & U. Schnyder (Eds.), *Reconstructing early intervention after trauma: Innovations in the care of survivors* (pp. 14–23). Oxford, UK: Oxford University Press.

Gillespie, K., Duffy, M., Hackmann, A., & Clark, D. M. (2002). Community based cognitive therapy in the treatment of post-traumatic stress disorder following the Omaha bomb. *Behaviour Research and Therapy, 40*, 345–357.

Hoven, C. W., Duarte, C. S., Lucas, C. P., Mandell, D. J., Cohen, M., Rosen, C., et al. (2002). *Effects of the World Trade Center attack on New York City public school students: Initial report to the New York City Board of Education.* New York: Applied Research and Consulting LLC, Columbia University Mailman School of Public Health, and New York State Psychiatric Institute.

Jones, E., & Wessely, S. (2003). "Forward psychiatry" in the military: Its origins and effectiveness. *Journal of Traumatic Stress, 16*, 411–419.

Kaniasty, K., & Norris, F. (1993). A test of the support deterioration model in the context of natural disaster. *Journal of Personality and Social Psychology, 64*, 395–408.

Kilpatrick, D. G., Edmunds, C. N., & Seymour, A. K. (1992). *Rape in America: A report to the nation.* Arlington: National Victims Center and Medical University of South Carolina.

McFarlane, A. C. (2003). Early reactions to traumatic events: The diversity of diagnostic formulations. In R. Orner & U. Schnyder (Eds.), *Reconstructing early intervention after trauma: Innovations in the care of survivors* (pp. 45–56). Oxford, UK: Oxford University Press.

McNally, R. J., Bryant, R. A., & Ehlers, A. (2003). Does early psychological intervention promote recovery from posttraumatic stress? *Psychological Science in the Public Interest, 4*, 45–77.

Norris, F. H., Friedman, M. J., Watson, P. J., Byrne, C. M., Diaz, E., & Kaniasty, K.

(2002). 60,000 disaster victims speak: Part I. An empirical review of the empirical literature, 1981–2001. *Psychiatry, 65,* 207–239.

North, C. S., Nixon, S. J., Shariat, S., Mallonee, S., McMillen, J. C., Spitznagel, E. L., & Smith, E. M. (1999). Psychiatric disorders among survivors of the Oklahoma City bombing. *Journal of American Medical Association, 282,* 755–762.

Perrin, S. (2003). Learning theory perspectives on early reactions to traumatic events. In R. Orner & U. Schnyder (Eds.), *Reconstructing early intervention after trauma: Innovations in the care of survivors* (pp. 65–71). Oxford, UK: Oxford University Press.

Pitman, R. K. (1989). Posttraumatic stress disorder, hormones, and memory. *Biological Psychiatry, 26,* 645–652.

Resnick, J., Acierno, R., Holmes, M., Kilpatrick, D. G., & Jager, N. (1999). Prevention of post-rape psychopathology: Preliminary findings of a controlled acute rape treatment study. *Journal of Anxiety Disorders, 13,* 359–370.

Rothbaum, B. O., Foa, E. G., Riggs, D. S., Murdock, T. B., & Walsh, W. (1992). A prospective examination of post-traumatic stress disorder in rape victims. *Journal of Traumatic Stress, 5,* 455–475.

Ruzek, J. I., & Cordova, M. J. (2003). The role of hospitals in delivering early intervention services following traumatic events. In R. Orner & U. Schnyder (Eds.), *Reconstructing early intervention after trauma* (pp. 228–235). Oxford, UK: Oxford University Press.

Ruzek, J. I., Young, B. H., Cordova, M. J., & Flynn, B. W. (2004). Integration of disaster mental health services with emergency medicine. *Prehospital and Disaster Medicine, 19,* 46–53.

Shalev, A. Y. (2003). Psychobiological perspectives on early reactions to traumatic events. In R. Orner & U. Schnyder (Eds.), *Reconstructing early intervention after trauma: Innovations in the care of survivors* (pp. 57–64). Oxford, UK: Oxford University Press.

Shalev, A. Y., & Ursano, R. J., & (2003). Mapping the multidimensional picture of acute responses to traumatic stress. In R. Orner & U. Schnyder (Eds.), *Reconstructing early intervention after trauma: Innovations in the care of survivors* (pp. 118–129). Oxford, UK: Oxford University Press.

Solomon, Z., Shklar, R., & Mikulincer, M. (2004, November 14–18). *A window of opportunity for psychological first-aid: PIE revised 20 years after the Lebanon War.* Paper presented at the annual meeting of the International Society for Traumatic Stress Studies, New Orleans.

Steil, R., & Ehlers, A. (2000). Dysfunctional meaning of posttraumatic intrusions in chronic PTSD. *Behaviour Research and Therapy, 38,* 537–558.

Taylor, S., Koch, W. J., & McNally, R. J. (1992). How does anxiety sensitivity vary across the anxiety disorders? *Journal of Anxiety Disorders, 6,* 249–259.

Ullman, S. E., & Filipas, H. H. (2001). Predictors of PTSD symptom severity and social reactions in sexual assault victims. *Journal of Traumatic Stress, 14,* 369–389.

Ursano, R. J., Norwood, A. E., Fullerton, C. S., Holloway, H. C., & Hall, M. (2003). Terrorism with weapons of mass destruction: Chemical, biological, nuclear, radiological, and explosive agents. In R. J. Ursano & A. E. Norwood

(Eds.), *Annual review of psychiatry* (Vol. 22, pp. 125–154). Washington, DC: American Psychiatric Association Press.

Weisaeth, L. (2001). Acute posttraumatic stress: Nonacceptance of early intervention. *Journal of Clinical Psychiatry, 62,* 35–40

Young, B. H., Ford, J. D., Ruzek, J. I., Friedman, M., & Gusman, F. D. (1998). *Disaster mental health services: A guide for clinicians and administrators.* Palo Alto, CA: National Center for Post-Traumatic Stress Disorder.

Zoellner, L. A., Foa, E. B., & Brigidi, B. D. (1999). Interpersonal friction and PTSD in female victims of sexual and nonsexual assault. *Journal of Traumatic Stress, 12,* 689–700.

PART II

PREPARATION, TRAINING, AND NEEDS ASSESSMENT

Improving Resilience Trajectories Following Mass Violence and Disaster

PATRICIA J. WATSON, ELSPETH CAMERON RITCHIE,
JAMES DEMER, PAUL BARTONE, and BETTY J. PFEFFERBAUM

Recently, interest in resilience-building interventions that help individuals prepare for and recover from disasters and terrorism has surged. Unfortunately, the constructs used to define resilience are often extrapolated loosely and/or interchangeably. Program recommendations often lack a sound empirical and theoretical base. Research in resilience, hardiness, stress resistance, and recovery from trauma has been conducted within the fields of developmental pathology, trauma, and positive psychology, with little cross-referencing among fields (Luthar & Zelazo, 2000).

First we define a few core constructs related to resilience, with a discussion of their possible contributions to intervention strategies to foster resilience and recovery.

CORE CONSTRUCTS

Resilience

The American Psychological Association Task Force on Promoting Resilience in Response to Terrorism defines resilience as "the process of adapting well in the face of adversity, trauma, tragedy, threats, or even significant sources of stress." It cites many studies showing that the primary factors in resilience are (1) caring relationships within and outside the family that create love and trust, provide role models, and encourage and reassure; (2) the capacity to make realistic plans and implement them; (3) self-confidence; (4) communication and problem-solving skills; and (5) the capacity to manage emotions. It is generally accepted that resilience is common and derives from the basic human ability to adapt to new situations (Masten, 2001).

Most writings on resilience have come from developmental psychopathology, where initially researchers tried to identify general characteristics associated with resilient recovery from stressors: resourcefulness, hardiness, self-efficacy, and flexibility (Luthar & Cicchetti, 2000). Currently, there is a trend toward further refining the constructs of adaptation to stress and traumatic stress. For instance, whereas stress-"resistant" individuals may not exhibit any change in functioning or distress after exposure to a stressor, resilient individuals may exhibit an initial decremental response, followed by an accelerated or positive recovery (Steinberg, 2004). This distinction is functional in that the processes that foster resistance may be different from those that foster resilience.

Resilience is generally considered to be "multidimensional" (Luthar & Cicchetti, 2000), with different characteristics expressed variably across many areas of the individual's life (e.g., occupation and social). These "resilient trajectories" may be uneven (Luthar & Cicchetti, 2000; Tusaie & Dyer, 2004); for example, an individual may function adequately in work settings following a trauma but suffer from interpersonal numbing or withdrawal. Furthermore, the expression of resilience is influenced by context: the quality of the stressor, the individual's traits, and the surrounding culture (Tusaie & Dyer, 2004). Many researchers in this area conclude that resilience is not a fixed attribute but a type of "functional trajectory" dependent on circumstances and individual variations (e.g., vulnerability and protective mechanisms) in response to risk. If circumstances change, resilience trajectories can change (Luthar & Cicchetti, 2000; Rutter, 1993).

The literature delineates some caveats regarding the application of resilience research to practical interventions. First, few longitudinal prospective studies track resilient trajectories in adulthood. In addition, it is rare to delineate the interplay between multiple risk and protective factors at individual, family, and broader social level. Multidimensional analysis indicates that resilient behavior in one domain may extract a price in another; for example, competence in work domains may involve emotional detachment from family problems (Anthony & Cohler, 1987; Werner & Smith, 1992), and at-risk individuals with exemplary behavior may experience internal distress (Cohler, Stott, & Musick, 1995; Luthar, 1991). Finally, there has been some acknowledgment that the factors that bolster both resistance and resilience may not be adaptive in all domains (i.e., sociopathy and narcissism) (Bonanno, 2004).

Experts in the field of resilience hold that all plans for research and intervention should clearly define resilience as a state, not a trait (Luthar & Cicchetti, 2000). Therefore, they recommend avoiding the term "resiliency," with its connotation of a trait. Rather, it is recommended to use the phrase "resilient trajectory or adaptation," explaining that these trajectories vary across situations and within individuals at different times (Luthar & Cicchetti, 2000).

Resilience researchers have moved from producing relevant lists of protective factors to attempting to prioritize domains most likely to yield robust benefits in interventions. For instance, the child/family literature demonstrates that resilience-based interventions must address the quality of parent–child relationships and well-being of caregivers. Many intervention programs have sought to increase coping and parenting skills, as well as to foster improved social networks and to build resources. As expected, social support appears to play a strong role. When resilient children, youth, and adults in Werner and Smith's (1992) longitudinal study were asked who helped them succeed, they credited extended family, neighbors, mentors in voluntary associations, and teachers who were confidants and role models. Support from such an informal network was more often sought and appreciated than that of mental health professionals (Werner, 1990a, 1990b, as cited in Werner & Johnson, 1999).

Other Factors Contributing to Resilience

A number of other theoretical constructs have overlap with resilience. They include hardiness, coping self-efficacy, posttraumatic recovery, posttraumatic growth, and biological processes related to resilience.

Hardiness is a characteristic that has been shown to neutralize the negative effects of stress. Similar to the findings in the resilience literature, research with hardy individuals suggests that they often employ multiple strengths that foster resilient recovery: (1) They seek help and build large support networks and reframe their experiences more positively (e.g., difficulties as leading to benefits); (2) they believe they can change a stressor or recover from its detrimental effects; (3) they focus selectively on the positive effects of a trauma; (4) they view themselves as controlling their fate, are committed to meaningful goals, and view stress as a surmountable challenge; and (5) they are less likely to use behavioral disengagement, denial, mental disengagement, and alcohol to confront stress and more likely to try to solve problems (Kobasa, Maddi, & Kahn, 1982; Maddi & Hightower, 1999; Waysman, Schwarzwald, & Solomon, 2001).

Coping self-efficacy (CSE), a specific form of self-efficacy, is defined as "the perception of one's capability for managing stressful or threatening environmental demands." Self-efficacy accounted for 25% of the variance in psychological distress in individuals affected by Mount St. Helens (Murphy, 1987). Benight and colleagues (1999) found that the capacity for optimism and social support was significantly mediated through victims' confidence in their own restorative capabilities. In the aftermath of disasters, they have recommended that individuals be taught to set achievable goals, enabling them to have repeated success experiences, and helping to reestablish a sense of environmental control. Moreover, teaching new problem-solving skills can increase an individual's sense of problem-solving efficacy.

Posttraumatic recovery has been charted within the more specific realm of traumatic stress, rather than in ongoing chronic stress. The empirical literature shows that recovery following traumatic stress is promoted by a sense of relationship with the divine, trauma-focused treatment (e.g., cognitive-behavioral therapy), individually chosen disclosure and social support, the perception that the social milieu accepts one's reactions and welcomes disclosure, and seeing oneself as hero or survivor rather than victim (Bonnano, 2004). Among adult trauma survivors, posttrauma social support and relatively fewer posttrauma negative events may serve as protective factors mediating posttrauma recovery (Brewin, Andrews, & Valentine, 2000; King, Fairbank, Keane, & Adams, 1998).

Beyond successful return to adequate functioning following trauma, positive adaptation has been called "*posttraumatic growth*," or "adversarial growth." Posttraumatic growth tends to fall into three broad domains: changed sense of self, changed relationships, and changed philosophy of life (Calhoun & Tedeschi, 2001; Linley & Joseph, 2004.). For instance, a substantial percentage of people who have faced a major loss find some positive aspect, such as viewing themselves as stronger by continuing to go on despite the loss (Aldwin, Levenson, & Spiro, 1994; Davis, Nolen-Hoeksema, & Larson, 1998). As with resilience trajectories, those who report growth do not necessarily experience it in all areas, and the presence of growth does not mean the absence of pain and distress (Tedeschi & Calhoun, 1995). All researchers in this area indicate that it is still too early to make prescriptive recommendations about how to promote posttraumatic growth and caution against rushing individuals toward growth. Research participants repeatedly note that even well-intentioned efforts are frequently interpreted as an unwelcome attempt to minimize the unique burdens and challenges (King & Miner, 2000). They prefer responses that highlight growth in character and gain of skills only *when already exhibited* (Lehman, Ellard, & Wortman, 1986).

Understanding and working with *biological components of resilience* is an area with great potential for intervention. In an extensive review of the biological literature related to resilience (Charney, 2004), the evidence posits that resilient individuals will score in the highest range for measures of dehydroepiandrosterone (DHEA), neuropeptide Y, galanin, testosterone, as well serotonin (5-HT1$_a$), and benzodiazapine receptor function; and in the lowest range for hypothalamic–pituitary–adrenocortical (HPA) axis, corticotropin-releasing hormone (CRH), and locus–cereleus–norepinephrine activity, with opposite findings for those individuals vulnerable to stress. Studies in genetics currently suggest that the genetic basis of vulnerability to anxiety may relate to gastrin-releasing peptide, gastrin-releasing peptide receptor, and gamma-aminobutyric acid (GABA), and that depression following stressful events may be related to a polymorphism of the short allele of the 5-HTT promoter gene compared to individuals homozygous for the long allele (Caspi et al., 2003).

INTERVENTIONS

Fostering resilience can occur in many different ways and with different goals. Interventions may be designed to prepare individuals and to facilitate recovery immediately following trauma, or tailored for individuals who have experienced higher exposure levels or more debilitating reactions. Preparation fosters "resistance" to stress, which would result in the least decrements in functioning following adversity. Another strategy seeks to enhance recovery from traumatic situations (secondary prevention) by intervening shortly afterward to mobilize resilience among the general population. Finally, when there is either high exposure or intense psychological reaction, more formal interventions such as cognitive-behavioral trauma-focused treatments or pharmacotherapy may be indicated (tertiary prevention) in the weeks and months following the event, when other possible strategies have failed. These strategies are all discussed in light of research literature findings and exemplar programs.

Preparation and Prevention

It is unclear at present whether preparation is likely to inoculate individuals fully against severe trauma. A number of strategies extrapolated from different fields are described as possible components of preparation and prevention. One factor that needs consideration is that preparation requires motivation, foresight, and the resources of time and energy, which may not be realistic for most individuals. If preparedness is not feasible in situations of traumatic stress, research shows the importance of preventing or reducing risk exposure as a first-line course in improving recovery from traumatic stress (Brewin et al., 2000). For instance, in Israel people try to clear debris and any reminder of attacks as quickly as possible (Shalev, Tuval, Frenkiel, & Hadar, 2004). Research on resource loss suggests that preventing resource loss is a more efficient in promoting recovery than attempting to introduce additional resources following a traumatic event (Hobfall, 1989). Other programs designed to prepare individuals are discussed next.

Toughening

Can individuals become better prepared for the traumatic stress of disasters and mass violence? The literature on "toughness" suggests that under certain conditions, repeated episodes of challenge/threat followed by recovery periods (e.g., aerobic exercise and working in cold environments) can "toughen" neuroendocrine systems responsive to stress. People who undertook programs of aerobic training, for instance, were subsequently more energetic and more emotionally stable (Dienstbier, 1984). Better performance and learning in even complex tasks was associated with greater adrenergic responsivity in humans.

Toughness is less relevant, however, to situations experienced as harm or loss, where negative outcomes already have occurred, or where instrumental coping is considered useless (e.g., one can overwhelm organisms with excessively intense, extended, or unexpected training; even a single episode of a traumatic stressor can overwhelm). Combining unpredictability with great severity may overwhelm the organism's capacity to recover, leading to weakness rather than toughness (Dienstbier, 1989).

The Military

Very little research has been conducted on preparedness interventions with adults exposed to extremely adverse situations. The military provides one possible environment that might test the effectiveness of resilience-building strategies. Findings from the adult literature on resilience have often come from studies of men in combat. These studies indicate that resilience is often related to an ability to bond with a group with a common mission, a high value placed on altruism, the capacity to tolerate high levels of fear and still perform effectively, and psychobiological factors related to low tendency to dissociate (as cited in Charney, 2004). The following strategies of military training, designed to prepare personnel for deployment, are also applicable in civilian settings:

1. *Repetition and standardized measures of mastery* via field training exercises foster a sense of control for the service member. In the civilian sector, this component is most strongly observed in emergency services person-

nel who are key figures in community recovery following mass violence and disaster.

2. *Unit cohesiveness* serves as an extension of individual pride. The soldier's self-esteem becomes linked to the unit's reputation, providing additional motivation and also incorporating a collective identity that, when well developed, seems to be a protective factor. In the civilian world, a strong sense of group identity may also help in preparation and reaction to mass trauma.

3. *Physical fitness* prepares soldiers for the exertion necessary in battle. In the civilian sector, it has also been proven to reduce stress, anxiety, and depression (Dimeo, 2001).

4. *Drills and exercises* enhance cognitive knowledge and encourage bonding and a sense of mastery. However, recent experience has shown that many military members are not prepared for the sight and smells of atrocities or for the experience of handling bodies. The best stimuli to prepare, rather than oversensitize people, is still unknown. In the United States, schools in the Washington, DC, and other urban areas have regular drills in case of fire, shooting sprees, and other terrorist attacks. Israel differs from the United States in many ways. It has numerous mass casualty drills and all citizens are issued masks and are trained to use them in case of chemical or biological attacks. The civil preparedness drills are taken seriously and well attended.

5. *Leadership.* Military leaders are taught to foster hardiness, unit cohesion, and morale by (a) "leading by example," (b) facilitating open communication regarding planning of missions, (c) stating how mistakes or failures are corrected and learned from, (d) seeking out (and creating if necessary) meaningful and challenging group tasks, (e) remaining aware of one's team's basic needs (including rest), and (f) providing opportunities for each individual to use his or her unique coping skills (including prayer or letter writing home). During the World Trade Center tragedy the people of New York City appeared to find great comfort in the response of Mayor Rudolph Guiliani. One might postulate that New Yorkers observed hardiness in their leaders and responded in similar fashion.

6. *Preparation for deployment regarding the "state of affairs at home."* Emotional support has been shown to affect the impact of deployment (Bolton, Litz, Glenn, Orsillo, & Roemer, 2002). Recently the army has developed a vigorous deployment cycle support plan to assist returning soldiers to reintegrate into their families and society. In the civilian world, secondary stressors both before and after disasters have been one of the strongest predictors of the development of posttraumatic stress disorder (PTSD) and other trauma-related disorders (Brewin et al., 2000).

7. *Recognizing the deceased.* Proper burial gives soldiers a sense of control, sending the message to survivors that each life is valuable and will be treated with dignity, especially in death, and beginning the mourning process for those closely linked to people lost. In civilian settings, rituals to memorialize the dead are a common component of community recovery following mass trauma (Young, Ford, Ruzek, Friedman, & Gusman, 1998).

Self-Help Programs

The American Psychological Association has recently placed an online module on building resilience on its self-help website (www.apahelpcenter. org/featuredtopics/feature.php?id=6). Leading researchers in the field of resilience and posttraumatic growth formed the committee that created the module. The website explicates basic self-help steps for improving resilience, based on empirical and consensus information: increasing social support, optimism, realistic appraisal and goal setting, emotional and social balance, and a mix of both problem-focused and emotion-focused coping. Because literature on adult learning suggests that self-paced instruction is important to successful mastery of material, this dissemination strategy may be highly effective in assisting individuals with their own recovery course.

Building Strengths through Training Programs

A recent expert panel reached consensus that any intervention program designed for situations of ongoing threat should incorporate elements designed to foster hope, safety, efficacy, calming, and connectedness (Hobfall & Watson, 2005). The learned optimism and positive psychology models (Seligman, 1994; Seligman & Peterson, 2003) incorporate many of these components in order to build strengths in people at risk. The components they apply to strength building and prevention include (1) instilling hope; (2) building buffering strengths (i.e., interpersonal skill, optimism, perseverance, capacity for pleasure, and purpose); (3) narration, or the telling of stories about one's life to another; and (4) disputing—the skill of recognizing one's own catastrophic and exaggerated thinking and effectively disputing it.

Seligman has found that such training is self-reinforcing and prevents depression and anxiety in children and adults. This training is unique in that it focuses on building strength rather than repairing damage. Seligman's intervention programs are called "training programs" rather than therapy, and yet they have similar therapeutic effects to psychotherapy (Peterson, 2000; Seligman & Peterson, 2003; Seligman, Schulman, DeRubeis, & Hollon, 1999).

Preparing Individuals by Teaching Skills Commonly Utilized During Trauma Situations

Although this line of preparation has not been tested empirically, a recent case study (Ness & Macaskill, 2003) illustrates that the use of problem-solving techniques in trauma survivors enabled them to retain a sense of efficacy and control during life-threatening situations. Examples of strategies by survivors employed include the following:

- Recalling and practicing skills from previous education about the situation they were in (i.e., safety and breathing);
- Having confidence in friends to help;
- Analyzing everything closely, and demanding results;
- Dismissing thoughts of death as unconstructive;
- Concentrating on how to pacify the person making the threat;
- Feeling a sense of control;
- Remaining calm;
- Thinking of loved ones;
- Prayer;
- Concentrating on positive coping actions; and
- Not letting sounds or sights distract them.

Potential victims of major trauma may be better prepared if they have specific information to help them master their life-threatening situation, and they are instructed in how to use this as part of their problem-solving strategy. Importantly, in addition to teaching skills for specific situations, it may be important to prepare individuals in how to cope with unexpected situations where they may feel confused, bewildered, or helpless. For instance, skills can be taught that help them to identify barometers within which they can act rationally (A. Y. Shalev, personal communication, April 18, 2004). Carl Bell's (2001) resilience program seeks to address these issues through the use of esoteric training principles, including meditation exercises that develop steadiness, clarity, pliancy, mindfulness, and emotional endurance. Although these principles have not been tested in situations of traumatic stress, they are a rich heuristic to test within a largely untested aspect of traumatic stress preparation.

Secondary and Tertiary Prevention

Educating Individuals in Adaptive Coping Strategies

The American Psychological Association Task Force identifies both emotion-focused and problem-focused coping as one element of resilience. Unfortunately, research in the field of differential coping strategies in traumatic stress situations has been hampered by inconsistent definitions, as well as inaccurate generalization of findings across timelines and levels and types of traumatic stress exposure (Maguen & Litz, in press). Aldwin (1999) has identified four ways in which coping with traumatic stress differs from daily stress: Individuals may feel they have little control over their cognitions and behaviors, disclosure is more important for recovery, the process is more extended, and making meaning is more important.

One example of research following mass trauma indicated that within a U.S. sample, active coping following 9/11 was associated with lower levels of anxiety and stress than the emotion-focused strategies of disengagement and denial, and that focus on and expression of emotions was associated with increased anxiety and worry about future threat (Liverant, Hofmann, & Litz, 2004; Silver, Holman, McIntosh, Poulin, & Gil-Rivas, 2002). Some of these findings mirror risk findings for PTSD, in that development of PTSD has been associated with catastrophic thinking, self-blame, rumination, negative response to trauma symptoms, and anger. Some of the characteristics of effective trauma treatment may therefore be applied to educating individuals about effective coping following trauma. Individuals could be given strategies they could use to cope with specific events (i.e., authoritative, concise information on how to wear a gas mask or inject antidotes), as well as providing targeted information on the importance of more general coping strategies (social support, disclosure, problem-solving steps, etc.).

One approach to understanding effective coping strategies is to survey individuals who have coped with severe stress, as well as differential coping strategies over time. In Israel, for example, the four most helpful *short-term* coping strategies used by Israelis 4 to 5 days after a bus explosion were self-distraction through activity, active search for social support, faith in God, and checking on the whereabouts of family and friends following terrorist attacks (Bleich, Gelkopf, & Solomon, 2003). *Long-term* strategies in light of ongoing threat include actively seeking information, planning for travel, diverting attention (reframing, humor, acceptance), having their apprehensions circumscribed to actual threat rather than generalizing to similar situations, shifting expectations about day-to-day expectations and about what is considered a "good day," shifting focus more to quality family time, creating specific routines of living and not worrying beyond those routines, proceeding with life's necessities, and maintaining an "unyielding attraction for life" (A. Y. Shalev, personal communication, April 18, 2004). Until these coping strategies are more directly and temporally linked to mental health outcomes, these findings are limited in their applicability. However, they provide a starting point for developing interventions, which can then be correlated to outcome.

Because the resilience literature suggests that the educational approach most likely to result in behavior change is designed to tailor the information to the individual's specific situation, as well as offering opportunities for practice and mastery (Beardslee et al., 1999), it may be important to offer tertiary prevention in the form of individualized intervention for a subset of the population who are most strongly affected. Cognitive-behavioral techniques (involving exposure, cognitive restructuring, and anxiety management) currently have the strongest empirical support for preventing long-lasting psychiatric conditions following psychological trauma. Interventions adapted from cognitive-behavioral treatment are additionally being incorporated into secondary prevention in the immediate and intermediate phases posttrauma to reduce anxiety and promote more adaptive recovery. These interventions are described in detail in Chapters 9 and 10 of this book.

Community Resilience Programs

Recent reviews of research on disaster point to the central role of psychosocial resources in accounting for resilience and protecting disaster victims' mental health (Norris et al., 2003) and support a community resilience approach as the most effective form of intervention (Padgett, 2002). One example of a community resilience program has been delineated by Landau and Saul (2004), who note that any attempt to increase individual resilience in the wake of a large-scale disaster must take into account the larger societal context. In this model, representative members of the community develop their own concept of resilience, develop overarching goals for the different sections of the community, recruit support from ministry professionals and paraprofessionals, identify workable tasks from their goals, arrange work groups to achieve them, and provide daily brief bulletins on the results of the workgroups.

In the process of community building, the members of the workgroups help community members identify their resources, engage them in some form of creative expression to rebuild what has been destroyed, ensure continuity of the family, help families and communities work through grief and loss, gather people together, establish a balance of agency and communion, foster natural support systems, value the inherent competence of the community, and work with natural change agents to access families or communities that would normally, due to their culture and/or circumstances, not invite or welcome outsiders.

Because of the complexity of social resilience programs, their effectiveness has received limited empirical support. However, Nation and colleagues (2003) identified nine characteristics consistently associated with effective community prevention programs: They use varied teaching methods, give sufficient dosage to meet population needs, are research-based/ theory-driven, foster positive relationships, are appropriately timed, seek to be socioculturally relevant, include outcome evaluation, and have well-trained staff. Although these components may require additional time and resources, varied research evidence and expert opinion across a variety of resilience-fostering programs clearly support them.

SUMMARY AND CONCLUSIONS

The construct of resilience represents a dynamic process involving protective and vulnerability factors in different risk contexts and developmental stages. We still need to determine which interventions are likely to improve resilience for which individuals and when to intervene in the early to intermediate phases postincident. Few empirical data currently exist on resilience-building interventions following disasters and terrorism. Fostering resilience can occur in many different ways and with different goals. Interventions may be designed to prepare individuals, to facilitate recovery immediately following trauma, or to be introduced within a clinical treatment context for individuals who have experienced higher exposure levels or more debilitating reactions. Each strategy has benefits and detriments that need consideration in overall planning.

Preparation is most likely effective with those individuals frequently subject to high-risk situations. Primary prevention involves interventions such as teaching problem-solving skills or toughening exercises like those in military training. Because this form of stress inoculation is designed to foster "resistance," it would be expected to produce the fewest decrements following adversity. However, it requires motivation, foresight, and resources of time and energy and therefore may have limited application with unmotivated individuals. It is also unclear whether it might inoculate against the impact of severe trauma. Stress inoculation can only protect if it has been accurately calibrated to the severity and quality of the stressors. However, the nature of traumatic stress is unpredictability or uncontrollability. Therefore, although stress resistance is related to specific or probable stressors, traumatic stress preparation may be more geared toward preparing individuals for the unexpected, when they may not yet understand what is going on, when conditions are new, and when they may feel confused, bewildered, or helpless. It would rather help them to identify barometers within which they can act rationally (A. Y. Shalev, personal communication, April 18, 2004).

Another strategy seeks to enhance recovery from traumatic situations (secondary prevention) by intervening shortly afterward to facilitate accelerated resilient trajectories to most of the population, such as by teaching the importance of enhancing social support and self-efficacy or positively changing beliefs or actions following trauma. It may involve building restorative, replenishing activities into the posttrauma schedule, having individuals try to find what might restore their inherent capacity to thrive, and raising awareness about the cost and benefit of denial at different phases postincident. Unfortunately, after a disaster, survivors may already be taxed, and any program that requires time and energy may feel like an additional drain on those already struggling to recover. Therefore, programs need to prepare to assist in recovery and resilience for weeks and months following a disaster or mass violence event.

Finally, when there is either high exposure or high levels of distress, and other possible strategies have failed to achieve an adequate response, more formal interventions such as cognitive-behavioral trauma-focused treatments (tertiary prevention) may be indicated in the weeks and months following the event. The shortcoming of this model is that individuals often resist more formal treatment because of fear of stigma. This model also requires resources of the community, such as trained practitioners. Furthermore, strong motivation may be required of the survivor, as cognitive-behavioral treatment takes time, energy, and a willingness to face memories of the traumatic event.

Experts in the field of developmental psychopathology recommend that because resilient trajectories vary across situations and timelines, searching for unifactorial solutions to fostering resilient recovery is unlikely to yield satisfactory results (Luthar, 2000). What works for individuals in one context may not work for the same or other groups in others. A sensible strategy for maximizing resilient trajectories following mass violence would be multidisciplinary, multifaceted, and sensitive to the cultural and event context, as well as to differential exposure and response, and would include multiple intervention possibilities, both before the event and after. The programs should have an empirical or theoretical basis and be realistic in their expectations and claims. Because more research is needed in this field, there is also a strong need to partner clinicians and researchers in designing and evaluating programs (Luthar & Cicchetti, 2000; Luthar & Zelazo, 1987).

Finally, society as a whole, not just mental health providers or leaders, has an enormous role in enhancing resilience. Advances in the empirical literature are expected to facilitate a more effective strategy for communities to promote both individual and societal resilience.

AUTHOR NOTE

The opinions expressed in this chapter are those of the authors and do not represent the official views of the Uniformed Services University of the Health Sciences, the Department of the Army, or the Department of Defense.

REFERENCES

Aldwin, C. M. (1999). *Stress, coping, and development: An integrative approach.* New York: Guilford Press.

Aldwin, C. M., Levenson, M. R., & Spiro, A. (1994). Vulnerability and resilience to combat exposure—can stress have lifelong effects. *Psychology and Aging, 9,* 34-44.

Anthony, E. J., & Cohler, B. J. (Eds.). (1987). *The invulnerable child.* New York: Guilford Press.

Beardslee, W. R., Versage, E. M., Salt, P., & Wright, E. (1999). The development and evaluation of two preventive intervention strategies for children of depressed parents. In D. Cicchetti & S. L. Toth (Eds.), *Rochester Symposium on Developmental Psychopathology: Volume 9. Developmental approaches to prevention and intervention* (pp. 223–234). Rochester, NY: University of Rochester Press.

Bell, C. C. (2001). Cultivating resiliency in youth. *Journal of Adolescent Health, 29*(5), 375–381.

Benight, C., Ironsen, G., Klebe, K., Carver, C., Wynings, C., Burnett, K., et al. (1999). Coping self-efficacy as a predictor of psychological distress following a natural disaster: A causal model analysis. *Anxiety, Stress and Coping, 12,* 107–126.

Bleich, A., Gelkopf, M., & Solomon, Z. (2003). Exposure to terrorism, stress-related mental health symptoms, and coping behaviors among a nationally representative sample in Israel. *Journal of the American Medical Association, 290,* 612–620.

Bolton, E., Litz, B. T., Glenn, D. M., Orsillo, S., & Roemer, L. (2002). The impact of homecoming reception on the adaptation of peacekeepers following deployment. *Military Psychology, 14,* 241–251.

Bonanno, G. A. (2004). Loss, trauma, and human resilience. Have we underestimated the human capacity to thrive after extremely aversive events? *American Psychologist, 59*(1), 20–28.

Brewin, C., Andrews, B., & Valentine, J. (2000). Meta-analysis of risk factors for posttraumatic stress disorder in trauma exposed adults. *Journal of Consulting and Clinical Psychology, 68,* 748–766.

Calhoun, L. G., & Tedeschi, R. G. (2001). *Posttraumatic growth: The positive lessons of loss.* Washington, DC: American Psychological Association.

Caspi, A., Sugden, K., Moffitt, T. E., Taylor, A., Craig, I. W., Harrington, H., et al. (2003). Influence of life stress on depression: Moderation by a polymorphism in the 5-HTT gene. *Biological Psychiatry, 54*(10), 1087–1091.

Charney, D. S. (2004). Psychobiological mechanisms of resilience and vulnerability: Implications for successful adaptation to extreme stress. *American Journal of Psychiatry, 161,* 195–216.

Cohler, B. J., Stott, F. M., & Musick, J. S. (1995). Adversity, vulnerability, and resilience. Cultural and developmental perspectives. In D. Cicchetti & D. J. Cohen (Eds.), *Developmental psychopathology: Vol. 12. Risk, disorder and adaptation* (pp. 753–800). New York: Wiley.

Davis, C. G., Nolen-Hoeksema, S., & Larson, J. (1998). Making sense of loss and benefiting from the experience: Two construals of meaning. *Journal of Personality and Social Psychology, 75,* 561–574.

Dienstbier, R. A. (1984). The effect of exercise on personality. In M. L. Sachs & G. B. Buffone (Eds.), *Running as therapy: An integrated approach* (pp. 128–135). Lincoln: University of Nebraska Press.

Dienstbier, R. A. (1989). Arousal and physiological toughness: Implications for mental and physical health. *Psychological Review, 96,* 84–100.

Hobfall, S. E. (1989). Conservation of resources: A new attempt at conceptualizing stress. *American Psychologist, 44,* 513-524.

Hofball, S. E., & Watson, P. J. (2005). *Five essential elements of immediate and mid-term mass trauma treatment: Empirical evidence.* Manuscript in preparation.

King, D. W., King, L. A., Fairbank, J. A., Keane, T. M., & Adams, G. A. (1998). Resilience-recovery factors in posttraumatic stress disorder among female and male Vietnam Veterans: Hardiness, postwar social support, and additional stressful life events. *Journal of Personality and Social Psychology, 74,* 420–434.

King, L. A., & Miner, K. N. (2000). Writing about the perceived benefits of traumatic life events: Implications for physical health. *Personality and Social Psychology Bulletin, 26,* 220–230.

Kobasa, S. C., Maddi, S. R., & Kahn, S. (1982). Hardiness and health: A prospective study. *Journal of Personality and Social Psychology, 42*(1), 168–177.

Landau, J., & Saul, J. (2004). Facilitating family and community resilience in response to major disaster. In F. Walsh & M. McGoldrick (Eds.), *Living beyond loss* (pp. 327–343). New York: Norton.

Lehman, D. R., Ellard, J. H., & Wortman, C. B. (1986). Social support for the bereaved: Recipients' and providers' perspectives on what is helpful. *Journal of Consulting and Clinical Psychology, 54,* 438–446.

Linley, P. A., & Joseph, S. (2004). Positive change following trauma and adversity: A review. *Journal of Traumatic Stress, 17,* 11–21.

Liverant, G. I., Hofmann, S. G., & Litz, B. T. (2004). Coping and anxiety in college students after the September 11th terrorist attacks. *Anxiety, Stress, and Coping, 17,* 127–139.

Luthar, S. S. (1991). Vulnerability and resilience: A study of high-risk adolescents. *Child Development, 62,* 600–616.

Luthar, S. S. (2000). The construct of resilience: A critical evaluation and guidelines for future work. *Child Development, 71,* 543–562.

Luthar, S. S., & Cicchetti, D. (2000). The construct of resilience: Implications for interventions and social policies. *Development and Psychopathology, 12,* 857–885.

Luthar, S. S., & Suchman, N. E. (2000). Relational psychotherapy mother's group: A developmentally informed intervention for at-risk mothers. *Development and Psychopathology, 12,* 235–253.

Luthar, S. S., & Zelazo, L. B. (1987). Research on resilience: An integrated review. In S. S. Luthar (Ed.), *Resilience and vulnerability: Adaptation in the context of childhood adversities* (pp. 510–549). New York: Cambridge University Press.

Maddi, S. R., & Hightower, M. (1999). Hardiness and optimism as expressed in coping patterns. *Consulting Psychology Journal, 51,* 95–105.

Maguen, S., & Litz, B. T. (in press). Coping with the threat of terrorism: A working model. In Y. Neria, R. Gross, & R. Marshall (Eds.), *September 11, 2001: Treatment, research and public mental health in the wake of a terrorist attack.* New York: Cambridge University Press.

Masten, A. S. (2001). Ordinary magic: Resilience processes in development. *American Psychologist, 56*(3), 227–238.

Murphy, S. (1987). Self-efficacy and social support mediators of stress on mental health following a natural disaster. *Western Journal of Nursing Research, 9,* 58–86.

Nation, M., Crusto, C., Wandersman, A., Kumpfer, K. L., Seybolt, D., Morrisey-Kane, E., et al. (2003). What works in prevention programs. *American Psychologist, 58,* 449–456.

Ness, G. J., & Macaskill, N. (2003). Preventing PTSD: The value of inner resourcefulness and a sense of personal control of a situation: Is it a matter of problem-solving or anxiety management? *Behavioural and Cognitive Psychotherapy, 31,* 363–486.

Norris, F. H., Friedman, M. J., Watson, P. J., Byrne, C. M., Diaz, E., & Kaniasty, K. (2002). 60,000 disaster victims speak: Part I. An empirical review of the empirical literature, 1981–2001. *Psychiatry, 65,* 207–239.

Padgett, D. K. (2002). Social work research on disasters in the aftermath of September 11 tragedy: Reflections from New York City. *Social Work Research, 26,* 185–192.

Peterson, C. (2000). The future of optimism. *American Psychologist, 55,* 44–55.

Rutter, M. (1993). Resilience: Some conceptual considerations. *Journal of Adolescent Health, 14,* 626–631.

Seligman, M. E. P. (1994). *What you can change and what you can't.* New York: Knopf.

Seligman, M. E. P., & Peterson, C. (2003). Positive clinical psychology. In L. G. Aspinwall & U. M. Staudinger (Eds.), *A psychology of human strengths: Fundamental questions and future directions for a positive psychology* (pp. 195–305). Washington, DC: American Psychological Association.

Seligman, M. E. P., Schulman, P., DeRubeis, R. J., & Hollon, S. D. (1999). *The prevention of depression and anxiety: Prevention and Treatment, 2.* Retrieved December 10, 2004, from journals.apa.org/prevention/volume2/pre0020008a.html

Shalev, A. Y., Tuval, R., Frenkiel, S., & Hadar, H. (2004). *Psychological reactions to continuous terror.* Manuscript under review.

Silver, R. C., Holman, E. A., McIntosh, D. N., Poulin, M., & Gil-Rivas, V. (2002). Nationwide longitudinal study of psychological responses to September 11. *Journal of the American Medical Association, 288,* 1235–1244.

Steinberg, A. (2004, March). *A conceptual framework for stress-related concepts and community resilience.* Paper presented at the National Center for Child Traumatic Stress, University of California, Los Angeles.

Tedeschi, R. G., & Calhoun, L. G. (1995). *Trauma and transformation: Growing in the aftermath of suffering.* Thousand Oaks, CA: Sage.

Tusaie, K., & Dyer, J. (2004). Resilience: A historical review of the construct. *Holistic Nurse Practitioner, 18,* 3–8.

Waysman, M., Schwarzwald, J., & Solomon, Z. (2001). Hardiness: An examination of its relationship with positive and negative long term changes following trauma. *Journal of Traumatic Stress, 14*(1), 531–548.

Werner, E. E. (1990). Protective factors and individual resilience. In S. J. Meisels & J. P. Shonkoff (Eds.), *Handbook of early childhood intervention* (pp. 97–116). Cambridge, UK: Cambridge University Press.

Werner, E. E., & Johnson, J. L. (1999). Can we apply resilience? In M. D. Glantz & J. L. Johnson (Eds.), *Resilience and development: Positive life adaptations* (pp. 259–268). New York: Kluwer Academic/Plenum.

Werner, E. E., & Smith, R. S. (1992). *Overcoming the odds: High risk children from birth to adulthood.* Ithaca, NY: Cornell University Press.

Young, B. H., Ford, J. D., Ruzek, J. I., Friedman, M. J., & Gusman, F. D. (1998). *Disaster mental health services: A guidebook for clinicians and administrators.* Menlo Park, CA: National Center for Post-Traumatic Stress Disorder.

CHAPTER 4

Disaster Mental Health Training

Guidelines, Considerations, and Recommendations

BRUCE H. YOUNG, JOSEF I. RUZEK, MARLEEN WONG,
MARK S. SALZER, and APRIL J. NATURALE

Disaster mental health (DMH) training necessarily takes into account the scope and complexity of disaster mental services delivery from the perspective of preparedness planning/training and training in the wake of a disaster. DMH service delivery and related training vary widely, according to when, where, by whom, and to whom DMH services are delivered. Comprehensive training should include instruction about navigational, engagement, screening/assessment, referral, and other intervention strategies that help the effort to respond to the needs of survivors of all ages (including emergency responders) who are seen either on- or off-site at various points in time (ranging from hours to months after the event). Moreover, in multicultural societies, ethnic diversity must be taken into account if mental health services are to be accepted and efficacious. Aggregate groups (e.g., families, communities, schools, and organizations) present unique system-level access, assessment, and intervention challenges that can be addressed in training. Preexisting community conditions, resources, and history (e.g., political, economic, and cultural), preexisting individual resources and history (e.g., mental health, medical, and economic), and the severity of the impact of the disaster on the community and helpers must also be taken into account to make training relevant.

GUIDELINES AND CONSIDERATIONS
FOR DMH TRAINING

DMH training is shaped primarily by seven factors: (1) trainees' credentials, roles, and experience; (2) when the training is delivered; (3) topics and learning objectives; (4) the training process; (5) the time available for training; (6) background and teaching experience of the trainer; and vii) available funding.

Trainees

Training may be delivered to a wide range of individuals, who by their credentials, job, or wish to volunteer are put in contact with survivors and disaster workers. Trainees should be sanctioned to operate within officially recognized structures. Trainees may include mental health professionals (e.g., social workers, psychologists, marriage and family therapists, psychiatric nurses, and psychiatrists), medical professionals (e.g., physicians, physician's assistants, nurses working in primary care, family practice, and pediatrics), clergy, fire department and police personnel, school personnel, and paraprofessionals (e.g., staff of helping organizations, community volunteers, and graduate students).

When Training Is Delivered

Of course, predisaster training is optimal as it can facilitate efforts to coordinate and integrate a system-level response as well as provide professional trainees with opportunities to learn about the significant differences between DMH services and conventional clinical services. Predisaster training and drills should be offered that, ideally, involve numerous community emergency services. Combining classroom teaching with participation in disaster simulations provides opportunities for operating within an incident command system, networking, operational testing, team building, and skill building. In lieu of more comprehensive training, a series of focused and specialized trainings can be provided to address a wide range of topics specific to DMH service delivery.

When training takes place in the aftermath of disaster, the content is shaped by the temporal phase of the disaster and the topics associated with relevant learning objectives. For example, topics specific to "just-in-time" training given in the immediate aftermath may include psychological first aid, common stress reactions, navigational and engagement strategies, grief work, and identification of high-risk individuals. Training given in the second to fourth week might include topics of acute stress disorder, early-intervention modalities, working in the schools, outreach strategies, brief education delivery, and cross-cultural issues. Training in the later stages following disaster might include topics of posttraumatic stress disorder (PTSD) and other chronic reactions to trauma, comorbidities (e.g., depression and substance abuse), treatment protocols, vicarious traumatization, outreach strategies, and helper self-care.

Training Topics and Learning Objectives

Much of the disaster-related research over the past two decades has focused on the *impact* of disasters, with relatively little research on *interventions* (Norris et al., 2002). A recent report (Young, Ruzek, & Pivar, 2001) reviewed available training materials related to the systematic mental health response to disaster and community violence, describing the content of existing training materials, commenting on strengths and weaknesses of training in this arena, and making recommendations for more effective training methods. The reviewers found that although the training materials adequately cover a broad range of topics, they make too little reference to empirical evidence examining the effects of disaster and to procedures and tools for screening and assessment, devote little attention to problematic intervention issues, and provide insufficient guidance regarding planning for long-term follow-up services. Until specific DMH interventions are examined, the existing literature can be used to inform and guide training in disaster-related assessment with regard to individuals at risk for adverse mental health outcomes (e.g., Young, 2002), and as noted in the next section, the findings in other areas of research (e.g., early intervention) can be reasonably generalized and applied to DMH training.

We recommend multiple trainings to prepare mental health professionals and paraprofessionals to effectively respond to the varying needs of survivors and disaster-related personnel. Figures 4.1–4.5 present a comprehensive outline of training modules, designed and organized to take into account the training needs of mental health practitioners and administrators during preparedness and throughout the temporal phases after a disaster. Drawing from these fundamental modules, preparedness and postdisaster training coordinators can develop programs specific to practitioner and administrator needs.

Specific learning objectives are determined by who is being trained, the identified learning needs, and when the training is delivered. The trainer often must make this judgment, informed by his or her own professional experience. Table 4.1 on page 61 presents a generic list of learning objectives.

MODULE I. DMH SERVICES: A CONCEPTUAL FRAMEWORK

A. *Natural and Human-Caused Disasters*
   • Typology and Traumatic Stressors
   • Associated Risks
   • Service Delivery Issues: Key Concepts

B. *Effects of Disaster on Communities*
   • A review of the literature

C. *Effects of Disaster on Individuals*
   • Conservation of Resources and Other Paradigms
   • Common Stress Reactions
     • Adults
     • Children
   • Emergency Responders and Other Helpers
     • Stressors Associated with Disaster Work
     • Service Delivery Issues
   • Risk Factors Associated with Adverse Mental Health Outcomes
   • Acute Stress Disorder
   • Posttraumatic Stress Disorder and Comorbidities

FIGURE 4.1. DMH training curriculum: *Universal* module for practitioners and administrators.

Processes of Training

In addition to the content of training materials, it is important to consider the *process* of training. Much of the material in the existing training manuals is dedicated to explaining their topics or content (Young et al., 2001). The complexity of the skills involved in delivering DMH services suggests that the best training must go beyond simply describing the array of disaster reactions, coping behaviors, and various methods of intervention. Two recent studies of involving mental health practitioners who provided services to individuals affected by either the Oklahoma City or the World Trade Center bombings (Norris, Watson, Hamblen, & Pfefferbaum, 2005) found that the majority of these practitioners preferred to observe the demonstration of helping interventions. Allowing trainees to rehearse interventions and receive feedback should also be helpful in regard to their gaining mastery of essential helping skills. Videotapes can be used to enable trainees to see and hear disaster-related stories, survivor/responder reactions and coping efforts, and examples of helping behaviors. Using improvised vignettes, helping skills can be demonstrated with opportunities to practice them with performance feedback.

MODULE II. PRACTITIONER GUIDELINES

A. *Overview: Disaster Mental Health Services*
- Objectives: Micro/Macro
- Methods
  - Outreach, Engagement Strategies, Building Rapport and Casefinding
  - Assessment
  - Brief Survivor Education
  - Referral
  - Follow-Up
- Interventions
  - Early Intervention Modalities
  - Group and Individual Treatment Modalities, Etc.
- Temporal Phases
  - Preparedness
  - Emergency
  - Early Post-Impact
  - Recovery
  - Restabilization
  - Matching methods/ interventions to temporal phase
- Service Delivery Settings
  - Nontraditional Community Settings
    - Relief Centers
    - Family Assistance Centers
    - Shelters
    - Commercial
    - Residential, Etc.
- Consumers
  - Survivors

B. *DMH Practitioner Preparedness*
- DMH Training Guidelines
  - Training Content (content of other modules)
  - Training Processes
  - Recruitment, Selection of Team Members, Operational Procedures, Team Readiness Maintenance
  - Networking, Systems, Memorandums of Understanding
  - Training Paraprofessionals

*Sections "C" and "D" share some similar topics as each is designed to be used separately with Section A and Module I. In cases of comprehensive training, that is, training about emergency and crisis counseling program services, eliminate redundant topics.

C. *DMH Emergency Services**
- Practice Objectives
  - Micro (specific to)
    - Temporal Phase (emergency, early post-impact)
    - Consumers (identification of survivors, helpers, and special-needs groups at risk for continuing problems)
    - Service Delivery Settings (relief centers, family assistance centers, shelters, etc.)
  - Macro (specific to)
    - Communities (public health)
- Micro Practice Methods
  - On-Scene Support
  - Psychological First Aid
  - Key Processes in Recovery: Basic principles of care and helping skills
  - Stress Reactions: What survivors should expect
  - Social Support
  - Outreach and Casefinding Methods
    - One-Contact Protocols
    - Two-Contact Protocols
    - Three-or-more-Contact Protocols
    - Working Large-Group Settings
    - Working Commercial and Residential Settings
  - Assessment (common stress reactions; acute stress reactions; risk factors for adverse outcomes; long-term effects of disaster; screening methods and tools)
  - Referral Protocols (securing linkage)
  - Bereavement Support
  - Age-Specific Interventions
  - Pharmacotherapy
  - Individual and Group Education: Content— understanding trauma reactions, self-care strategies, active problem solving, maladaptive coping

D. *DMH Crisis Counseling Services and Programs**
- Practice Objectives
  - Micro (specific to)
    - Temporal Phase (transition from early post-impact to recovery and restabilization)
    - Consumers (identification of survivors, helpers, and special-needs groups at risk for continuing problems)
    - Service Delivery Settings (community, school, workplace, etc.)
  - Macro (specific to)
    - Communities
- Professional Practice Methods
  - Outreach and Casefinding Services
    - One-Contact Protocols
    - Two-Contact Protocols
    - Three-or-more-Contact Protocols
    - Working Large-Group Settings Working Commercial and Residential Settings
  - Assessment
  - Referral Protocols (securing linkage)
  - Screening tools
  - Early Intervention Modalities
    - Brief Interventions to Reduce Alcohol Consumption
      - Assessing alcohol consumption
      - Brief advice about moderate drinking
      - Increasing motivation to reduce consumption
  - Group and Individual Treatment Modalities: Cognitive Therapy Methods
  - Trauma-Focused Treatment
  - Problem-Solving-Oriented Treatment
- Paraprofessional Practice Methods
  - Outreach and Casefinding
  - Service General Helping Behaviors
  - Assessment and Referral Protocols
- Consumer-Directed Services
- Special Service Delivery Issues

FIGURE 4.2. DMH training curriculum: *Practitioner* modules.

MODULE III. ADMINISTRATIVE GUIDELINES

A. *Overview: Multivariate and Contextual Integration*
- Objectives: Micro/Macro
- Methods: Community-wide assessment strategies and tools, interagency planning, program development
- Temporal Phases: Preparedness, Emergency, Early Post-Impact; Recovery, Restabilization
- Settings: Nontraditional
- Consumers: Survivors, Helpers, Special Populations
- Resources: Internal/External
- Services: Integration of Multiple Variables

B. *DMH Planning*
- Administrative Objectives
  - Micro Specific to
    - Temporal Phase
    - Consumers (survivors, helpers, high-risk and special-needs groups)
    - Service Delivery Settings
  - Macro Specific to
    - Communities
      - Media utilization (e.g., information dissemination)
      - Events
- Administrative Methods: Guidelines for Developing DMH Plans
  - Involving Community and Cultural Stakeholders (e.g., service providers, businesses, faith communities, primary care professionals and other stakeholder groups) in Planning and Infrastructure Development Activities
  - DMH Plans: General Contents
    - Authority and Mission statement
    - Linkage of Agency Level Planning to Federal, State, Regional, County, and Community-Based Organizations
    - Staffing Roles, Responsibilities, and Training
    - Involving Key Stakeholders
    - Disaster Management Strategies
      - Community-wide Assessment Strategies and Tools
      - Risk Communication Guidelines
      - Procedures for Delivering and Providing Care to Survivors
      - Procedures for Delivering and Providing Care to Local and State Emergency Response Personnel During and Following Disaster Operations
      - Educational Materials for Survivors and Emergency Responders
  - Budgeting for Emergency Management Services
  - Quality Assurance and Program Evaluation

C. *DMH Emergency Services*
- Administrative Objectives
  - Micro Specific to
    - Temporal Phase (emergency, early post-impact)
    - Consumers (survivors, helpers, high-risk and special-needs groups)
    - Service Delivery Settings
  - Macro Specific to
  - Communities
- Administrative Methods
  - Technical Assistance and Grant Applications
  - Community-wide Assessment Strategies and Tools
  - Risk Communication Guidelines
  - Procedures for Delivering and Providing Care to Survivors
  - Procedures for Delivering and Providing Care to Local and State Emergency Response Personnel During and Following Disaster Operations
  - Procedures for Obtaining and Distributing Educational Materials for Survivors and Emergency Responders via Media

D. *DMH Crisis Counseling Services and Programs*
- Administrative Objectives
  - Micro Specific to
    - Temporal Phase (transition from early-post impact to recovery)
    - Consumers (survivors, helpers, high-risk and special-needs groups)
    - Service Delivery Settings
  - Macro Specific to
    - Communities
      - Media campaigns
      - Event planning
- Administrative Methods
  - Program Formation, Implementation, and Maintenance
  - Linkage of Services and Programs to Federal, State, Regional, County, and Community-Based Organizations
  - Staffing Roles, Responsibilities, and Training
  - Contracting for Service Locations
  - Involving Key Stakeholders
  - Fiscal Mechanisms
  - Staff Health Care
  - Quality Assurance and Program Evaluation
  - Closing Programs

FIGURE 4.3. DMH training curriculum: *Administrative* modules.

MODULE IV. SPECIAL POPULATIONS

A. *High-Risk, Ethnic, and Special-Needs Groups: Service Considerations*
- Injured
- Bereaved
- Children
- Ethnic Minorities and Cross-Cultural Competency
- Older Adults
- Chronically Mentally Ill
- Displaced Individuals
- Emergency Workers: Self-Care before, during, and after an Assignment
- Mental Health Workers: Self-Care before, during, and after an Assignment

FIGURE 4.4. DMH training curriculum: Special-populations module for practitioners.

Time Allotted for Training

The amount of time allotted for training is determined by many variables, however, most trainings fall into 4-, 8-, 12-, or 16-hour programs. Longer programs can use the extended time to create opportunities for planning, team building, networking among participants, role playing, exercises, and demonstrations of helping behaviors.

Trainers

Generally speaking, most trainers are licensed mental health clinicians or administrators who have disaster experience that includes responding to a range of disasters (natural, human-caused, mass casualties) and communities (urban, rural, ethnic diversity). Exceptions to this rule are speakers who can address specific topics (e.g., resources, administrative methods, cultural

MODULE V. RESPONSE STRUCTURES, PROCESSES, AND ORGANIZATIONS

A. *The Big Picture: Response Structures, Processes, and Organizations*
- Federal Response Plan
- National Disaster Medical System
- Federal Resources
- State Resources
- Community Resources
- Nonprofits
- Professional Organizations
- New Developments and Future Directions

FIGURE 4.5. DMH training curriculum: Response structures, processes, and organizations module for practitioners and administrators.

TABLE 4.1. Generic Practitioner Learning Objectives of DMH Emergency Response Training

Upon completion of training, participants will be able to:

- Identify the conceptual framework of emergency/DMH services.
- Identify DMH response structures, processes, and organizations.
- Identify fundamental components to an emergency mental health response plan.
- Identify common survivor stress reactions.
- Identify predisaster, within-disaster, and postdisaster risk factors associated with adverse mental health outcomes.
- Identify at-risk groups and individuals in the wake of disaster.
- Target phase-specific interventions to match needs of specific at-risk groups and individuals.
- Identify guidelines for delivering psychological first aid.
- Identify strategies of engagement and building rapport with non-treatment-seeking and treatment-seeking survivors.
- Identify guidelines for working in large-group settings.
- Identify guidelines for brief one-on-one supportive counseling (one contact; two contacts; three or more).
- Identify guidelines for delivering brief education packages.
- Identify guidelines for delivering stress management skills.
- Identify guidelines for securing referral linkages.
- Identify intervention considerations specific to disaster workers, children, minority groups, and older adults.
- Identify guidelines for emergency mental health provider stress management and self-care.

characteristics of the community, spirituality, bereavement, and treatment modalities). The characteristics of an effective instructor have been delineated in the *American Red Cross Instructor Candidate Training Participant's Manual* (American Red Cross, 1990). These characteristics include possessing good communication skills, in-depth knowledge of the subject, a positive attitude, appropriate attire, patience and flexibility in responding to trainee's learning needs, and skills to manage class and motivate trainees. In addition, having a conceptual and practiced understanding of the learning process is essential. From classroom setup to conducting a course, skills such as good "climate setting," bridging ideas from one section of training to another, facilitating discussion, guiding student practice, clarifying, using interactive learning, and knowing current media presentation technology are important instructor qualities for achieving learning objectives.

Funding

Funding for DMH training may come from many sources, depending on whether the program is sponsored by the government, nonprofit, or private sectors. Funding from the federal government is overseen primarily by the Department of Homeland Security, Federal Emergency Management Agency (FEMA), the Substance Abuse and Mental Health Services Administration, and the Center for Mental Health Services (CMHS), through various grant mechanisms. Nonprofit funding and private-sector funding may involve pharmaceutical company or local institutional support.

POSTTRAUMA EARLY-INTERVENTION RESEARCH: IMPLICATIONS FOR TRAINING

As indicated in this book, research on early posttrauma interventions is increasing rapidly. Although this field of research is relatively new and does not yet offer up strong directives regarding postdisaster practice, such intervention research can inform our design of DMH training.

An encouraging development in this regard is the increasing attention to new cognitive-behavioral treatment "packages" directed at individuals diagnosed with acute stress disorder. The pertinent outcome studies have all been targeted at assault and accident survivors, and the extent to which findings will generalize to disaster-affected populations is not yet clear. However, similarities in acute stress response across traumatized populations, correspondence of the package components to empirically validated treatments for chronic PTSD, and theory-based construction of these methods suggest that these treatment packages will be applicable for severely affected disaster-exposed groups 2–3 months after the event.

Less encouraging is the controversy regarding the utility of "psychological debriefing," a face-valid small-group method that as been widely used following disasters. Recent studies of the efficacy of debriefing methods call into question its usefulness in preventing psychopathology (Bisson, McFarlane, & Rose, 2000; Litz, Gray, Bryant, & Adler, 2002); however, the quality of these studies has been viewed as poor by the International Society for Traumatic Stress Studies (ISTSS) and to date, researchers have not been able to examine how debriefing is commonly used following disasters.

Survivor Education

While little is known about the impact of postdisaster education, there is reason to believe that when delivered alone, some forms of education have limited effectiveness in preventing the development of PTSD in those most at risk following motor vehicle accident and assault (Bryant & Harvey,

2000; Bryant, Harvey, Dang, Sackville, & Basten, 1998; Bryant, Sackville, Dang, Moulds, & Guthrie, 1999). Given the evident need for individual and group survivor education services following disasters, it is important that DMH workers be trained in education targeted at those factors that are both thought to affect recovery (on the bases of empirical findings and current theory) and that may be influenced via brief provision of information (Ruzek, 2002; Young & Gerrity, 1994)

Skills Training

Little is known about the effectiveness of our ability to increase adaptive coping in DMH service environments and whether such changed coping is associated with better outcomes. Nonetheless, research has suggested that several kinds of coping may be associated with reduced post-trauma problems (e.g., social support, anxiety management, and problem solving), and much postdisaster care involves education about coping. Methods used in skills training, such as modeling, behavior rehearsal, self-monitoring, repetitive practice in the real-world environment, and multisession instruction can be expected to enhance the impact of disaster-related education.

Brief Psychological Interventions to Reduce Traumatic Stress Reactions

The success of brief (i.e., 4–5 sessions) cognitive-behavioral treatment (CBT), comprised of education, breathing training/relaxation, imaginal and *in vivo* exposure, and cognitive restructuring, delivered within weeks of the traumatic event, with both acute stress disorder (Bryant et al., 1998, 1999) and chronic PTSD (Foa & Rothbaum, 1997; Resick, Nishith, Weaver, Astin, & Feuer, 2002) suggests that it may be appropriate to deliver aspects of these interventions to severely impaired disaster survivors.

The most powerful elements of effective CBT interventions are thought to involve exposure therapy and cognitive restructuring. Exposure therapy holds significant promise as an early intervention, but because of its potential to exacerbate short-term distress and the fact that most practitioners have not received training in its application, research must be conducted to determine whether and under what conditions it can be recommended for use with disaster survivors. Cognitive restructuring is an intervention that may be less emotionally provocative. Because disaster counselors often encounter negative cognitions, they should receive education about the role of cognition in development of PTSD (Ehlers & Clark, 2000) and training in more systematic approaches to modification of distressing disaster-related beliefs (e.g., misinterpretations of acute stress reactions, guilt and shame, and negative beliefs about the future).

Brief Alcohol Interventions

Research on brief alcohol interventions has shown that such services can lower alcohol consumption (e.g., Heather, 1995). Particularly relevant is a demonstration that a single session of counseling can reduce drinking in patients recently treated in hospital trauma centers (Gentilello et al., 1999). Although this body of research has not been brought to bear on DMH practice, it is reasonable to hope such interventions will reduce the likelihood of problem drinking postdisaster. Given their robustness even as brief interventions, alcohol-abuse interventions should be incorporated into training.

Identification of Survivors at Risk
for Longer-Term Problems

One of the key functions of DMH workers is referring "at-risk survivors" for mental health treatment. Ideally, training would also include a module on screening. Research has much to say about pre-, within-, and post-disaster risk factors affecting development of PTSD and other negative sequelae in the contexts of disaster (e.g., Galea et al., 2002; Norris et al., 2002) and traumatic stress (see Ørner, Kent, Pfefferbaum, Raphael, & Watson, Chapter 7; Bryant & Litz, Chapter 9; Young, Chapter 8; and Raphael & Wooding, Chapter 10; this volume).

However, identification of the most vulnerable people during the immediate posttraumatic period is very difficult at this time. Experts in the field are currently grappling with the multiple issues that make screening in the early phases after mass trauma difficult.

Referral: Reducing Obstacles to Use
of Mental Health Services

Though it is often reported by DMH practitioners that most survivors do not seek post-disaster-related mental health services, to date, there is no published research examining survivors' attitudes toward the use of such services. Many factors, such as having to attend to basic needs and imminent problems, avoidance, fear of stigmatization, misunderstanding of the nature of counseling, and cultural norms about coping, may all limit motivation to pursue a referral. Discussing these attitudes and employing motivational interviewing techniques (Rollnick, Heather, & Bell, 1992) may enable outreach workers and other DMH counselors to increase rates of referral acceptance.

DMH TRAINING IN SCHOOLS

In times of disasters, schools are the primary, *de facto* provider of mental health services in the community. Even without a disaster, the school is often a source of social support through parent and teacher activities and associations, which are familiar, customary, and accepted conduits of information and assistance. Utilization studies have shown that up to 80% of children who receive some form of mental health intervention or treatment access those services from a school counselor, school psychologist, school social worker, or a community mental health professional assigned to a school-based program (Burns et al., 1995).

Few mental health programs have been rigorously designed, implemented, and evaluated in the real-world setting of schools (Hoagwood & Erwin, 1997), and even fewer are designed, implemented, and evaluated specifically for ethnic minority children (Kataoka, Zhang, & Wells, 2002) or for large-scale incidents of disaster or terrorism (Norris et al., 2002). However, there is a literature that is relevant to school interventions. For example, several studies (Almqvist & Brandell-Forsberg, 1997; Malmquist, 1986; Rigamer, 1986; Sack, Angell, Kinzie, & Rath, 1986) suggest the value of psychoeducation for parents and teachers based on their findings that parents and teachers tend to minimize children's trauma-related reactions. Such findings point to the importance of teaching school mental health staff about why and how to deliver psychoeducational programs for parents and teachers.

Training and Access to Schools

In general, board members, superintendents, and educators in management vary greatly in their understanding of DMH training for schools, and likewise, community mental health professionals vary greatly in their understanding of how schools operate. Consequently, schools and community mental health agencies can benefit from establishing predisaster working relationships and trainings-in-common to help each learn about their respective personnel and operations. Without predisaster planning, coordination, and training, well-intentioned mental health professionals can compound the chaotic environment after a disaster.

For example, after one tragic school shooting that received national media attention, 250 "counselors" from a variety of city and county, private and public agencies flooded the high school campus of 1,900 students to offer help. The principal wanted to know the counselors' credentials. Were they licensed? Were they experienced with children or adults? Because state education law required background checks of adults, including volunteers, working with students in a school, some of the questions were answered. During the process of screening, many of the volunteers disclosed that they had never worked at a school or provided crisis counseling services to adolescents. Some became highly emotional about the death and injury of the students and needed support themselves. Some volunteers had no degrees but worked as gang or drug peer counselors. School administrators were grateful for the overwhelmingly positive response of the volunteers but did not fully realize the implications of having to screen, train, feed, house, and organize a volunteer group that was larger than the total number of employees in the school. Developing partnerships with appropriate, child-serving mental health agencies before a crisis allows all parties to plan ahead for these contingencies.

DMH training for schools must be geared toward implementing school-based mental health services that enhance classroom management and demonstrate benefits to children's health, mental health, and learning. The challenge is to establish school/DMH partnerships to ensure that mental health interventions result in the least disruption to the work of the classroom and the routines of the schoolday.

Once training is approved, the first step is delivering multidisciplinary staff training to develop sufficient skills and resources to implement specialized DMH services. Preparing school and district staffs to respond requires increasing their level of information and awareness and building skills necessary to develop disaster-related roles and responsibilities. Work to ameliorate the negative effects of disasters on children begins with the adults in the school family. Teachers, principals, school nurses, counselors, and others at the school must be encouraged to take the time to address their own disaster experiences and any related trauma effects.

Training for Individuals in Positions of School Leadership

Community and school-based mental health professionals may be in the best position to mentor school leadership through the unfamiliar landscape of creating postdisaster school-based recovery programs that enhance classroom management and demonstrate benefits to children's health, mental health, and learning, All school personnel operate within a hierarchical system of governance from school sites to the "central office" or executive staff of the school district. At the highest levels of leadership in schools, the Board of Education and the Superintendent of Schools represent the ultimate authority to approve the provision of all training, programs, and services in the schools of the district.

Training for Teachers

After disasters, the classroom teacher is not only the instructional leader of the classroom but also the caregiving adult well acquainted with the cognitive, social, and emotional status of students. Teachers require training about the disaster-related behaviors that are common among school-age children (e.g., impaired concentration and learning; regression; and altered behavior such as aggression, recklessness, reduced inhibitions, somatic complaints, and school attendance refusal).

Teacher training should also include opportunities to practice new methods of intervening with disaster-related anxiety, withdrawal, anger, or uncooperative student behavior. Mental health professionals can "coach" teachers on how to speak with students about disaster-related fears and experiences in a manner appropriate to age and developmental level. For example, teachers can help students identify traumatic reminders or encourage them to alert the teacher when intrusive thoughts and/or anxious feelings overwhelm their ability to cope in the classroom (Pynoos & Nader, 1988).

Training for "Nonteaching" School Personnel

In all school districts, there is an array of nonteaching staff members of all ages, often reflecting the community surrounding the school. They are paraprofessionals who may speak a second language, in addition to English, or share the same ethnicity, culture, religion, or place of birth of the students. As such, after a disaster, they are an important linguistic, cultural, and emotional bridge to students and their families. The office manager, secretary or clerical staff, custodians, cafeteria staff, and bus drivers should all receive training with appropriate levels of content and demonstrations of supportive actions and interactions with students and adults.

Training for School Nurses

Beyond their extensive education and health-related skills, school nurses can benefit from training that provides them with additional skills to assess medical problems that may be caused by disaster-related stress and educate students, parents, and staff about disaster-related stress and coping skills. As key members of the school crisis team, nurses can enhance their work in triage and psychological first aid with DMH training.

Training for School Mental Health Staff

The school counselor, the school psychologist, and the school social worker represent the "in-house" mental health professionals of the school. Obviously, each should be included in community mental health training for response and recovery work with children. It is not uncommon across school-based disciplines that professional training and experiences widely vary.

An additional step is to combine the training of school mental health professionals with community mental health professionals (before and after a disaster). Joint training can provide opportunities to strengthen partnerships and develop an integrated, coordinated DMH response in the school and community. Most "school crisis training" typically focuses on the immediate response phase, emphasizing checklists, psychological first aid, psychoeducation, and community referral. Training with community mental health professionals gives school-based practitioners the opportunity to gain a more comprehensive view of DMH needs over time, including assessments and interventions appropriate to the intermediate and long-term mental health needs of students and staff.

DMH TRAINING TO PROMOTE SELF-HELP/MUTUAL AID FOLLOWING A DISASTER

Self-help/mutual aid (SH/MA) interventions in response to disasters refer to a set of approaches for increasing personal coping through informal sources, and specifically peers (i.e., those who share firsthand knowledge associated with a particular circumstance or event), in some structured way. Postdisaster SH/MA interventions could include peer-led community-wide meetings that allow members to share stories and provide support and promotion of self-help groups for persons experiencing posttraumatic distress or grieving the loss of a loved one, as well as versions of these approaches offered over the Internet. The promotion of SH/MA interventions before a disaster occurs could include establishing the groundwork for community meetings to take place in the event of future national, state, or local events that affect local communities.

Training

DMH practitioners generally have little experience in helping establish SH/MA interventions. Furthermore, overinvolvement, control, and direction by mental health professionals might coopt the SH/MA ethos (Constantino & Nelson, 1995). Table 4.2 presents an outline of training, designed and organized to be consistent with the SH/MA ethos and methods.

TABLE 4.2. DMH Practitioner Training: How to Help Establish Disaster-Related Self-Help Groups

- Rationale and theoretical foundation of self-help groups
- Specific issues about self-help groups in response to disasters
- Self-help groups: Mental health professional roles
- Promoting the formation of self-help groups
- Allocation of resources for training of self-help group leaders
- Encouraging participation in self-help groups as a coping strategy
  —Media campaigns (newspapers, radio, television)
  —Referrals
- Encouraging the development of a broad range of groups (parenting, displaced families, bereavement, cultural groups, etc.)
  —Partnering with community groups (e.g., ethnic, disability and elderly groups) to encourage them to develop groups
- Assistance to group leaders in identifying meeting places
- Advisory/consultant role
- Group types (e.g., long-term support vs. single or short-term groups)
- Leadership skills
  —Starting and ending groups
  —Listening skills
  —Effective group leadership skills
  —Dealing with difficult situations (e.g., hostility and extreme emotional distress)
  —Confidentiality
- Special issues

An innovative example of SH/MA disaster preparedness is the Disaster Community Support Network of Philadelphia (DCSN), a program established by the Mental Health Association of Southeastern Pennsylvania (MHASP). A document describing the DCSN in greater detail can be found online at www.mhasp.org/help/dcsn.pdf.

Theory and Research on SH/MA

The potential benefits associated with SH/MA interventions in which peers provide support and assistance to one another are based on a wide range of theories presented in Table 4.3 (Salzer & Mental Health Association of Southeastern Pennsylvania Best Practices Team, in press).

REAL-WORLD ISSUES: DMH TRAINING IN NEW YORK STATE FOLLOWING 9/11

Determining and meeting the training needs of large numbers of crisis counselors most of whom were not experienced in the delivery of DMH services, who were working with different populations in different stages of

TABLE 4.3. Theories Underlying Benefits of Peer-Delivered Services

Social comparison theory

- People seek out interactions with others who have similar experiences.
- Upward comparisons increase self-improvement (e.g., develop skills) and self-enhancement (e.g., increase sense of hope and decrease fears) efforts.
- Downward comparisons are ego enhancing and maintain positive affect by providing examples of how bad things could be.

Social learning theory

- Behavior change is more likely when modeling is provided by peers than nonpeers.
- Peers model coping and health-enhancing behaviors.
- Peers enhance self-efficacy that one can change behavior.

Social support theories

- Consumer-directed services increase support networks, receipt of supportive behaviors, and perceptions of support.
- There are five types of support: (1) emotional (someone to confide in, provides esteem, reassurance, attachment and intimacy); (2) instrumental (services, money, transportation); (3) informational (advice/guidance, help with problem solving and evaluation of behavior and alternative actions); (4) companionship (belonging, socializing, feeling connected to others); and (5) validation (feedback, social comparison).

Experiential knowledge

- Experience leads to an understanding and knowledge base that is different from that acquired through research and observation (i.e., professional knowledge).
- Experiential knowledge leads to different intervention approaches.

Helper-therapy principle

- Helping others is beneficial: (1) increased sense of interpersonal competence as a result of making an impact on another's life; (2) development of a sense of equality in giving and taking between himself or herself and others; (3) helper gains new personally relevant knowledge while helping; and (4) helper receives social approval from the person they help and others.

disaster recovery in a densely populated area, was a significant and never-ending challenge following 9/11. Of primary importance in training crisis counselors is imparting the philosophical underpinnings of the Federal Emergency Management Agency (FEMA) Crisis Counseling Program (CCP). Briefly, the CCP is designed to address short-term mental health needs of communities affected by disasters through public education, outreach, and crisis counseling. In contrast to traditional clinical practice, such programs assume that (1) disaster victims are normal people responding normally to very abnormal situations, and services should be directed at normalizing individuals' experiences and distress; (2) crisis counselors can help reduce distress, restore preevent functioning, prevent chronic dysfunction and distress, facilitate community recovery, and provide comfort and support through empowerment and skills building, education, resource referral, support, outreach, and community capacity building; (3) services may be provided appropriately by trained paraprofessionals; (4) people prefer natural sources of assistance, and services should be provided in schools, churches, and places of work; and (5) people who need help the most may not necessarily seek it, and services must assume a proactive posture to reach out to vulnerable groups. Because of their emphasis on normalizing responses, CCPs have traditionally avoided diagnosis and psychological assessment.

The considerations regarding whom to recruit and train as part of the DMH response were, in large part, forced by the huge scope of the disaster. The immediate need for thousands of crisis counselors and hundreds of supervisors and managers from almost 200 provider agencies shaped many decisions. To uphold a reasonable level of quality management while attending to a sense of urgency in the Immediate Services Program, the New York City Department of Mental Health (as it was known at the time) required that provider agencies be licensed by New York State Office of Mental Health. Working directly with only licensed mental health provider agencies largely determined the staff who would be working in the program and eliminated the huge and time-consuming process of credentialing staff and/or verifying the quality, credibility, and sustainability of service providers largely unknown to the state or the city departments of health.

The FEMA CCP model recommends caution in diagnosing in the immediate aftermath of the disaster unless an individual is in severe psychotic or functional distress that impairs daily activities (Center For Mental Health Services, 2001). The mental health community wanted a highly prescriptive model of crisis counseling service delivery, symptom checklists, and PTSD scales. Outside a limited number of disaster experts, a significant paradigm shift was required for almost all involved. Many community members expressed disappointment that several models of crisis intervention and trauma treatment that they utilized were not supported by the project due to the controversy surrounding their efficacy. The significant differences between conventional clinical practice and a DMH conceptualization of service delivery remained a training issue throughout the disaster.

Moreover, the notion of using paraprofessionals, such as psychiatric interns, emergency room residents, psychology students, caseworkers, and indigenous community members vital to disseminating services in closed communities (Everly, 2002; North & Hong, 2000), was aggressively shunned by the mental health professional community, whose members felt that mental health professionals would be better equipped to make more subtle clinical judgments about the need for targeted education, coping skills training, and referral to more intensive services. This reinforced the recommendation of the state mental health authority and the consulting CMHS staff that training was needed in the basic crisis counseling model during the initial phase and that supervision also needed to occur frequently at this stage (Holloway & Neufeldt, 1995; Najavits, 2000). The FEMA CCP model also emphasizes that crisis counselors provide a supportive presence in the community, where survivors normally gather, not in mental health counseling offices. This, too, was contrary to how most mental health clinicians conceptualized and traditionally delivered mental health services.

In an attempt to lessen the anticipated resistance of the mental health professional community to this "nontraditional" model of care, FEMA CCP model trainings were scheduled almost immediately and were offered often to large audiences. At the trainings, the differences between the FEMA model and the existing mental health structure were highlighted. The New York City disaster response unit mandated the FEMA overview training for all crisis counselors.

A significant training need was related to outreach, which was an unfamiliar mode of service delivery to most of the licensed mental health agencies and their staff of licensed clinicians. Some agencies began by attempting outreach services to community members unknown to them. Other, more community-rooted agencies looked to hire larger numbers of paraprofessionals and indigenous workers from within their communities to deliver services. This plan resulted in the need to train nonlicensed interns, bachelor's-level workers, and students from mental health fields such as psychology or nursing. Other paraprofessionals in need of training included clergy, caseworkers, community leaders, and peer counselors. Indigenous workers such as laborers, clerks, caregivers, and shopkeepers were seen as important for providing crisis counseling in ethnic communities where culture and language barriers existed (Aguilera & Planchon, 1995; Diaz-Lazaro & Cohen, 2001).

Trainers

The New York community was privileged to have many experts in disaster and trauma volunteer to participate in the necessary trainings. Due to large numbers of self-identified experts, cross-scheduled trainings, and the need to ensure a consistent, appropriate approach that followed the CCP model, it was determined that all training activities funded by the FEMA grant would need to be approved centrally, at the state level, rather than at the local provider level. This determination also prompted New York's Bureau of Training and Workforce Development to organize a training task force of representatives from the organizations participating in any mental health training activities in the overall disaster relief response.

As the disaster response project moved into the regular services program phase, the state and city staff intensified training in outreach strategies, identifying hidden populations, expanding the understanding of cultural competence, and using marketing strategies and geomapping to assist in targeted outreach planning.

Challenges Associated with Training in the Aftermath of 9/11

After 9/11, disaster workers had to overcome many obstacles:

- Translating what was heard in terms of training needs into the next set of training workshops with expert, tailored materials within short time frames;
- Attending both to high-risk groups that may benefit from referral for treatment and to the general public, who are less likely to need (or accept) long-term, formal mental health treatment;
- Effectively tailoring each segment of the program by working with community groups and providers to develop the specific training needs that address their populations, organizational structure, and cultural norms.

TOWARD IMPROVING DMH TRAINING

In this concluding section, we offer a number of recommendations toward improving DMH training as it applies to content and procedures; identifying how new technologies can advance the efficacy, availability, and efficiency of training; and developing future research.

Content and Procedures

Because a significant amount of training and services takes place under the auspices of FEMA/CMHS, our recommendations begin with how the FEMA model of crisis counseling is taught.

1. The potential for resistance to the model (by those with minimal experience in crisis counseling experience as well as by highly trained psychotherapists) suggests that in-depth review of the conceptual framework is needed. In addition, role-plays enabling trainees to practice necessary helping skills (e.g., strategies of engagement, rapport building, administering psychological first aid, delivering brief survivor education, skills training, and reducing and managing stress reactions) can help to overcome precon-

ceptions that trainees might hold about the conceptual framework of the FEMA model.

2. The FEMA/CMHS model does little to train counselors to meet the mental health service needs of the severely affected (i.e., survivors who may benefit from treatment). Whereas, the current model emphasizes psychoeducational-oriented interventions, we propose that FEMA/CMHS training be broadened to include evidence-based interventions for disaster-related PTSD, depression, and substance abuse. Specifically, it may be useful to incorporate some parts of CBT intervention packages into training, after adapting them for disasters (i.e., for delivery by nonspecialists, or in briefer formats, for use with individuals who are at high risk for problems following disaster).

3. The state Offices of Emergency Management may be the most suited lead organizations for coordinating local community efforts toward recruiting indigenous workers to join with the paraprofessionals and professionals participating in disaster relief training. With the state's coordination of the potential workforce, the development of a database of these available resources may yield the largest numbers of prepared individuals for deployment over long periods in the advent of large-scale disasters.

4. Including DMH training as a component of the academic curriculum across mental health disciplines in academic institutions can boost the number of trained paraprofessionals (and future professionals). Curricula can include the key concepts of disaster recovery, the strategic use of indigenous and paraprofessionals helpers as well as professional staff, and the importance of interdisciplinary coordination. Schools of medicine, psychology, social work, nursing, and counseling can also be a significant and immediate source of paraprofessional staff to rely on after disaster.

5. Standing DMH response teams may periodically need to take new courses and visit settings (e.g., hospital trauma centers) where acutely traumatized individuals are seen and offered services in order to minimize skill decay (Hagman & Rose, 1983) and to learn about advancements in the field.

6. It may be helpful to develop training "tracks" for specific helper audiences that require special skills or who encounter disaster survivors in settings different from the emergency response setting. DMH team leaders may benefit from specific training in the skills need to organize and lead their disaster team. Psychiatrists and other physicians who may be called on to medicate survivors of traumatic disaster may benefit from training in up-to-date pharmacotherapeutic management of acute stress responses. "Indigenous" primary care physicians/nurses who receive training in screening, brief intervention, and referral may significantly improve their ability to be of service to survivors. Local mental health clinicians may benefit from learning about newer treatment approaches.

7. One desirable outcome of training coordination between the state, localities, and voluntary agencies assigned to the immediate disaster response is a statewide certification in disaster response, encompassing those concepts most common across localities in any type of disaster. Compulsory DMH training for clinical licensure renewal should also be considered.

8. It is highly recommended to invite DMH training experts from nonaffected areas.

9. Future work is needed to develop and disseminate a wide range of SH/MA intervention modes.

10. Specification and standardization of training procedures can ensure quality control and set the stage for more careful evaluation of the impact of training. Greater detailed instruction in how to conduct a course (including instructor scripts to introduce sections and promote discussion, and procedural guidelines regarding use of slides, videotapes, role-plays, and skills demonstration) is needed.

New Technologies

Despite new preparedness initiatives, one aspect of DMH training improvement relates to the need to train DMH workers quickly in the aftermath of a disaster. A potential new technology for "just-in-time" training is the use of personal digital assistants (PDA) and tablet-size computers. Pocket-size computers can now hold detailed training content, algorithms for procedural decisions, and video (visual) demonstrations of helping behaviors. A recent study (Wisher, Sabol, & Ozkaptan, 1996) showed that job aids predicted improvement and increased performance by nearly 25% on seven critical tasks. Another major option for "just-in-time training" is use of Web-facilitated training. In addition, Web-based training may ultimately be the most optimal form of training in the event that a community is quarantined and there is limited access to those in need of training. Another strength of Web-based curricula is that it could potentially be used for many different applications: preparations/credentialing, periodic upgrade of skills, just in-time training, or on-the-ground guidance.

Research

For the content of DMH training to become more evidence-based, a DMH research–training interface must continue to develop. Empirical investigations of interventions, intervention timing, intervention–survivor matching, intervention with individuals versus groups, intervention by professionals versus paraprofessionals, consumer-directed services, optimum administrative service-delivery networks, types of training procedures, the efficacy of specific training modules, and other topics will, in effect, help training content and procedures to become more extensive and precise. It will be important to design a system for periodically updating DMH practice guidelines and associated training content based on emerging empirical findings and theoretical developments.

Just as it is important to move toward evidence-based DMH services, it is important to use evaluation to guide the evolution of DMH training procedures. However, there are significant challenges to determining the efficacy of disaster-related training because of the inherent "distance" between training and clinical outcomes. Even so, valuable information could be gained from studies comparing the efficacy of various teaching procedures (lecture, role-play, "teachbacks," knowledge-based tests, trainer demonstrations, self-guided software programs, etc.) and the efficacy of specific training modules for a controlled application.

CONCLUSION

In this chapter we have delineated the content and procedures for DMH training for clinicians, administrators, school personnel, and paraprofessionals. Factors related to training such as trainees' credentials, roles, and experience; when the training is delivered; topics and learning objectives; the training process; the time available for training; background and teaching experience of the trainer; and available funding were discussed. The implications of posttrauma early-intervention research for DMH training was presented, along with considerations for training school personnel and mental health professionals to help in the development of disaster-related self-help groups. In addition, the real world challenges of assessing and meeting the learning needs of mental health professionals and paraprofessionals in the aftermath of 9/11 was described. Finally, we presented recommendations about improving DMH training with regard to content, procedures, research, and new technologies.

REFERENCES

Aguilera, D. M., & Planchon, L. A. (1995). Disaster response project: Lessons from the past, guidelines for the future. *Professional Psychology: Research and Practice, 26,* 550–557.

Almqvist, K., & Brandell-Forsberg, M. (1997). Refugee children in Sweden: Posttraumatic stress disorder in Iranian preschool children exposed to organized violence. *Child Abuse and Neglect, 21,* 351–366.

American Red Cross. (1990). *American Red Cross instructor candidate training participant's manual* Washington, DC: Author.

Bisson, J. I., McFarlane, A. C., & Rose, S. (2000). Psychological debriefing. In E. B.

Foa, T. M. Keane, & M. J. Friedman (Eds.), *Effective treatments for PTSD: Practice guidelines from the International Society for Traumatic Stress Studies* (pp. 39–59). New York: Guilford Press.

Bryant, R. A., & Harvey, A. G. (2000). *Acute stress disorder: A handbook of theory, assessment, and treatment.* Washington, DC: American Psychological Association.

Bryant, R. A, Harvey, A. G., Dang, S. T., Sackville, T., & Basten, C. (1998). Treatment of acute stress disorder: A comparison of cognitive-behavioral therapy and supportive counseling. *Journal of Consulting and Clinical Psychology, 66,* 862–866.

Bryant, R. A., Sackville, T., Dang, S. T., Moulds, M., & Guthrie, R. (1999). Treating acute stress disorder: An evaluation of cognitive behavior therapy and supportive counseling techniques. *American Journal of Psychiatry, 156,* 1780–1786.

Burns, B. J., Costello, E. J., Angold, A., Tweed, D., Stangl, D., Farmer, E. M., et al. (1995). Children's mental health service use across service sectors. *Health Affairs, 14,* 147–159.

Center for Mental Health Services. (2001). *An overview of the crisis counseling assistance and training program* (CCP-PG-01). Rockville, MD: Author.

Constantino, V., & Nelson, G. (1995). Changing relationships between self-help groups and mental health professionals: Shifting ideology and power. *Canadian Journal of Community Mental Health, 14,* 55–70.

Diaz-Lazaro, C. M., & Cohen, B. B. (2001). Cross-cultural contact in counseling training. *Journal of Multicultural Counseling and Development, 29,* 41–56.

Ehlers, A., & Clark, D. M. (2000). A cognitive model of posttraumatic stress disorder. *Behaviour Research and Therapy, 38,* 319–345.

Everly, G. S., Jr. (2002). Thoughts on peer (paraprofessional) support in the provision of mental health services. *International Journal of Emergency Mental Health, 4,* 89–92.

Foa, E. B., & Rothbaum, B. O. (1997). *Treating the trauma of rape: Cognitive-behavioral therapy for PTSD.* New York: Guilford Press.

Galea, S., Resnick, H. S., Ahern, T., Gold, J., Buevvalas, M. J., Kilpatrick, D. G., et al. (2002). Posttraumatic stress disorder in Manhattan, New York City, after the September 11th terrorist attacks. *Journal of Urban Health, 79,* 340–353.

Gentilello, L. M., Rivara, F. P., Donovan, D. M., Jurkovich, G. J., Daranciang, E., Dunn, C. W., et al. (1999). Alcohol interventions in a trauma center as a means of reducing the risk of injury recurrence. *Annals of Surgery, 230,* 473–483.

Hagman, J., & Rose, A. (1983). Retention of military tasks: A review. *Human Factors, 25,* 199–213.

Heather, N. (1995). Brief intervention strategies. In R. K. Hester & W. R. Miller (Eds.), *Handbook of alcoholism treatment approaches* (2nd ed., pp. 105–122). New York: Pergamon Press.

Hoagwood, K., & Erwin, H. D. (1997). Effectiveness of school-based mental health services for children: A 100 year research review. *Journal of Child and Family Studies, 6,* 435–451.

Holloway, E. L., & Neufeldt, S. A. (1995). Supervision: its contributions to treatment efficacy. *Journal of Consulting and Clinical Psychology, 63,* 207–213.

Kataoka, S. H., Zhang, L., & Wells, K. B. (2002). Unmet need for mental health care among US children: Variation by ethnicity and insurance status. *American Journal of Psychiatry, 159,* 1548–1555.

Litz, B. T., Gray, M. J., Bryant, R. A., & Adler, A. B. (2002). Early intervention for trauma: Current status and future directions. *Clinical Psychology: Science and Practice, 9,* 112–134.

Malmquist, C. (1986). Children who witness parental murder: Posttraumatic aspects. *Journal of the American Academy of Child Psychiatry, 25,* 320–325.

Najavits, L. M. (2000). Training clinicians in the seeking safety treatment protocol for posttraumatic stress disorder and substance abuse. *Alcoholism Treatment Quarterly, 18,* 83–98.

Norris, F. H., Friedman, M. J., Watson, P. J., Byrne, C. M., Diaz, E., & Kaniasty, K. Z. (2002). 60,000 disaster victims speak, Part I. an empirical review of the empirical literature: 1981–2001. *Psychiatry, 65,* 207–239.

Norris, F. H., Watson, P. J., Hamblen, J. L., & Pfefferbaum, B. J. (2005). Provider perspectives on disaster mental health services in Oklahoma City. In Y. Danieli, D. Brom, & J. B. Sills (Eds.), *The trauma of terrorism: Sharing knowledge and shared care, an international handbook* (pp. 649–662). Binghamton, NY: Haworth Press.

North, C. S., & Hong, B. A. (2000). Project CREST: A new model for mental health intervention after a community disaster. *American Journal of Public Health, 90,* 1057–1058.

Pynoos, R. S., & Nader, K. (1988). Psychological first aid and treatment approach to children exposed to community violence: Research implications. *Journal of Traumatic Stress, 1,* 445–473.

Resick, P. A., Nishith, P., Weaver, T. L., Astin, M. C., & Feuer, C. A. (2002). A comparison of cognitive-processing therapy with prolonged exposure and a waiting condition for the treatment of chronic posttraumatic stress disorder in female rape victims. *Journal of Consulting and Clinical Psychology, 70,* 867–879.

Rigamer, E. F. (1986). Psychological management of children in a national crisis. *Journal of American Academy of Child Psychiatry, 25,* 364–369.

Rollnick, S., Heather, N., & Bell, A. (1992). Negotiating behaviour change in medical settings: The development of brief motivational interviewing. *Journal of Mental Health, 1,* 25–37.

Ruzek, J. I. (2002). Providing "Brief Education and Support" for emergency response workers: An alternative to debriefing. *Military Medicine, 167*(Suppl.), 73–75.

Sack, W. H., Angell, R. H., Kinzie, J. D., & Rath, B. (1986). The psychiatric effects of massive trauma on Cambodian children, II: The family, the home, and the school. *Journal of American Academy of Child Psychiatry, 25,* 377–383.

Salzer, M. S., & Mental Health Association of Southeastern Pennsylvania Best Practices Team. (2002). Consumer-delivered services as a best practice in mental health care and the development of practice guidelines. *Psychiatric Rehabilitation Skills, 6,* 355–382.

Wisher, R. A., Sabol, M. A., & Ozkaptan, H. (1996). *Retention of "peace support operations" tasks during Bosnia deployment: A basis for refresher training* (special report). Alexandria, VA: U. S. Army Research Institute for the Behavioral and Social Sciences.

Young, B. H. (2002). Emergency outreach: Navigational and brief screening guidelines for working in large group settings following catastrophic events. *National Center for PTSD Clinical Quarterly, 11,* 1–6.

Young, B. H., & Gerrity, E. (1994). Critical incident stress debriefing (CISD): Value and limitations in disaster response. *National Center for Post-Traumatic Stress Disorder Clinical Quarterly, 4,* 17–19.

Young, B. H., Ruzek, J. I., & Pivar, I. (2001). *Mental health aspects of disaster and community violence: A review of training materials.* Menlo Park, CA: National Center for PTSD and Washington, DC: Center for Mental Health Services.

CHAPTER 5

Immediate Needs Assessment Following Catastrophic Disaster Incidents

ANTHONY H. SPEIER

Disasters are complex events that affect untold numbers of persons and communities through the catastrophic loss of loved ones, destruction of property, dissolution of economic security, or, for many disaster survivors, the loss of their psychological well-being. Disaster incidents are also public health incidents that threaten the general well-being and survivability of communities. This discussion of disaster incidents attempts to identify a number of issues associated with needs assessment and intervention strategies. As illustrated in the following three examples from Louisiana, New York, and Virginia, each approach to assess the needs of survivors and the affected communities depends on the resources available and the character of the incident.

The conceptual needs assessment model set forth in this chapter specifies the importance of gathering information from various sources: survivors, media, and traditional bureaucratic sources. The model also emphasizes the importance of recognizing the interaction between the incident response and survivors' ongoing recovery. By establishing information feedback loops within the disaster mental health (DMH) program design, one is more likely to access both qualitative and quantitative information sources reflecting the changing needs of survivors. Utilizing such an approach will result in the development of intervention services that remain consistent with the stages of recovery within affected communities.

BACKGROUND

Catastrophes disrupt the entire fabric of communities. Irrespective of origin, the potential for loss to individuals is pervasive and potentially enduring across the remainder of their lifespan. The consequences of the psychological impact of disasters has spawned much speculation about mitigation, the development of intuitively derived interventions, and a variety of evaluation and research studies of varying quality (Norris, 2001).

A few Web-based inquiries regarding disaster and mental health consequences and one is quickly overwhelmed with theory and services/approaches to dealing with disasters and associated trauma reactions. Even with all the discussions of the physical and psychological impact in the scientific, professional, and conventional media, people and communities are often ill prepared to deal with catastrophes. Lack of adequate preparation by communities and individuals before the disaster often results in disaster response activities implemented as reactive planning during the incident and not as a systematic implementation of a proactive incident response strategy.

Ideally, when a disaster happens, a series of preplanned community response activities are mobilized: highly disciplined responses by cadres of first-responder units such as police, fire, emergency management units, and medical emergency units. Their collective response goals are to protect persons and property and to preserve the community infrastructure of roads, communications, utilities, and so on.

Recently the Federal Emergency Management Agency (FEMA) and the National Emergency Management Association (NEMA) initiated a strategy for assisting states and local communities with an ongoing assessment of response capabilities. The Capabilities Assessment for Readiness (CAR) initiative assists states in assessing their capability for response in 13 core areas: (1) laws and authorities; (2) hazard identification and risk assessment; (3) hazard management; (4) resource management; (5) planning; (6) direction and control; (7) communications and warning; (8) operations and procedures; (9) logistics and facilities; (10) training; (11) exercises, evaluations, and corrective actions; (12) crisis communications, public education, and information; and (13) finance and administration. The state/region self-assessment process seeks to answer three very basic questions:

1. Is the emergency management program comprehensive for the state's needs?
2. Are the objectives and mission of the organization being achieved?
3. Is the state able to redirect strategic deployment of resources and help communities and citizens avoid becoming disaster victims?

Preincident self-assessment by states and local communities is well developed compared to preparedness and mitigation efforts involved with responding to the psychological impact of catastrophes. Disaster response scenarios and planning efforts have traditionally recognized mental health areas as an aspect of the primary health care response. Disaster incidents of natural and terrorist origin over the last decade (e.g., Hurricane Andrew in Florida and Louisiana, 1992; the Alfred P. Murrah Federal Building bombing in Oklahoma City, 1995; the events of September 11, 2001, in Pennsylvania, New York City, Virginia, and Washington, DC; and Hurricane Katrina in New Orleans, 2005) demonstrated the pervasiveness of disaster stressors of both a social and psychological nature on communities and their residents.

It is still not uncommon for emergency response officials to view the assessment of the mental health needs of their communities as a secondary activity. The psychological impact of disaster incidents often becomes a consideration only after its symptoms appear in individuals and those symptoms place a subsequent strain on public and other community resources.

Immediate postincident mental health interventions are frequently triggered by the disruptive impact of overt psychological sequelae. Either response actions are linked to the American Red Cross and other shelter and relief operations, providing brief interventions of psychological first aid, or the public mental health system is asked to respond to persons who emerge from the incident gravely disabled, or a danger to self or others, and meet the standard for involuntary psychiatric hospitalization. As the literature documents, unresolved psychological distress can grow into varying states of emotional and cognitive dysfunction in individuals for weeks, months, and even years following exposure to trauma (Kalayjian, 1995; Kaniasty & Norris, 2000).

In the United States, the William T. Stafford disaster response legislation provides for crisis counseling to assist communities in addressing the psychological impact of disaster incidents. The focus of federal crisis counseling programs authorized under the Stafford Act is to determine who is at risk and what the identified strategy is for assisting communities and individuals to move through response and recovery. Funding for crisis counseling grants is contingent upon affected communities providing broad-based needs assessment data, which specifies who needs help and how much.

A recent analysis by Norris (2003) of the Center for Mental Health Services (CMHS) needs assessment methodology identified five implicit assumptions associated with estimating the scope of DMH recovery needs following a major disaster:

1. Mental health needs vary according to the severity and scope of the disaster.
2. Individual disaster victims are at risk according to their own se-

verity of exposure; some stressors create more problems than others.

3. Exposure of an individual affects the whole household.
4. A calculation based solely on the numbers of direct victims cannot capture the full impact of the disaster.
5. Certain subpopulations are more at risk for mental health problems than others, and if such groups are present in significant numbers in the community, the plan should address this.

Norris's review of the CMHS approach generally validates the aforementioned assumptions with some added caveats. Norris recommends including the following additional factors in future CMHS needs assessments:

- Assessment of available community resources, not just assessment of loss indicators.
- Assessment of additional categories of impact from terrorist incidents, such as indicators of evacuation due to imminent danger and indicators of the number of persons involved in rescue/recovery activities.
- Assessment of special circumstances associated with the disaster, including questions specific to the degree of human causation, indirect impact on the community, and the extent of ongoing threat and uncertainty.

Determining who is affected directly or indirectly and to what degree is always related to the unique character of each disaster. The assessment of vulnerability for delayed emotional and instrumental recovery and/or the manifestation of significant indicators of psychological trauma within a community and its inhabitants is not yet fully documented. Evidence in the literature suggests that most people recover without assistance and that only a relatively small number experience enduring clinical symptoms from trauma exposure (Benight & Harper, 2002; McFarlane, 1996).

Experience with disaster survivors in Louisiana specifically, and similar informal reports to the author from other public mental health administrators throughout the country, repeatedly suggest that only a few survivors ever seek mental health assistance, and that virtually no one directly seeks services immediately following a disaster. Services, if sought out at all, are requested or implicitly accepted by survivors dealing with the immediacy of the circumstances. Persons most likely to seek services have just experienced a significant personal loss: the death of a loved one, the loss of possessions and resources such as their residence, a separation from loved ones, or direct exposure to disturbing sights, smells, and sounds of the catastrophe. Disaster survivors are seldom aware of its impact and are instead consumed with the business of survival.

During the first days and weeks following a major disaster event, individuals and communities are usually overwhelmed with activities involving debris removal, restoration of basic services from public utilities, and securing temporary solutions for housing/home repair. During this period, residents of communities are very visible to each other. One of the paradoxical impacts of a disaster is that through devastation and loss, individuals bond together, building common solutions for meeting basic needs.

Simultaneous with the activity of survival is the process of absorbing the breadth of loss. The literature on sudden loss and trauma is replete with accounts of individuals performing extraordinary acts of kindness and heroism. Brende (1998) described the first two of five phases of emotional and physiological response as (1) immediate coping and (2) early adaptation, where individuals exhibit clear thinking and much organized effort, coupled with a sense of fearlessness and cooperation. There appears to be a will among survivors not to be defeated. These early response phases give way to (3) mid-phase adaptation, with alternating states of denial and emotionally numbness, to (4) late-phase adaptation characterized by anger and stress-related physical symptoms. In Brende's final phase, (5) resolution or symptom development, individuals either move onward or become enmeshed with stress- and trauma-related symptoms.

This characterization of the process of emotional response is consistent with Cohen and Ahearn's (1980) seminal description of emotional processes in response to a catastrophe. When initiating a mental health response, Cohen and Ahearn emphasize a model of intervention that considers the interaction between the survivor's personal characteristics, history with dealing with loss/catastrophe, the environment, the impact and type of disaster event, and personal degree of loss. This intervention model emphasizes the following principles (Cohen & Ahearn, 1980, p. 39):

- Bereavement and loss reactions follow individuals when they affect an individual through a loss of person, property, or environment.
- Individuals vary in levels of adaptation to new situations and environments.
- Crisis symptoms are produced by and in turn affect social, psychological, and physiological disorganization.
- Postdisaster victims need social, psychological, physiological, and economic help.
- The aftereffects of crisis resolution can be long term, moderate, minimal, or severe, depending on the adaptive/nonadaptive resolution of demands the disaster places on the individual.

Interventions recognized by Franklin (1983) are consistent with response strategies implemented in crisis counseling programs funded through FEMA by the CMHS (2003). The basic approach emphasizes strategies based on the assumptions that the traumatized have histories of ongoing adaptive behavior and are basically resilient in their ability to overcome adversity. Hence, intervention strategies should assume that the symptoms expressed by persons are principally disaster related and not symptoms of mental illness requiring diagnosis and therapeutic intervention.

PLANNING FOR INTERVENTIONS

So how do we begin to initiate a response to persons traumatized by a disaster? Assume the following:

- People go through phases of psychological and emotional adjustment to crisis and trauma.
- The chaos associated with catastrophes leads to a disorganization in both the individual's and community's routine coping strategies.
- An individual's response is a function of personality, history of psychological and emotional response strategies, degree of the disaster's impact, breadth of loss (perceived and actual), and the environment.
- Emotional and physiological distress are normal and expected reactions to catastrophes.
- Emotional impact is not immediately expressed, as survivors and responders are busy with the immediacy of response; it may be weeks or months after the incident before such an impact is recognized.

To build an effective response strategy, which remains sensitive to the subtle issues and response characteristics of survivors, discussed previously, we must carefully assess socioenvironmental factors and unique features of the incident's impact on communities and individuals. To accomplish such a needs assessment, attention must focus on several things.

Location of the Disaster

The terrain in which a disaster occurs is important in developing a response. For instance, working through the FEMA Human Services Officer at the Disaster Field Office (DFO), state and local DMH staff can acquire site maps, which identify the path of the storm and the specific areas of impact. Street maps of affected communities contain census tract data describing the demographics of each area. FEMA also provides maps detailing the geographic location of claims for assistance filed through the teleregistration center. This information, plus damage estimates available from the American Red Cross, will let the DMH team target high- and low-disaster-impact areas. Location information and impact data are available through the FEMA website (www.fema.gov).

People Impacted by the Disaster

Once the DMH operations team has identified communities directly affected, the process of understanding the unique features of each community and its inhabitants can begin. During the earliest stages of incident response, the major objective of DMH operations is to mobilize available staff at shelters and other mass care facilities. This response tends to be more generic, with tailoring resources to the characteristics of the population being a secondary concern. During this stage, getting support to responders and survivors has priority. Within the first 2 weeks following the incident the primary response phase subsides and a more enduring method of operations is necessary. The DMH staff person charged with managing the continuing response must build an enduring response based on a thorough assessment of the disaster environment and the detrimental impact that will remain over several months and years.

Following is an extensive but by no means exhaustive list of factors that may influence the depth of a disaster's impact and the relative resilience of individuals and communities in their recovery. Staff tasked with conducting disaster-related needs assessment should consider such factors when gathering data, which will influence future response and recovery strategies.

- Demographic characteristics of affected community members.
- Racial and ethnic distribution of the various neighborhoods, villages, townships, and metropolitan areas.
- Primary languages spoken by the residents of the different communities.
- Age distribution among survivors.
- Range of family composition within neighborhoods.
- At-risk and medically fragile special populations groups.
- Structure of the local economy and range of jobs lost and those still available.
- Specific populations with limited resources, such as migrant farm workers living in the area.
- Educational resources in the area.
- Elementary and high schools located in the area.
- Resources for child care among the communities.
- Spiritual life of the community.

- Churches and church schools destroyed.
- Churches as part of the primary community infrastructure for community neighborhoods.
- Resources for the elderly.
- Nursing homes, retirement communities, and community centers.
- Educational level and professional training within the communities.
- Number of insured versus uninsured homes and businesses.
- Number of rental properties as primary residences versus owned/ mortgaged homes.
- Number and locations where residences are primarily trailers and mobile homes.
- Availability of temporary housing stock.
- Number of whole communities relocated.
- Number of survivors displaced and living with relatives or living in temporary housing in other communities.
- Number of survivors relocating to other areas. Stakeholder groups with a vested interest in community recovery such as the local ministerial alliance, school board, mayor's office, local universities, and medical schools.
- Previous community experience with catastrophes such as major disasters.
- Individual and community expectations about the occurrence of hurricanes, floods, tornadoes, and/or earthquakes.
- Awareness of population with the response and recovery process due to the frequency of natural disasters or terrorist attacks.

NEEDS ASSESSMENT FOLLOWING A NATURAL DISASTER INCIDENT: HURRICANE LILI

As mentioned previously, FEMA-funded crisis counseling programs are based on a thorough needs assessment. An example of the limitations of relying simply on a quantitative needs assessment is illustrated in the assessment conducted by the Louisiana Office of Mental Health (2002) following Hurricane Lili in October 2002. Table 5.1 lists the number affected based on the CMHS categories for quantitative needs assessment.

The data in Table 5.1 are specific to number of dead, injured, and homeless but do not reflect other geographic, psychosocial stressors, and socioeconomic factors, which interact with the incident impact and complicate individual and community recovery. Examples of additional qualitative indicators of need expressed by Louisiana residents following Hurricane Lili include the following:

TABLE 5.1. Traditional Quantitative Needs Assessment

Loss categories	Number of persons	ANH (annual number per household)	Range estimated	Total[a]
Dead	1	2.7	100%	2.7
Hospitalized	4	2.7	35%	3.8
Nonhospitalized injured	60 (carbon monoxide poisoning from generators)	2.7	15%	24.3
Homes destroyed	243	2.7	100%	656
Homes with "major damage"	2,012 (American Red Cross) estimate	2.7	35%	1,904
Total				2,591

[a]Total number of persons targeted per loss category = number of persons × ANH × range estimated (at-risk multiplier).

1. FEMA human services activity through October 10, 2002, indicated a total of 66,646 teleregistrations, with an anticipation of over 100,00 registrants.
2. Through October 10, 2002, only $2,762,200 in emergency housing checks had been issued; $14.8 million had been approved.
3. The Small Business Administration had received 16,508 home and business referrals from FEMA registrations for individual assistance. In addition, 33,000 home inspections had been returned to FEMA by October 14, 2002.
4. There were 235 frail elderly housed in a special needs shelter in Lafayette Parish.
5. Farm and fishery reports from the agricultural communities indicated significant loss of crops due to flooding and wind damage. Louisiana State University estimated damage to crops as high as $242 million.
6. Large numbers of snakes, mosquitoes, fungi, molds, and mildew became more prevalent and presented a very real as well as perceived threat to survivors.
7. A tremendous amount of waste materials was released into homes and private water wells flooded by overrun sewage systems.
8. There were special population issues unique to rural southwestern and southeastern Louisiana, such as the number of older persons of French–Cajun heritage who are functionally monolingual in

French and functionally illiterate. In addition, Iberia Parish and Terrebonne/Lafourche Parishes have indigenous populations of The Houma Indian Nation, as well as many Vietnamese immigrants. These persons are suspicious of government programs and will only seek much needed assistance if they trust the source.

9. A wide range of marginal living conditions and ongoing or disaster-related stressors interact, complicating recovery from the disaster. Following are selected case examples reflective of these conditions:

- A mother, father, and two children are living in their storm-damaged and unlevel mobile home. They fear snakes, spiders, and alligators coming on the porch again. The two children are terrified, not sleeping and noncommunicative. The husband and wife both have histories of clinical depression.
- A 5-year-old boy has not spoken since the hurricane; fire destroyed his house after a power line fell on it.
- Two families were removed from homes to a motel after a pack of 100 opossums claimed their trailers following the storm when they had been forced to evacuate.
- A woman with pressured speech is nervous and anxious about her husband who works in Atlanta, and she tries to clean up debris and mud on weekends.
- The impact of previous floods and now two in one week caused an older woman to feel trapped in Louisiana; she won't leave due to family and memories.
- A 52-year-old grandmother is depressed and without resources to repair her trailer. She recently lost both her son and daughter to suicide, was abused by her father and grandfather, and was stalked by first husband. She possesses limited resources and is trying to raise her 6- and 8-year-old grandchildren.

The quantitative needs assessment suggested 2,591 persons most at risk. The inclusion of additional quantitative and qualitative indicators unique to the incident indicated that 23,464 residents in Louisiana needed assistance from the FEMA-funded crisis counseling program. In sum, the comprehensive assessment submitted by the state relied on data representative of persons directly experiencing loss of loved ones, property, and jobs as well as general indicators of distress among residents of the affected communities. Longer-term assessment of ongoing recovery needs and resources to respond to these needs should reflect both quantitative and qualitative aspects of the individuals and communities in areas of the greatest physical destruction.

NEEDS ASSESSMENT FOLLOWING A TERRORIST-INITIATED CATASTROPHE WITH MASS CASUALTIES: THE PENTAGON AND WORLD TRADE CENTER BOMBINGS

Assessment of disaster-related mental health needs following September 11, 2001, in the states of Virginia and New York reflect two different assessment approaches to terrorist incidents that were of the same origin but resulted in distinct disasters.

The Virginia Needs Assessment

The plane crash into the Pentagon in Arlington, Virginia, was in one respect a terrorist act on a military installation but, from a broader perspective, a bombing incident impacting nine counties in northern Virginia and the metropolitan Washington, DC, area. Accounts of the response produced by the Virginia Community Resilience Crisis Counseling team show the complexity of variables involved when assessing the needs for response and recovery operations. The Pentagon sustained major damage from the terrorists' using American Airlines Flight 77 as its weapon of mass destruction. Three of the five rings of the Pentagon were damaged, killing 189, including the 64 persons on the aircraft. Over the days and weeks after the attack, the Virginia response teams were confronted with numerous needs:

1. *Sociodemographic and cultural*
   - Counseling needs of families and friends of the dead, first responders, schoolchildren, airport employees, commuters who witnessed the attack, and immigrants who had fled their own war-torn countries.
   - The unique impact of job loss, fear of subsequent attacks, loss of colleagues, and personal safety on the 23,000 Pentagon employees, 10,000 airport employees in the region, and 70,000 individuals in the hotel, restaurant, and travel industries.
   - Regional demographic factors implicit within nine governmental jurisdictions encompassing 1.8 million persons, speaking over 100 languages in the sixth largest immigrant metropolitan area in the United States.
   - Twenty percent of the Arlington County population is foreign-born and 20,000 residents are of the Muslim faith.
2. *Initial incident response*
   - Resource cost (psychological and instrumental) on the public mental health system, law enforcement agencies, fire and rescue operations, emergency medical services, hospitals, state medical

examiners office, emergency management agencies, public health departments, military, and volunteer agencies.

3. *Covariables influencing response and recovery*
   - Constrained interagency information exchange between military and civilian agencies due to the Pentagon's high security as a military facility.
   - Variability among the numerous media reports of the incident, response, and recovery operations.
   - Subsequent anthrax attacks within governmental facilities in the area.
   - Ongoing reporting of the likelihood of more terrorist attacks on area bridges and public facilities.

The Virginia experience demonstrates the numerous factors that must be considered when assessing the mental health needs of communities affected by catastrophe. Even at the most cursory level of assessment, the interaction between the existing characteristics of the community and the nature of the incident exposes numerous risk factors that create a psychological impact.

The CMHS funded a comprehensive mental health needs assessment for states affected by September 11, 2001. As part of its needs assessment methodology, the Virginia Department of Mental Health (VADMH; 2001) conducted key-informant interviews and focus groups. Through this and other estimation processes the VADMH identified an unduplicated count of 3,223 persons receiving services in the 6- to 8-week period following September 11. Initial estimates indicated that 4,700 persons (duplicated count) received mental health services and 17,000 accessed 72 community service agencies, including mental health agencies. An important aspect of any needs assessment is to account for individuals accessing many services multiple times as distinct from persons who access services only once. Similar needs assessment activities in Louisiana following Hurricane Lili suggest the importance of separating intensity of service utilization by any given individual from the number of individuals in need of assistance.

In Virginia, within the first 6–8 weeks postincident the following groups received services:

- Direct survivors
- Families, friends, and neighbors of those killed
- Emergency personnel and their families who responded to the incident
- Emergency personnel and their families who did not respond to the incident
- Those unemployed as a result of terrorist activities

- Individuals living near terrorists targets or the Pentagon
- Persons who because of their nation of origin or Islamic faith feel themselves targets of misplaced anger
- Immigrants who had come to Virginia to escape danger
- School-age children

Indicating the variability among needs assessment estimation techniques, the number of persons identified as in need of services was different for each of the three estimation methodologies that the VADMH used. The local mental health community service board estimated 35,776 persons in need; the FEMA approach estimation technique showed a "low" estimate of 165,706 and a "high" estimate of 170,581; an extrapolation of the Oklahoma City approach estimated 32,376 in need of mental health services. The VADMH needs assessment staff highlighted the limitations of current needs assessment methodologies to estimate postincident DMH needs following September 11. VADMH's final report recommends a national needs assessment model and that methodology be established to answer the following:

- Who needs services (e.g., age, gender, race, and population group)?
- What services are needed for different types of recipients?
- What is the distribution of service need by geographic location?

New York State Needs Assessment

The New York State Office of Mental Health (2001) defines needs assessment as

> a set of tools designed to provide accurate and reliable population-based information to emergency managers. The objective is to obtain information about the disaster mental health needs of the community. Specific needs assessment may be conducted for determining disaster mental health needs of children and families. In assessing need, it is important to get that information directly from the population you are trying to help and from persons directly responding to the needs of the particular population. . . .

However, estimating techniques used by staff following September 11 were inconsistent with the approach specified in the aforementioned definition. As the New York Office of Mental Health staff reported, the singularity of the event overwhelmed the needs assessment process as a systematic activity. Incident data and indicators of future needs of the persons affected were confounded by factors that introduced inconsistencies, hence unreliability, into the information. And, due to the complexity, sources were not always directly linked to those needing assistance.

The experience in New York, although unique, resembles experiences with needs assessment approaches in Louisiana and Virginia in that the FEMA/CMHS loss categories of (1) missing or dead, (2) hospitalized, (3) nonhospitalized injured, (4) homes destroyed, and (5) homes major/minor damage did not reflect all factors influencing the need for mental health assistance. Regarding New York City, continuous efforts to refine estimates of need resulted in the use of the foregoing five categories with an enhanced "at-risk" multiplier for 28,047 persons.

Expanding the needs estimation indicators to include (6) disaster-displaced employed/unemployed, (7) World Trade Center (WTC) emergency and recovery workers, (8) WTC evacuees, (9) WTC workers absent at time of attack, (10) schoolchildren and teachers in evacuated area, (11) New York City schoolchildren at high risk, (12) preschool and school-age children, and (13) global community outreach expands the estimated need to 2,109,762 persons. Global outreach (655,391), preschool and school-age children (690,400), and New York City schoolchildren at high risk (206,000) account for 1,551,791 of those with ongoing mental health needs (New York State Office of Mental Health, 2002). Of special interest are other more subtle factors identified within the New York needs assessment that reflect the fabric of communities and directly inform the structure of mental health services provided in both 60-day postincident and long-term (1–3 years postincident) recovery efforts.

In sum, the assessment of need throughout New York City's five boroughs underscores the necessity of considering population and community factors that place various subgroups within a community at risk. Examples unique to the WTC bombing include the impact on the first-responder community, notably police and fire departments, the thousands of disaster workers, and other public servants and volunteers who experienced the incident at either a primary or a secondary level. New York City residents who work or live in the area continued to experience many weeks and months of ongoing exposure to the sights and smells of the disaster. Identifying the unique stressors associated with this level of incident exposure as well as the intra- and interpersonal resources and vulnerabilities and cultures of the population is essential information in formulating an effective response and recovery strategy. The New York example suggests that for man-made terrorist attacks, the "at-risk" multipliers for estimation of need significantly increase above those from natural disasters.

Techniques used to assess level of need for mental health services as reported included:

- A random-digit telephone survey of residents ($n = 494$) living below 110th Street utilizing a questionnaire identifying respondent demographics, trauma event experiences, lifetime stressors, substance abuse, posttraumatic stress disorder, and depression. The survey was conducted by the New York Academy of Medicine (Rudenstine, Galea, Ahern, Felton, & Vlahov, 2003).
- The Rapid Assessment Survey by the New York Department of Health and the Centers for Disease Control and Prevention (New York City Department of Health, 2001) to assess the need for assistance in home, medical, and behavioral health. Residents of housing projects in Battery Park, Southbridge, and Independence Plaza were the respondents ($n = 414$).
- Identification of diversity in ethnicity, language, primary spoken language, literacy, religious practices, attitudes toward health care and help-seeking behaviors by borough.
- Recognition of special population groups: children, adolescents, older adults, people with physical and mental disabilities, disaster workers, culture and ethnic groups, and people of low socioeconomic status.
- Degree of exposure interacting with special population status such as exposure to direct life threat, witnessing mutilating injuries, hearing cries for help, brutality of violence, unexpectedness and duration of the incident, and separation from family.

Based on the needs assessment, which informed the degree of exposure experienced by the population, a two-tiered response plan was developed. Tier one population subgroups include family members of the deceased, survivors, evacuees, and rescue workers. Tier two subgroups include coworkers of the deceased; persons displaced from their homes; special populations; children in foster care; severely disturbed children; college students living away from home; elderly individuals; individuals with alcohol and other substance abuse, serious and persistent mental illness with developmental disabilities, and physical disabilities; and Arab/Moslem Americans.

NEEDS ASSESSMENT STRATEGIES: INTERNATIONAL EXAMPLES

As evident, many factors unique to a disaster influence its psychological impact on individuals and communities. A recently released position paper by the World Health Organization (2003)—*Mental and Social Aspects of*

Health Populations Exposed to Extreme Stressors—suggests that interventions following a disaster be preceded by:

- Careful planning and broad assessment of setting, culture, history and nature of problems, local perceptions of distress and illness, ways of coping, community resources, etc.
- Qualitative assessment of context.
- Quantitative assessment of disability or daily functioning.
- Identification of unmet needs and urgency of needs.
- Local resources and potential external resources.

A CONCEPTUAL MODEL FOR ASSESSING DISASTER MENTAL HEALTH NEEDS FOLLOWING A DISASTER

The proposed model for assessing DMH needs (see Figure 5.1) illustrates how survivors and community stakeholders affected by the disaster become the repositories of significant sets of information, which ultimately influence intervention strategies. DMH personnel must continue to gather data pertinent to response and recovery needs throughout the incident.

One seeks safety and security for one's self and significant others; as a community stakeholder (e.g., school principal, fire chief, pastor, or news reporter), one responds to the disaster within the context of one's duty. All these respondents are in all respects disaster survivors; some are both survivors and responders. The immediate and potential long-term successful impact of disaster needs assessment strategies involves the acquisition of multiple levels of information regarding the demographics and socioeconomic and environmental factors, which interact with the geographic location of the incident.

Reliable data better inform the needs assessment. Is the goal to determine the segments of the population in need of nonclinical crisis counseling and support, or is it to identify those groups and individuals most at risk for acute posttraumatic stress disorders? Analysis of the data should be consistent with the goals of the needs assessment, which in turn informs the DMH program intervention design.

In summary, the needs assessment process is an ongoing activity throughout the recovery cycle. A well-planned needs assessment continually redefines stakeholder groups most relevant to the phase of disaster response and recovery. Stakeholders represent resources integral to providing services as well as those most in need of services. From the program design emerge program goals of addressing the needs identified through the

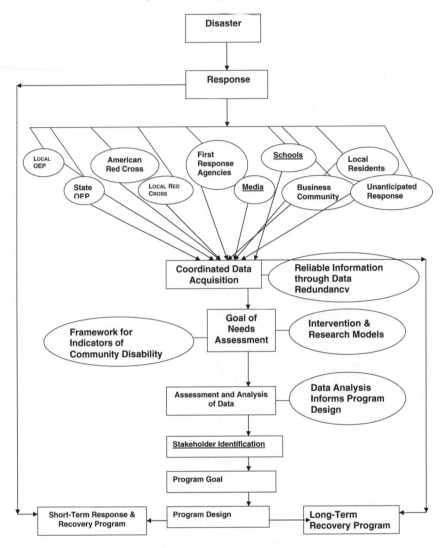

FIGURE 5.1. Conceptual model of disaster incident needs of assessment.

assessment process. Program design is what ultimately leads to both the short-term and long-term intervention services, and we hope the successful recovery of the individuals and communities affected by the disaster.

LINKING RESPONSE ARCHITECTURE TO NEEDS ASSESSMENT

Once the DMH operations team has established specifically where the disaster occurred and who was affected, the next step is to determine how the scope of impact informs the range of mental health resources required to respond to the emerging needs of the population. Successful response strategy involves the careful analysis of (1) present and future needs of individuals, (2) instrumental supports available in relationship to the degree of recovery activity necessary to return individuals and communities to their predisaster status, and (3) continuing reassessment of factors on which response strategies were based. The necessary structural elements in a response strategy include

- Veteran mental health professional staff familiar with the supervision and delivery of community-based services.
- Access to mental health experts with topical knowledge on grief and sudden loss, posttraumatic stress and other dissociative disorders, critical incident stress, child and lifespan developmental issues, gender-specific issues, and cultural competency (individual differences).
- Representatives of social service and community action groups that have been identified as core community stakeholder groups.
- NVOAD (National Voluntary Organizations Active in Disaster) groups, and other national, state, or local voluntary organizations.
- Representatives of politically active indigenous groups including the NAACP and labor unions.
- Job pool of potential outreach workers, primarily native to the area.
- Target goals for project activities in terms of the number of survivors (primary and secondary), communities, responders, and response agencies that the project will target for intervention and support.
- Specific number of outreach teams needed, including the range of expertise among the teams. The teams must include persons who have a basis of common identification/alliance with the survivors/ communities they are trying to help. Examples include multilingual individuals, race, age, and ethnic diversity consistent with survivor groups to be served, or history with the community across multiple generations

CONCLUSION

The foregoing list is representative of the many factors that come into play when designing and building a long-term DMH response strategy. The method best used for understanding what the crucial elements are in responding to any particular event is simply to talk to many people in many different settings. Convene, for example, small brainstorming groups of people active in response operations, persons who are veteran service delivery representatives in nondisaster times. Most important, remain aware of who "just naturally" emerges through the response process: "Who" is always being quoted in the press as the "expert" on various aspects of the impact of the disaster on different constituent groups?

The process of service delivery informs the needs assessment process as new stakeholders emerge. Individuals functioning in the role of survivor or helper are key to the ongoing interactive process of needs assessment and program design. Knowledge of who was affected and where they live and work, although essential, only represents the basic building blocks of comprehensive long-term mental health response and recovery operations. Irrespective of one's efforts to conduct a broad-based and careful needs assessment, more issues relevant to community recovery will continue to emerge. Identifying them in a proactive way gives the DMH teams an opportunity to organize and implement an integrated response strategy early in the response phase of disaster recovery.

ACKNOWLEDGMENTS

I gratefully acknowledge the contributions of Diana Nordboe, Director of Virginia Community Resilience Crisis Counseling Project, in the preparation of sections of this chapter. Additional thanks are extended to Chip Felton, Deputy Chief Commissioner, New York State Office of Mental Health, and members of his staff for their many helpful comments and suggestions. Contents of this chapter and any misstatements in the text remain the responsibility of the author.

REFERENCES

Benight, C., & Harper, M. L. (2002). Coping self-efficacy perceptions as a mediator between acute stress response and long-term distress following natural disasters. *Journal of Traumatic Stress, 15*(3), 177–186.

Brende, J. O. (1998). Coping with floods: Assessment, intervention, and recovery processes for survivors and helpers. *Journal of Contemporary Psychotherapy, 28*(2), 107–139.

Center for Mental Health Services. (2003). *Emergency Mental Health and Traumatic Stress Services Branch fact sheet.* Substance Abuse and Mental

Health Services Administration, Center for Mental Health Services, Division of Prevention, Traumatic Stress, and Special Programs. Retrieved December 31, 2003, from www.mentalhealth.org/publications/allpubs/KEN95-0011/default.asp

Cohen, R. E., & Ahearn, F. L. (1980). *Handbook for mental health care of disaster victims.* Baltimore: Johns Hopkins University Press

Franklin, T. (1983). Crisis intervention in community disasters. In L. Cohen, W. Claiborn, & G. A. Specter (Eds.), *Crisis intervention* (2nd ed., pp. 147–163). New York: Human Sciences Press.

Kalayjian, A. S. (1995). *Disaster and mass trauma.* Long Branch, NJ: Vista.

Kaniasty, K., & Norris, F. (2000). Help-seeking comfort and receiving social support: The role of ethnicity and the context of need. *American Journal of Community Psychology, 28*(4), 545–581.

Louisiana Office of Mental Health. (2002). *Louisiana crisis counseling immediate services application* (FEMA-DR-1435/37-LA). Baton Rouge: Louisiana Department of Health and Hospitals, Office of Mental Health.

McFarlane, A. C. (1996). Resilience, vulnerability, and the course of posttraumatic reactions. In B. A. van der Kolk, A. C. McFarlane, & L. Weisaeth (Eds.), *Traumatic stress: The effects of poverwhelming exoerience on the mind, body, and society* (pp. 155–181). New York: Guilford Press.

New York City Department of Health. (2001, December). *A community needs assessment of lower manhattan following the World Trade Center attack.* New York: Community Health Works, New York City Department of Health.

New York State Office of Mental Health. (2001). *Crisis counseling guide.* New York: Author. Retrieved February 2, 2001, from www.omh.state.ny.us/omhweb/crisis/crisiscounseling4.html

New York State Office of Mental Health. (2002, July 18). *Project Liberty* (Regular Services Program Application Supplemental Report, FEMA-1391-DR-NY). New York: Author.

Norris, F. (2001). *50,000 disaster victims speak: An empirical review of the empirical literature, 1981–2001* (Report prepared for The National Center for PTSD and The Center for Mental Health Services). Retrieved December 31, 2003, from www.ncdpt.org/docs/Norris.pdf

Norris, F. (2003). *A critique of the CMHS immediate services program needs assessment procedures.* Unpublished manuscript, Center for Mental Health Resources, National Center for Post Traumatic Stress Disorders.

Rudenstine, S., Galea, S., Ahern, J., Felton, C., & Vlahov, D. (2003). Awareness and perceptions of a communitywide mental health program in New York City after September 11. *Psychiatric Services, 54,* 1404–1406.

Virginia Department of Mental Health, Mental Retardation and Substance Abuse. (2001). *Virginia terrorism-related mental health needs assessment.* Manuscript submitted to the Center for Mental Health Services of the Substance Abuse and Mental Health Administration, Richmond, VA.

World Health Organization. (2003). *Mental health in emergencies: Mental and social aspects of health of populations exposed to extreme stressors.* Geneva, Switzerland: Author. Retrieved December 31, 2003, from www.who.int/disasters/repo/8656.pdf

PART III

MENTAL HEALTH INTERVENTIONS

Interventions for Traumatic Stress

Theoretical Basis

ARIEH Y. SHALEV

When he who walks in the dark whistles . . .

Knowledge about early interventions for survivors of traumatic events is scant because of the paucity of research, the complexity of the problem, and mechanistic approaches to recommending solutions. Other chapters in this volume masterfully depict the few paths to be seen in this gloom. Notwithstanding, the current "state of the art" recalls Freud's (1917/1963) comment: "When he who walks in the dark whistles, he feels better but doesn't see better." That is not enough.

True, postdisaster research is difficult. The complexity of mass trauma, the variety of potential victims, and the array of eventual outcomes are daunting. However, the main difficulty is conceptual: a lack of good theory of trauma and recovery. Without theory, the list of unanswered questions becomes endless, not for lack of knowledge but because there is no good conceptual framework to organize it. Much has already been learned, but most of the knowledge is descriptive (e.g., percentage of recovery from acute stress disorder [ASD] or prevalence of symptoms in a population). Theory development has been less energetically pursued.

Lack of theory hinders understanding the acute responses to traumatic events. The cost of being nontheoretical and descriptive is reasonable

103

with relatively stable phenotypes. Therefore in chronic posttraumatic stress disorder (PTSD), studies concurrently validated the construct, which sufficed to guide research and practice. However, in the case of the "polymorphous and labile" (Yitzhaki, Solomon, & Kotler, 1991) expressions of the acute response to stress, descriptions are inadequate. This condition is better captured by its organizing principles than by its myriad evolving expressions.

A theory of acute response must differ from that of PTSD. The latter is a theory of disease, where symptoms persevere despite the absence of current stressors. The former should encompass the entire range of reactions to adversity, from adaptive responses to preludes of mental disorders (Galea et al., 2002).

A theory of chronic PTSD can assume that observations (such as activation of specific brain areas) are only marginally contaminated environmental "noise." Although generally true, inconsistencies in some findings are attributed to the experimental context (e.g., startle responses in reassuring vs. ambiguous environment) (Grillon, Morgan, Davis, & Southwick, 1998). Nonetheless, we read an article on brain imaging in PTSD without attributing the effect to background noise or needlestick. A theory of acute stress, in contrast, must address the essential interaction between harmful agent, reacting host, and social or group context. A theory of acute stress must also include a proposition about time and distance from a triggering event. Interventions based on such theory must consider these dimensions or else their effects are unpredictable and erratic.

Figure 6.1 offers a schematic three-dimensional space in which early responses occur. The figure comprises a stressor severity ("demands"), a

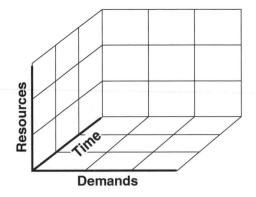

FIGURE 6.1. Three-dimensional depiction of the interaction between stressor ("demands"), resources, and time soon after a traumatic event.

time progression, and availability of resources. It illustrates the idea that the responses to a traumatic event are stress dependent, resource dependent, and time dependent. Because the linearity of each axis is not assured, and there might be other relevant dimensions, one can appraise the potential complexity of predicting the outcome of unidimensional interventions.

Another luxury of looking into chronic PTSD is that at such distance from a triggering trauma, the difference between normal and abnormal outcome (between survivors with and without PTSD) is salient. Differentiating normal and abnormal responses soon after a traumatic event is harder. Research outlined in the other chapters in this volume depicts two approaches to differentiating the two: (1) a quantitative approach that showed that in groups of survivors, higher initial responses generally predict subsequent disorders; and (2) a qualitative approach that postulates a link between distinct attributes of the initial response (e.g., dissociation, low plasma cortisol, and elevated heart rate; Resnick, Yehuda, Pitman, & Foy, 1995; Shalev, Peri, Canetti, & Schreiber, 1996; Shalev, Sahar, et al., 1998) and subsequent PTSD. Both approaches yielded productive approximations: They identified probabilities (e.g., of having PTSD following ASD); but they did not uncover necessary paths of disease, which early interventions must address (e.g., dissociation is not a necessary antecedent of PTSD; Shalev, Sahar, et al., 1998); and they have not delineated a reliable threshold of early response, above which intensive and costly treatment is indicated.

The lack of specific indications for treatment at the early stages of the responses to trauma leaves us with two competing and contradicting practices: a controversial "intervention for all" (e.g., group debriefing) and a "wait, see, and intervene later" strategy (i.e., do nothing before time segregates real patients from those who recover). All the arguments for or against one form of practice are essentially rhetorical, because there are no comparative studies of the two.

Another problem is how one defines the early interventions. Adopting a narrower view, an intervention can be defined as a *deliberate, evidence-based, and planned activity by professional helpers, conducted according to recognized standards of care and aimed at treating or preventing mental disorders.* This approach has many advantages, the most important being its adherence to the relatively well regulated and somewhat better charted areas of formal clinical interventions and diagnosis. The latter may serve for both prescribing treatment and evaluating its outcome—hence the powerful research methodology that these interventions allow (within-subjects repeated measure design). Providing cognitive-behavioral treatment (CBT) for survivors with ASD to prevent PTSD exemplifies this approach (Bryant, Harvey, Dang, Sackville, & Basten, 1998; Foa, Hearst-Ikeda, & Perry, 1995). The problems with this approach are that it requires significant and often unavailable resources. Additionally, so soon after a traumatic event, case definition is problematic and treatment desirability might be low.

At the other end, everything may be construed as being an intervention: consulting with leaders, conferring with the media, providing food and shelter, making survivors narrate their recent experience, or distributing leaflets with lists of "expected but normal" symptoms. While such steps may affect survivors (for better or worse), it is difficult to systematically describe them, other than through "laundry lists"—"wish lists" of all the good deeds that one may imagine following adversity. This is eminently problematic, because many such interventions, including those better planned, managed, and executed, can have unpredictable effects. For example, limiting the tour of duty in Vietnam to 1 year, intended to reduce individual exposure and thereby lower the number of stress casualties. However, the effect of an individually timed tour of duty on unit cohesion might have been negative (Marlowe, 1986).

Similar bidirectional effects can be expected from interventions such as educating survivors about PTSD (because the "preparedness" component might be confounded by a "modeling" effect; i.e., by suggesting symptoms) or educating military commanders about PTSD (because better perception of distressed soldiers might be confounded by scapegoating of undesired ones). Bidirectional effects were, almost predictably, seen in debriefing—a treatment protocol offered to all cases of "critical stress" and provided regardless of context, trauma severity, and survivors' specific experiences or intensity of early response (Rose, Bisson, & Wessely, 2002).

Returning to the need for theory, the core question is whether one can productively generalize from current knowledge. I believe this is the case, and risking another "whistle in the dark," this chapter outlines two generic dimensions of the response to traumatic stress and defines specific targets for interventions. The context of this chapter is mass trauma, but the chapter is meant to instruct clinicians for all traumatic situations.

TRAUMATIC STRESS: BETWEEN TWO THEORIES

The term "traumatic stress" links *stress* and *trauma* and thereby refers to two theoretical bodies: stress theory and the partially formulated theory of psychological trauma. The interface between the two has not been convincingly articulated, but it is vaguely assumed that the "stressfulness" of an event will affect the likelihood of "psychological trauma." Ample research shows, however, that the stressfulness of events provides but partial explanation of subsequent stress disorders (e.g., Brewin, Andrews, & Valentine, 2000), hence the need for a *theory of trauma* on top of *stress theory*.

The two theories differ: *Stress theory* is essentially homeostatic, postulating dynamic interaction between stressor and defending (coping) host. The construct of *trauma*, in contrast, refers to a breakdown, a breach in the homeostatic rules, causing survivors to carry long-term sequelae of their encounter with "stress." Equating "trauma" with a breach of homeostasis is not new: Following World War I, Freud (1920/1955) pointed out that traumatic neurosis, unlike other neuroses, defies (demolishes) the homeostatic interplay between drives and defenses. Bruce McEwen (e.g., 1999) uses a similar template when he proposes that prolonged exposure to stress may end by creating "allostatic" wear and tear of the body, including damage to specific brain structures. In other words, stress theory pertains to resisting pressure: How much weight can a bone bear? Trauma theory, by analogy, introduces the concept of fracture. The early aftermath of trauma involves both, and this has caused confusion between two categories of early intervention: stress management and prevention of PTSD. *A priori*, stress management is not a treatment for PTSD. Similarly, genuine prevention of PTSD might focus on other elements of the traumatic experience and the early reactions. The following two sections address this distinction.

STRESS, STRESS RESPONSE, AND STRESSFUL EVENTS

Demands, Responses, and Resources

Stress theory assumes that external demands evoke responses in the receiving host, and these responses draw on the host's inner and external resources. Disasters may also reduce the availability of external (e.g., community) resources (Figure 6.2). Some responses may reduce demands (e.g., by fighting back or withdrawing from danger) and increase resources (e.g., by seeking help). Other responses can increase the demands (e.g., by unnec-

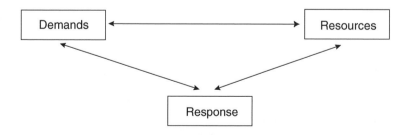

FIGURE 6.2. Interaction between demands, resources, and response at the early aftermath of traumatic events.

essarily remaining exposed) or deplete community resources (by providing individual treatment following a disaster; Norris et al., 2002).

Figure 6.2 delineates the resulting interaction and outlines three core targets for early interventions: demands, responses, and resources. It also reiterates the consistent observation that survivors are active participants in disaster scenarios. Helpers must assess these three dimensions. They should not consider survivors as being passive recipients (of harm or of help) but, rather, identify and support their clients' ways of coping with adversity. Survivors who wish to share their experiences should find a listening ear, whereas those who opt to remain silent should not be required to narrate their experiences.

Primary, Secondary, and Tertiary Stressors

Shortly after the impact of an event, the prevalent demands are those created by the primary stressor (e.g., destruction and injury); the initial response is driven by survival needs and resources go to rescue. Later, demands might stem from secondary stressors (e.g., relocation, pain, or uncertainty) and resources are allocated to damage control and stabilization (including medical). Only later do recovery and reconstruction become the focus. Survivors' own responses (e.g., anxiety, insomnia, and depression) may tax survivors' resources and become tertiary stressors.

Reality and Perceived Reality

Developing this view, one must consider the human mind's capacity for appraisal and evaluation. Appraisal colors experience, provides meaning to situations and events, guides behavior, and evaluates its outcome. In potentially traumatic situations, appraisal concerns imminence of the threat, availability of inner resources, and likelihood of successful action (Lazarus & Folkman, 1984).

Thus, each of the three components of Figure 6.3 should include both "real" and "perceived" quality. Threats can be real or perceived, resources real or perceived, responses real or perceived. We (Shalev, Schreiber, & Galai, 1993) described an incident in which a bus overturned in a valley en route to Jerusalem and demonstrated major differences in appraisal, despite similar exposure to the traumatic event. Ehlers and Steil (1995) show that survivors' perception of their symptoms predicts subsequent PTSD. Kaniasty and Norris (2004) have outlined a major role of perceived social support in shaping communities' responses to disasters.

To illustrate the importance of appraisal, consider the following: Upon admission to an emergency room, one terror survivor might be convinced another attack is imminent and will kill him, whereas another knows he

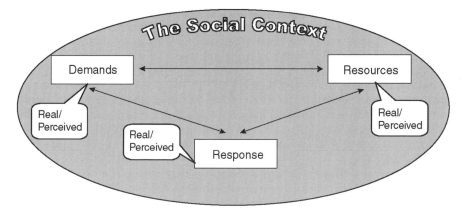

FIGURE 6.3. Early responses to "embedded in context."

has reached safety in a hospital. The two behave differently, appraise signals differently (e.g., the beeps of a close-by respirator), and might have different levels of physiological arousal.

Feeling better following trauma may shape one's perception of the trauma, one's own responses, and one's belief in a positive outcome of the situation. Inversely, a self-reinforcing cycle of negative appraisal, inflated risk-perception, and increased distress might be created. Early interventions must address this vicious cycle, perhaps by accessing any one component of this cycle (e.g., by reducing excessive responses, correcting catastrophic appraisal, or providing real and concrete resources).

Some way to help distressed survivors always exists. When little can be done to reduce the main stressor (as in the case of sudden traumatic loss), it is wise to reduce survivors' loneliness. When reality is truly terrible (repeated terror, torture, siege, or captivity), hope becomes a major resource. We can do much before, and often instead of, formal treatment interventions. Professionals may find themselves in situations in which being a therapist is not the required skill and should humbly accept other roles.

The Social Context

In an era of abundant communication, appraisal is rarely individual. Survivors and witnesses are affected by what they see, hear, understand, or derive from the news, Internet, and rumor. The social context operates as narrated and not as actually present: A horrific picture on the front page of a newspaper may affect risk perception more than columns of balanced estimates. Peritraumatic appraisals are embedded in group perception and narrative.

Survivors and helpers are part of that narrative and embedded in the same social context. A military psychiatrist in war cannot escape conflicting roles as healer on one hand and, on the other, a member of the military institution (e.g., Camp, 1993). After 9/11 or during the Gulf War missiles attacks in Israel, survivors and helpers were similarly affected. Sharing the same reality presents an opportunity for intuitive understanding, empathy, and connectedness. It can also overwhelm helpers and reduce their efficiency (e.g., Shalev et al., 2003).

The Individual Context:
Prior Trauma, Life Trajectory, and Attachment Bonds

Also relevant is the survivor's own context (i.e., personal history, current life situation, and trajectory). *Prior events* and their resolution are background for appraising current adversity. *Life situations* include recent events and specific details of the traumatic exposure. Was the survivor traveling with his family? Exposed as a professional? Recently divorced? Immigrated?

Trauma engages survivors' bonding and attachment (e.g., in their last minutes of life, victims of 9/11 phoned home for a few more words with loved ones). Desperate survivors of an earthquake (or the Oklahoma bombing) might have stared at the rubble for hours and days, expecting to hear—almost hearing—a familiar voice. Clinicians may wish to remember that *what is threatened in mass disaster is not just the individual but the integrity of his or her living network*. The triangle of demands, responses, and resources should be extended to include a family, group, or community.

Controllability, Prediction, and Escape

Theory predicates that intense, uncontrollable, unpredictable, and inescapable stress is particularly harmful (Foa, Steketee, & Rothbaum, 1989). This applies to primary, secondary, and tertiary stressors. Thus, uncontrollable symptoms, such as repeated episodes of dissociation, should become specific and urgent targets for early interventions.

Time Course and Recovery

With time, the direct effects of the acute event cease, the balance between demands and resources eventually favors the latter, and most survivors show a parallel decrease in distress. Recovery, therefore, is the expected outcome of time-limited exposure with conservation of resources. Secondary stressors, deterioration of resources, and self-perpetuating, distressing symptoms may hinder recovery. Thus, beyond heeding symptoms and complaints, clinicians should identify factors that are interfering with recovery (e.g., lack of supportive others, uncertainty about the safety of significant others, intolerable mental pain).

Evaluating the Early Responses: A Stress Management Perspective

Stress theory does not predict symptoms. Its inherent outcome is the quality of the balance achieved by the interplay between stressors and coping. Pearlin and Schooler (1978) identified four observable indicators of successful coping: (1) sustained task performance, (2) controllability of emotion, (3) sustained capacity to enjoy rewarding human contacts, and (4) sustained sense of personal worth. Failure to cope will show in deteriorated task performance, overwhelming emotions, inability to relate to others, and self-blame (or self-denigrating rumination). Early PTSD symptoms may or may not constitute a valid or desirable outcome of stress management, but improved coping efficacy *is* such an outcome.

To summarize, stress management includes reducing the stressor, optimizing resources, and managing survivors' reactions. Stress management encompasses real and perceived elements of this triad. It applies to individuals and groups. Its outcome is better judged by evaluating the resulting improvement in coping.

This is almost as far as stress theory can take us in guiding early interventions for traumatic stress. Stress theory does not explain why some stressful experiences never cease. This question requires a theory of trauma.

FROM STRESS TO TRAUMATIC STRESS

A time-honored understanding of traumatic events emphasizes their threatening nature and the resulting fear, emotional learning, and avoidance. Accordingly, fear-driven learning is a major etiological factor in traumatic stress disorders. This view, explored in prospective studies, shows a relationship between physiological parameters of early stress responses (e.g., heart rate) and subsequent PTSD (Shalev, Sahar, et al., 1998). Yet the contribution of early arousal to subsequent PTSD is negligible. Chemical prevention of the underlying adrenergic drive may not prevent PTSD—while reducing physiological responses to reminders (Pitman et al., 2002). The initial "stress response" is a necessary—but insufficient—cause of traumatic stress disorders.

Going beyond stress-driven learning, the etiology of PTSD can be sought in the domain of autobiographic memory, among factors that make some recollections incongruous, intrusive, distressful, and unremitting.

Incongruous Novelty and Intrusive Recollections

Severe traumatic events may be hard to grasp, understand, and accept. Immediate reactions to some traumatic events (e.g., surrendering to a rapist, or running away from a site or explosion) may contrast with what the survivor knows—or assumes to know—about him- or herself. The survivor has no inner schemas to deal with occurrences that are utterly unacceptable and forcefully present. They are not just stressful and signaling threat: They tax survivors' cognition. They also tax the cognition of witnesses—often regardless of direct exposure (e.g., responses to 9/11 in remote areas of the United States). In such events, people are not exposed in the sense of being there (e.g., Galea et al., 2002). Rather, they find the event personally relevant, shocking, salient, new, and incongruous.

In a *Newsweek* report from Iraq (Nordland & Gegax, 2004), an Army captain reports memories he will "never be able to purge: e.g., having buried babies caught in crossfire. The hardest," he continues, "was trying to resuscitate that fellow officer who died in the field." The captain was not under fire and did not report any threat to himself or others, but he *witnessed the unthinkable.*

Unthinkable memories do not simply "go away" when the stress is over. They are not amenable to "stress management." They do not stem from a life threat but from a threat to one's image of the world. They tax the brain's mapping of reality—rather than its alarm and survival machinery. They challenge rules, expectations, and assumptions and pose a different challenge to the brain. Specifically, these "unthinkable" experiences evoke intrusive recollections.

Not every stressful event comprises such challenges. One can escape a flood and be thankful to be alive. Yet, as soon as children's bodies are seen, floating in the stream, incongruity and horror surface (Stern, 1976). *Stressful events are traumatic when they include novel and incongruous experiences,* extreme brutality, exposure to disfigured dead bodies, major loss— any mentally unacceptable novelty.

Important information comes from listening to survivors. Careful observation of the early occurrence of intrusive recollections in survivors of terror in Jerusalem (Shalev et al., 2003) shows that the survivors may express extreme forms of intrusive recollections within an hour of the traumatic event, as soon as their initial survival-driven response (fight, flight) is over and they are brought to safety. Then some survivors become flooded by "flashbulb" recollections. Typically, repeated images of a fragment of the traumatic event appear, literally within the survivor's visual field, often with the intensity of an epileptic fit. Several survivors in our care found it difficult to close their eyes, because as soon as they did they were flooded by disturbing images. Others were so absorbed by these inner experiences that they could barely pay attention to external reality (e.g., to the emergency room situation). They responded to questions as if absorbed in some other mental activity, to which they immediately returned when left alone. Their faces continued to express horror and disarray. Their relatives found them "changed," or "shocked."

For some, the intrusive images concerned particularly gruesome experiences from the aftermath of the trauma. Some of the most severely disturbed survivors of terror are naive rescuers who, in trying to help, confronted the unthinkable and froze. For them the event becomes traumatic because of its informational load.

Brewin, Dalgleish, and Joseph (1996) theorized that traumatic memories in PTSD are encoded as images, are not amenable to voluntary control, do not decay with time, and must be further processed to become normal autobiographical recollections (i.e., amenable to voluntary recall and forgetfulness). This view approaches Lindemann's (1994) observation of reiterative and painful recall in processing the novelty of traumatic loss. Freud's construct of grief work, where recollections of the deceased must be recoded, through painful reiteration, as belonging to the past for the "psyche" to regain a sense of reality, is also in line with this observation. Lazarus's construct of "reappraisal" is also in line with these descriptions. However, the acute expression of intrusive experiences does not seem to allow the cognitive distancing subsumed under reappraisal. Instead, these are powerful sensory and emotional experiences, where the recent past is lived as being intensely present and little is left for elaboration and reflection.

To summarize, incongruous novelty requires serial mental processing, which, following mass disasters, is expressed as repeated intrusive recollections. The intensity of this phenomenon varies from mild and manageable reactions to dissociation, where recollections of the trauma dominate one's sense of reality. Uncontrollable dissociation is a defining feature of ASD and therefore a risk indicator of subsequent PTSD.

Memories Acquired during Stress

Perception is altered by stress, such that a threatening object becomes the focus and peripheral elements are neglected. In dire circumstances survivors may act and react without much reflection—or be driven by strong emotions: fear or an urge to flee, surrender, or fight back. Many survivors eventually question these experiences in the aftermath of events (e.g., "Have I done what I should have done?" "Could I have acted otherwise?"). Self-denigrating resolution of these questions may leave open wounds, often for years, along with a more general avoidance of recall and reflection.

Early Depressive Reactions

Studies show that depression at the early aftermath of trauma strongly predicts PTSD (e.g., Shalev, Freedman, et al., 1998). Depressed survivors might not try to regain territory lost to avoidance. Unless brought to therapy by others, they are poor help seekers. Depressive rumination may further enhance the intrusive activity of processing novelty—keeping a negative emotional tag attached to each recollection. Depressed patients generalize bad feelings and extend a negative perception to both inner and external reality. Early depression, therefore, is a prime target for intervention.

Processing Traumatic Reactions

Processing traumatic recollections requires time, reiteration, and good partners. Research (e.g., Pennebaker & Susman, 1988) can only replicate what has already been published for ages (Job 2:11–13):

> Now when Job's three friends heard of all this evil that had come upon him, they came each from his own place, Eli'phaz the Te'manite, Bildad the Shuhite, and Zophar the Na'amathite. They made an appointment together to come to condole with him and comfort him. And when they saw him from afar, they did not recognize him; and they raised their voices and wept; and they rent their robes and sprinkled dust upon their heads toward heaven. And they sat with him on the ground seven days and seven nights, and no one spoke a word to him, for they saw that his suffering was very great.

Later, these listeners might become responders and partners to the survivor's attempt to find new meaning. However, the core attribute of helpers at the early phase is the quality of their rapport with the survivor and, specifically, the extent to which his or her grief partially becomes theirs, to share and participate.

Good listeners may come from survivors' social network and family. A target of early interventions is to support these helpers. When the network of helpers is intact and functions well, professionals have little to do. At other times, professionals may be called on to transiently become such partners, and they should expect to truly participate in a traumatic experience—sometimes at a cost, and as an edifying experience for themselves.

But while one wishes to allow time for spontaneous recovery, allowing too much time will lead to intervening too late. The proper temporal boundaries of recovery from trauma are not known and may differ from one experience to the other and between individuals. Those who continue to express intense and uncontrollable symptoms should be advised to seek professional help.

IMPLICATIONS FOR EARLY INTERVENTIONS: A STABLE STRATEGY TO ADDRESS MOVING TARGETS

Therefore postdisaster interventions might include *stress management* and *treatment of traumatic responses*. Stress management involves all steps to reduce the intensity of environmental demands, enrich resources, and support adaptive responses; it is a generic approach, valid across traumatic situations. Trauma theory adds another dimension: the extent to which the encounter of specific individuals with a specific event includes an element of incongruous novelty, loss, major change, or other traumatic challenge. Trauma therapy should specifically address the processing of incongruous experiences.

Table 6.1 completes the previous three-dimensional schema by adding a dimension of severity to each axis and showing how they might interact to increase the risk for survivors. The table should be read as three-

TABLE 6.1. Severity of Responses, as Judged from Interactions between Demands, Resources, and Response

| | Social environment/resources | | |
	Stable	Unstable	Disrupted
Responses			
Mild	1	2	3
Intense	2	3	4
Uncontrollable	3	4	5
Demands			
Mild	1	2	3
Severe	2	3	4
Disruptive/incongruous	3	4	5

dimensional. It shows that survivors of disruptive stressors whose responses are uncontrollable and whose resources are depleted are at the highest risk for subsequent stress disorders. It also suggests that intervening to improve one dimension might reduce the pathogenic effect of others.

CLINICIANS AND HELPERS
DURING MASS TRAUMA

Clinicians may not be able to devise or provide sophisticated treatment during mass trauma. They may be called on to meet survivors' urgent needs. They often feel incompetent and overwhelmed. This feeling is their first enemy. Traumatized clients have the same basic needs that drive clients to seek treatment in other situations: They are anxious, depressed, detached, and lonely, and they cannot experience the full élan of life. Many cannot wait to talk about their traumatic experience but fear opening their "Pandora's box." They wish to rely on help offered but also to remain autonomic and empowered. None of this is new to clinicians. Trauma survivors need the same approach given to other clients: genuine interest in their case, good listening skill, empathy, emotional openness, and resonance. Clinicians must have a general understanding of traumatic experiences, yet in their management of specific cases they can rely on their professional skills.

Some dimensions of trauma can inhibit clinicians' intuition. Traumatic narratives communicate too well in that they evoke, in almost every listener, strong emotions. Recently one of our patients narrated, to a public, the tragic death of her friend in a terrorist attack in Jerusalem. Everyone in the audience wept as she described how everything suddenly became dark, how the ceiling was falling piece by piece, and how she escaped, immediately checked her body, happy to be alive, but then learned that her friend was dead.

Traumatic experiences can sweep therapists. They are intense and immediate and often breach our own defenses—we wonder whether we are therapists or participants. Add the often brief encounter with early survivors, who then move on to another facility, and the fact that early interventions cannot truly alleviate grief or fully address all levels of severe traumatic exposure and therapists may feel, similar to their clients' uncertainty, regret, and negative self-perception.

Stress management principles also apply to therapists: They might be under *excessive demands*, they need *resources*, and they must *manage their reactions*. Helpers have to have a group of reference, discuss their experiences, and eventually manage their exposure, or have their exposure managed by their leaders. To be manageable, helpers' own reactions must become controllable, escapable, and amenable to successful communication. One should not treat trauma survivors other than within supporting peer groups. Leaders of such groups must provide group sessions, supervision, and opportunity for sharing and disclosure and must monitor exposure to potentially traumatizing narratives.

At the initial stages of exposure one may have to curb one's emotional responses for the more urgent task of surviving adversity. This can be mistaken for emotional numbing, whereas it is often a protective shield—at least as long as adversities are expected. The relief of this protective veil is often gradual and in the best-case scenario occurs, as days pass, between survivors and their loved ones—or within survivors themselves, as they reflect and self-heal. Clinicians during traumatic circumstances may also find it difficult to access the full range of their emotional responses—and they should not always access them. Therapy at these early stages requires enough emotions for the encounter to be meaningful and enough distance to place the survivor away from his or her trouble.

TRAUMA, TREATMENT, AND TRANSCENDENCE

An illusion generated by dwelling too much in quantitative research is that solutions exist, just waiting discovery. Trauma, sometime, is insoluble, and leaves no path for escape.

Having lost her adult daughter on 9/11/2001, a mother cannot retrieve that missing part of herself. Turning to God, she finds comfort in believing that because of her daughter's natural goodness, and because what the daughter had suffered in earlier life, God would not have let her suffer. He might also have been merciful in delivering her from a life of misery.

Trauma can change survivors forever. Some traumatic situations confront survivors with evil, send them beyond the boundaries of civilization, evoke questions without answers. Some survivors may consume CBT to cope with such encounters, but even before the evidence-based interventions, Holocaust survivors and others coped by encapsulating the trauma, going back to living, bearing children, pretending to forget, and not letting memories dominate their lives. Many had PTSD symptoms 50 years later, but shouldn't experiencing genocide leave lifelong scars?

To some extent, and even soon after a traumatic event, therapists might identify survivors who encapsulate to survive. Some must simply go to work the next morning. Many may have PTSD symptoms years later, but it is the survivor's choice whether or not to construe the traumatic experience and his or her posttraumatic suffering within a classification of mental disorders.

Finally, a desire for life motivates survivors to recover. In our treatment of terror survivors in Jerusalem, we regularly address survivors' negativism, hoping that once the grip of such emotions loosens, the desire for life will put the trauma back into its right place as interference with life—rather than life-defining occurrence.

Most healing theories imply that a desire for life remains hidden behind inhibitions, symptoms, and anxiety. Thus most therapies do not foster positive emotions but tackle negativity. Trauma, however, might dampen survivors' desire for life. Helpers should not forget that healing trauma involves getting survivors to hope and prefer life to trauma. No manual can teach therapists this, but the human inclination to help others might.

REFERENCES

Brewin, C., Andrews, B., & Valentine, J. (2000). Meta-analysis of risk factors for posttraumatic stress disorder in trauma exposed adults. *Journal of Consulting and Clinical Psychology, 68,* 748–766.

Brewin, C. R., Dalgleish, T., & Joseph, S. (1996). A dual representation theory of posttraumatic stress disorder. *Archives of General Psychiatry, 50,* 294–305.

Camp, N. M. (1993). The Vietnam War and the ethics of combat psychiatry. *American Journal of Psychiatry, 150,* 1000–1010.

Ehlers, A., & Steil, R. (1995). Maintenance of intrusive memories in posttraumatic stress disorder: A cognitive approach. *Behavioural and Cognitive Psychotherapy, 23,* 217–249.

Foa, E. B., Hearst-Ikeda, D., & Perry, K. J. (1995). Evaluation of a brief cognitive-behavioral program for the prevention of chronic PTSD in recent assault victims. *Journal of Consulting and Clinical Psychology, 63,* 948–955.

Foa, E. B., Steketee, G., & Rothbaum, B. O. (1989). Behavioral/cognitive conceptualization of post-traumatic stress disorder. *Behavior Therapy, 20,* 155–176

Freud, S. (1955). Beyond the pleasure principle. In J. Strachey (Ed. & Trans.), *The standard edition of the complete psychological works of Sigmund Freud* (Vol. 18, pp. 1–64). London: Hogarth Press. (Original work published 1920)

Freud, S. (1963). Mourning and melancholia. In J. Strachey (Ed. & Trans.), *The standard edition of the complete psychological works of Sigmund Freud* (Vol. 14, pp. 237–260). London: Hogarth Press. (Original work published 1917)

Galea, S., Ahern, J., Resnick, H., Kilpatrick, D., Bucuvalas, M., Gold, J., et al. (2002). Psychological sequelae of the September 11 attacks in New York City. *New England Journal of Medicine, 346,* 982–987.

Grillon, C., Morgan, C. A., Davis, M., & Southwick, S. (1998). Effects of experimental context and explicit threat cues on acoustic startle in Vietnam veterans with PTSD. *Biological Psychiatry, 44,* 1027–1036.

Kaniasty, K., & Norris, F. (2004). Social support in the aftermath of disasters, catastrophes, and acts of terrorism: Altruistic, overwhelmed, uncertain, antagonistic, and patriotic communities. In R. Ursano, A. Norwood, & C. Fullerton (Eds.), *Bioterrorism: Psychological and public health interventions.* Cambridge, UK: Cambridge University Press.

Lazarus, R. S., & Folkman, S. (1984). *Stress, appraisal and coping.* New York: Springer.

Lindemann, E. (1994). Symptomatology and management of acute grief. *American Journal of Psychiatry, 151,* 155–160.

Marlowe, D. H. (1986). The human dimension of battle and combat breakdown. In R. A. Gabriel (Ed.), *Military psychiatry: A comparative perspective* (pp. 7–24). Westport, CT: Greenwood Press

McEwen, B. S. (1999). Stress and hippocampal plasticity. *Annual Review of Neuroscience, 22,* 105–122.

Nordland, R., & Gegax, T. T. (2004, January 12). Stressed out at the front. *Newsweek,* pp. 34–37.

Norris, F. H., Friedman, M. J., Watson, P. J., Byrne, C. M., Diaz, E., & Kaniasty, K. Z. (2002). 60,000 disaster victims speak: Part I, an empirical review of the empirical literature, 1981–2001. *Psychiatry, 65*(3), 207–239.

Pearlin, L. I., & Schooler, C. (1978). The structure of coping. *Journal of Health and Social Behavior, 22,* 337-356.

Pennebaker, J. W., & Susman, J. R. (1988). Disclosure of trauma and psychosomatic processes. *Social Science and Medicine, 26,* 327-332.

Pitman, R. K., Sanders, K. M., Zusman, R. M., Healy, A. R., Cheema, F., Lasko, N. B., et al. (2002, January 15). Pilot study of secondary prevention of posttraumatic stress disorder with propranolol. *Biological Psychiatry, 51*(2), 189–192.

Resnick, H. S., Yehuda, R., Pitman, R. K., & Foy, D. W. (1995). Effect of previous trauma on acute plasma cortisol level following rape. *American Journal of Psychiatry, 152,* 1675–1677.

Rose, S., Bisson, J., & Wessely, S. (2002). *Psychological debriefing for preventing post traumatic stress disorder (PTSD)* (The Cochrane Library, Issue 3). Oxford, UK: Update Software.

Shalev, A. Y., Addesky, R., Boker, R., Bargai, N., Cooper, R., Freedman, S., et al. (2003). Clinical intervention for survivors of prolonged adversities. In R. J. Ursano, C. S. Fullerton, & A. E. Norwood (Eds.), *Terrorism and disaster: Individual and community mental health interventions* (pp. 162–186). Cambridge, UK: Cambridge University Press.

Shalev, A. Y., Freedman, S., Peri, T., Brandes, D., Sahar, T., Orr, S. P., et al. (1998). Prospective study of PTSD and depression following trauma. *American Journal of Psychiatry, 155,* 630–637.

Shalev, A. Y., Peri, T., Canetti, L., & Schreiber, S. (1996). Predictors of PTSD in injured trauma survivors: A prospective study. *American Journal of Psychiatry, 152,* 219–225.

Shalev, A. Y., Sahar, T., Freedman, S., Peri, T., Glick, N., Brandes, D., et al. (1998). A prospective study of heart rate responses following trauma and the subsequent development of posttraumatic stress disorder. *Archives of General Psychiatry, 55,* 553–559.

Shalev, A. Y., Schreiber, S., & Galai, T. (1993). Early psychiatric responses to traumatic injury. *Journal of Traumatic Stress, 6,* 441–450.

Yitzhaki, T., Solomon, Z., & Kotler, M. (1991). The clinical picture of acute combat stress reaction among Israeli soldiers in the 1982 Lebanon war. *Military Medicine, 156,* 193–197.

CHAPTER 7

The Context of Providing Immediate Postevent Intervention

RODERICK J. ØRNER, ADRIAN T. KENT, BETTY J. PFEFFERBAUM, BEVERLEY RAPHAEL, and PATRICIA J. WATSON

The field of posttraumatic early intervention following mass violence has been the subject of great interest in the last few years. Interventions in the immediate aftermath of mass violence have received very little solid research support, and certain key questions are often raised by planners and providers following mass trauma

1. When should one provide intervention to traumatized individuals?
2. Who should receive services?
3. What evidence can we turn to for recommendations on what should be done?
4. What systems are in place in federal, state, and local government that can assist in preparing an organized mental, behavioral, and public health response to mass violence?

The overarching aim of early intervention is to improve the quality of survivors' recovery environment. This chapter offers a contextual frame and outline of structured approaches to planning and delivering early interventions to trauma survivors in the first week postevent. The guidance offered recognizes that no blueprint exists for all disaster and mass violence scenarios and that no interventions have proven to be appropriate and effective for all survivors of trauma.

THE RELEVANCE OF EARLY INTERVENTION

Early intervention programs can provide the basis of first response in terms of mental heath. Intermediate and longer-term interventions will inevitably relate to these in several different ways.

• Early intervention may *create a positive view* toward mental health and a willingness to continue with this type of support or to seek longer-term follow-up to deal with the issues identified. Alternatively, it may create distress and negative perceptions of helping agencies. A woman who was affected by the 1988 Locherbie disaster remarked that the mistreatment of her family in those 11 days remained with her and influenced her life.

• Early intervention may *begin a process* that is then continued into longer-term more specialized interventions for those who are identified as at risk or to need such follow-up.

• Early intervention may *provide a register* of those who have been affected and, with their consent, the capacity to link survivors to outreach and follow-up. This is important as the *names, addresses, and contacts* for those who are affected by such incidents may become an issue of privacy, and if used as the basis for an approach with outreach offered in the intermediate or longer term may become problematic. It may also provide, for those affected, the *capacity to identify* appropriate persons should the survivors need expert mental health interventions. This register also serves some protective function to deal with the *convergence* of those who would offer counseling perhaps without the necessary clinical expertise to deliver safe and effective care, as well as the knowledge of when to refer.

• Early intervention may provide an *educational function* about adaptive coping, expected positive outcomes, and how those affected may know when to seek help. This information may need to cover both physical and mental health consequences as both may coexist postdisaster. Early intervention may provide information on links to primary care providers and nongovernmental organizations. It may identify how to recognize a disaster affected person's needs and when to refer an individual for more specialized mental health interventions over the longer term, to mitigate risk.

• Early mental health intervention, both in terms of emergency response and its role in the first month of intermediate response, is provided *within a setting involving other agents who rapidly present to disaster-affected populations.* The challenge for specialist mental health response is to ensure that before any disaster or episode of mass violence occurs, (1) it has a defined and integral role in the emergency, intermediate and longer term; (2) this role and its importance is formally recognized by emergency and recovery organizations and the disaster response protocols; and (3) there are well-established protocols for interagency work, particularly as it is likely that practical, social, psychological, and health interventions will need to be effectively coordinated to meet affected persons and populations requirements.

STARTING PREMISES FOR EARLY INTERVENTION

Complex challenges face those who are responsible for planning early interventions for survivors of disasters and mass violence. In situations of mass violence, the expert consensus model (National Institute of Mental Health, 2002) assumes that many efforts can have a mental health impact on the community, even if not provided by mental health staff. For instance, the quality of national and local security has a profound impact on the populations' mental health. In addition, the quality of communication and coordination among responders, public confidence in leaders, and the accuracy and effectiveness of communications to the public about the risks and the appropriate actions to be taken can ameliorate anxiety and fear in communities. Expert panelists agree that mental health interventions cannot be isolated but must be embedded in an entire system with the recognition that each aspect of disaster response will affect mental health. As a result, there are many possible roles for mental health providers following mass violence. We delineate the following in this chapter.

REACTIONS OF INDIVIDUALS TO MASS VIOLENCE

A host of factors influence survivors' reactions to a disaster. These factors include, to name just a few, preincident history of trauma, psychiatric history, nature and duration of exposure to trauma, gender, age, and social support. Event characteristics and the manner in which events unfold also influence survivor responses (Wright & Bartone, 2002). More intense reactions are likely among survivors who experience prolonged and intense exposure. Reactions may also vary depending on the nature and source of the disaster. For example, trauma attributable to intentional human acts (e.g., war, terrorism, torture, and state-sponsored violence) or willful neglect (e.g., by individuals in positions of trust or public officials who fail to implement sufficient safety and maintenance programs) may have more severe consequences than trauma resulting from disasters construed as accidental or attributable to uncontrollable and unanticipated natural forces (e.g., volcanic eruptions and hurricanes) (Norris, Murphy, Baker, & Perulla, 2003).

BRINGING MODELS OF SERVICE DELIVERY
INTO LINE WITH EXPRESSED NEEDS

A key principle of informed service delivery is recognizing those who are in greatest need of service and abstaining from mandatory interventions where they are not welcomed or required (Ørner & Schnyder, 2003). The goal of early intervention is to provide psychosocial help and support that is responsive to the changing needs of survivors (Ajducovic & Ajducovic, 2003). Survivor behavior may be volatile, difficult, and unpredictable following a disaster. Therefore, it is important that planners and providers focus on providing care that is realistic and realizable in the short term.

Psychological debriefing has not been demonstrated to be effective in preventing postdisaster morbidity and may be associated with more adverse outcomes (Kenardy, 2000). Even so, it is still widely used because many believe in it, and see it as something active that can be done to help those in immediate need (see discussion in Raphael & Wilson, 2000; Rose, Bisson, & Wessley, 2003). Reviews of evidence-based studies relevant to early intervention have highlighted these problems of expectation, the need to act, and the dearth of studies that can inform action (National Institute of Mental Health, 2002). In the face of these findings, psychological first aid (Raphael, 1977) and triage have been recommended (Raphael, 1986), with a strong emphasis on the need to systematically evaluate and conduct research on these and other interventions.

The National Institute of Mental Health/Substance Abuse and Mental Health Services Administration expert panel on interventions following mass violence conducted a review of the empirical literature. It agreed that in the immediate phase postincident (0–7 days), universal interventions should be based on proven standards of care. That is, they warrant a low level of interference and a high level of choice to prevent possible negative effects. For instance, basic orienting information on trauma response and available resources should be offered, as well as education on parenting and friendship skills (Watson et al., 2003).

The expert panelists concluded that there is currently no empirical evidence to support any intervention that utilizes the components of trauma remembrance and emotional processing in the early phases following mass violence. For instance, there is currently no well-controlled studies supporting the use of psychological debriefing in preventing long-term negative outcomes, particularly in mass violence settings. Negative outcomes reported in some debriefing studies may be due to the psychological and physiological need for avoidant "downtime" immediately following traumatic events. Expert panelists agreed that the "systematic ventilation of feelings" is probably the most potentially harmful phase of debriefing. Because of the possible negative effects from this type of emotional processing, the chaotic and stressful nature of the postrecovery environment, these interventions are not generally recommended in the first 2–3 weeks postincident. However, for those individuals who develop psychiatric conditions such as posttraumatic stress disorder (PTSD), panic reactions, or depression, there is an obligation to treat these survivors in the weeks and months following the incident, utilizing the best empirically supported treatments to prevent long-term conditions (see Bryant & Litz, Chapter 9, and Raphael & Wooding, Chapter 10, this volume).

Those who are vicariously exposed to disaster may also be affected but their symptoms may differ in quality and/or duration (Robb, 1999). For example, first responders and members of the military may experience initial reactions of fear and shock but may recover quickly because of their training and experience in dealing with similar traumatic situations (see Watson, Ritchie, Demer, Bartone, & Pfefferbaum, Chapter 3, this volume). "Operational debriefing" in first responder settings is not a psychological intervention but a collection of shared information (minus emotional processing), and may be helpful in allowing the construction of a more coherent, shared narrative of the incident among those who have worked together or have a shared support system. For instance, in a description of an employee assistance program for British emergency services staff, Avery and King (2003) explain that the rationale for early diffusion meetings for officers called to nonroutine incidents is that they offer an opportunity to review the recent event, recognize that it may have been distressing to some, thank staff for their incident response, offer basic guidance on coping and adjustment strategies, and reassure those present that additional help and support can be made available on request.

The most positive results from early interventions are usually those that mobilize community support and address survivors' human affiliation needs (e.g., helping survivors establish contact with relatives) rather than interventions that focus on individual psychological reactions. Empirical evidence has shown that the recovery from disasters is facilitated by perceived social support, and that one of the best predictors of developing PTSD in the aftermath of trauma is a lack of meaningful social support (Brewin, Andrews, & Valentine, 2000; Norris, 2002). Therefore, facilitating social support should be a key objective for survivors of disaster.

EVALUATING THE DISASTER CONTEXT

Delivering immediate interventions to a particular locality is a function, in part, of the extent to which the social infrastructure has been damaged. If the infrastructure has been destroyed, the population may be displaced and may need to be relocated elsewhere before systematic psychosocial help and support is provided (Ajducovic & Ajducovic, 2003). If the infrastructure is intact, early intervention should proceed with minimal delay. Sometimes infrastructure reconstruction, such as an information center established postdisaster, can double as a venue for screening and family-focused public education (de Jong & Kleber, 2003).

The scale of the disaster and demographic characteristics of an affected community can shape the way in which immediate services are delivered. Some incidents may require international coordination. Further, the needs of those living in multicultural communities are expected to be more varied than needs arising in a homogenous population. For example, survivors may not share a common language; family structure and social networks may vary significantly; and customs and traditions pertaining to death, burial, and grieving may differ. Consultation with representatives of various ethnic groups in these types of settings is imperative.

Some affected communities will face the continuing threat of violence and destruction after an initial disaster. For example, those living near a volcano may have to flee to other locations more than once because of frequent volcanic eruptions; some cities may be vulnerable to repeated terrorist attacks. Any progress made with delivering initial early interventions may be compromised by further untoward events. Under such circumstances, immediate intervention programs may have to start anew time and time again (de Jong & Kleber, 2003).

History has shown that there is no set pattern for the occurrence of disasters and mass violence. Some crises have a definable beginning and progress in stages toward a point of closure. Others, as in war, may last for years and unfold in repetitive phases of destruction and reconstruction followed by further destruction and disruption. Thus, early intervention should be a resource on constant alert (Grieger et al., 2003; Myers, 1994).

UTILIZATION OF SCARCE RESOURCES

Providers of psychosocial services postdisaster are often faced with a seemingly limitless demand for assistance, which commonly can be matched with scarce resources. An inability to match resources with demand often accentuates the sense of crisis. However, scarcity of resources need not be an insurmountable obstacle if guided by two general principles. First, service providers should choose interventions based on the unique circumstances of each disaster scenario (Shalev & Ursano, 2003). Second, early interventions should have realistic aims and objectives and the types of services chosen should be based on need (Ørner & Schnyder, 2003). For instance, ensuring the safety of survivors, providing food and shelter, and then providing access to social support.

Mass media are a resource that should be used during a disaster as a key source of public information. Media resources and management are afforded unprecedented opportunities for addressing survivor needs. Reporting should include accurate and truthful public information based on what is known about unfolding events, the psychological reactions these can evoke, and coping strategies that may be used to minimize distress. Particularly important themes for the general public are descriptions of initial psychological reactions evoked by trauma, their likely time course, and details of services that are established to address the needs of survivors (Levant, Barbanel, & Delon, 2004).

KEY EARLY-INTERVENTION COMPONENTS

During the impact phase and rescue and recovery phase, survivors are faced with unique psychological tasks that must be mastered if they are to cope successfully with distress and fear. The premise for early interventions following a disaster, therefore, should be to view some reactions to abnormal events as natural and to focus on reinforcing positive adaptation mechanisms to lay the foundation for long-term recovery. Early interventions should be implemented with the knowledge that survivors maintain individual and collective competencies. The objective of initial support may be to consolidate these natural capabilities and to provide complementary assistance for their enhancement. Beyond the challenge of immediate survival, a core goal of early intervention is to promote survivor empowerment. Any early intervention should therefore not supplant or interfere with natural processes of adaptation and adjustment.

Shalev and Ursano (2003) have recently developed an excellent rationale to guide planning and delivery of early interventions postdisaster. Their model of "phased adaptive reactions" marks a significant development in the field. This model uses empirical evidence from intervention studies on a variety of survivor cohorts and offers practical suggestions for the planning and delivery of intervention services. Table 7.1 illustrates potential responses by survivors during the impact, rescue, and recovery phases of disasters or other major trauma.

In alignment with these phased interventions is a recommended list of early interventions, endorsed by the expert panel on mass violence (National Institute of Mental Health, 2003) to guide service providers, survivors, and the community in the context of disaster management. The appropriateness of some options is compelling even within the first week postdisaster, while others may be more appropriate in later phases. For planning purposes, however, there is no reason to exclude any of the listed suggestions because of the varying nature of unfolding disasters. To the extent possible, implementation should follow consultation with survivors and careful clinical judgment, to ensure that actions address actual need.

TABLE 7.1. Phased and Changing Responses to Disasters and Mass Violence

	Impact phase	Rescue phase
Principal stressor	Threat to physical and psychological integrity, separation, exposure	New external and internal realities
Concrete goals of behavior	Survival	Adjustment to new realities
Psychological tasks	Primary stress responses	Accommodation
Salient behavior pattern	Fight/flight, freeze, surrender	Resilience vs. exhaustion
Role of all helpers	Rescue and protection	Orient, provide for primary needs
Role of professionals	Secure primary needs, plan for appropriately phased psychosocial support	Offer flexible help and support in accordance with survivors' stated preferences, recognizing both resilience and fluctuating needs

Basic needs

- Provide safety and security.
- Provide food and shelter.
- Establish communication with family, friends, and community.
- Assess the environment for ongoing threats.

Early psychosocial interventions

- Protect survivors from further harm.
- Help reduce survivors' arousal and anxiety.
- Offer support for those in greatest distress.
- Keep families together and facilitate reunion with loved ones and chosen friends.
- Provide information and encourage communication and education.
- Use effective risk communication techniques.

Needs assessment and screening

- Assess current status and needs of survivors.
- Determine if immediate needs are being addressed.
- Enhance the immediate recovery environment.
- Consider whether additional interventions are needed for whole

groups or communities, particularly subpopulations or individual survivors.

Rescue and recovery

- Observe, listen to, and consult with those most affected.
- Monitor the environment for additional threats and stressors.
- Monitor past and ongoing threats.
- Monitor services that are being provided.
- Monitor media coverage and dispel rumors.

Outreach and information dissemination

- Use established community structures.
- Distribute information leaflets.
- Establish new websites.
- Prepare and distribute media releases.
- Participate in media interviews and public information programs.

Technical assistance, consultation, and training

- Improve capacity of organizations and caregivers to provide what is needed to reestablish community structures, support recovery in families, and safeguard community infrastructures.
- Offer technical assistance, consultation, and training for groups (e.g., professional responder groups, volunteers, leaders, and incident commanders) involved in disaster response.

Resilience, coping, and recovery

- Facilitate social interaction at family, group, and community levels.
- Offer structured modules for coping skills awareness training and procedures for conducting risk assessments.
- Provide education about stress responses, traumatic reminders, reducing impact of recent trauma, and differentiating normal and abnormal functioning.
- Provide education to survivors regarding potential risk factors for developing psychopathology and inform survivors of available support services and how to access them.
- Restore organizations to operational readiness.

Immediate need: Triage

- Conduct clinical assessment.
- Refer survivors to longer-term treatment programs when needed.
- Identify vulnerable, high-risk individuals and groups.
- Arrange emergency hospitalization if necessary.

Treatment

- Reduce or ameliorate symptoms to improve functioning using individual, family, and group psychotherapies.
- Consider pharmacotherapy.
- Offer and provide spiritual support.
- Provide short-term or long-term hospitalization.

SUMMARY OF GUIDING PRINCIPLES FOR EARLY INTERVENTION

For both planners and providers of immediate services to survivors of disasters and mass violence, a core guiding principle is that the planning for such events should be based on competence building and that maintaining general preparedness for future postincident response is of the essence. Immediate response should therefore be based on careful planning and preparation. As the case studies in Chapter 18 (Norris et al., this volume) illustrate, planning was strongly recommended by providers who had responded to terrorism in Oklahoma City and New York (Pfefferbaum, North, Flynn, Norris, & DeMartino, 2002). And when deployment occurs, response should be managed and coordinated within a preagreed framework of incident command and control.

In the immediate postdisaster phase, the principal challenges in survivor care tend to focus on survival, safety, security, and the most basic of human needs (see Tables 7.1 and 7.2). One of the crucial functions of frontline responders is offer reassurance until survivors have been moved to a secure containment area. Moving survivors to such an area ensures that they do not act in such a way as to further endanger themselves or others. Only when established in a secure environment is it reasonable to take further steps to try to lower levels of arousal and to facilitate social interaction with other survivors, family members, and friends. Speier (Chapter 5, this volume) offers more detailed information on how to provide psychological first aid to these populations.

Practical challenges to psychosocial adjustment during the earliest phases postdisaster do not typically require a high degree of therapeutic skill. Planners should anticipate a pressing need to address distress and concerns expressed by those affected by major incidents. A strategy for reliable public information sharing and mass media briefings is therefore a crucial component of immediate incident response. From this juncture forward it becomes possible to consult with survivors about their most pressing needs and to extend help or support. In so doing, it is useful to think of early-incident response as the initial step in a phased program of delivering inter-

TABLE 7.2. Summary of Early-Intervention Tasks

1. Provide for basic survival needs and comfort (e.g., liquids, food, shelter, clothing, and heat/cooling).
2. Help survivors achieve restful sleep.
3. Preserve an interpersonal safety zone protecting basic personal space (e.g., privacy, quiet, personal effects).
4. Provide nonintrusive ordinary social contact (e.g., a "sounding board," judicious uses of humor, small talk about current events, and silent companionship).
5. Address immediate physical health problems or exacerbation of prior illnesses.
6. Assist in locating and verifying the personal safety of separated loved ones/ friends.
7. Reconnect survivors with loved ones, friends, trusted other persons (e.g., AA sponsors and work mentors).
8. Help survivors take practical steps to resume ordinary day-to-day life (e.g., daily routines or rituals).
9. Help survivors take practical steps to resolve pressing immediate problems caused by the disaster (e.g., loss of a functional vehicle and inability to get relief vouchers). Consider ethnic and cultural preferences.
10. Facilitate resumption of normal family, community, work, and school roles.
11. Provide opportunities for grieving for losses.
12. Help survivors reduce problematic tension, anxiety, or despondency to manageable levels.
13. Support survivors' indigenous helpers through consultation and training about common stress reactions and stress management techniques.

mediate and longer-term assistance. The chapters in this volume on intermediate and long-term response will further clarify the coordinated, phased interventions that should ideally be facilitated by survivors' positive interactions with mental health personnel in the immediate phase.

REFERENCES

Ajducovic, D., Ajducovic, M. (2003). Systemic approaches to early interventions in a community affected by organized violence. In R. J. Ørner & U. Schnyder (Eds.), *Reconstructing early intervention after trauma innovations in the care of survivors* (pp. 82–92). Oxford, UK: Oxford University Press.

Avery, A., & King, S. (2003). The Lincolnshire Joint Emergency Services Initiative: An early intervention protocol for emergency services staff. In R. J. Ørner & U. Schnyder (Eds.), *Reconstructing early intervention after trauma innovations in the care of survivors* (pp. 212–219). Oxford, UK: Oxford University Press.

Brewin, C. R., Andrews, B., & Valentine, J. D. (2000). Meta-analysis of risk factors for posttraumatic stress disorder in trauma-exposed adults. *Journal of Consulting and Clinical Psychology, 68,* 748–766.

de Jong, K., & Kleber, R. (2003). Early psychosocial interventions for war-affected populations. In R. J. Ørner & U. Schnyder (Eds.), *Reconstructing early intervention after trauma innovations in the care of survivors* (pp. 184–192). Oxford, UK: Oxford University Press.

Grieger, T. A., Bally, R. E., Lyszczarz, J. L., Kennedy, J. S., Griffeth, B. T., & Reeves, J. J. (2003). Individual and organizational interventions after terrorism: September 11 and the *USS Cole*. In R. J. Ursano, C. S. Fullerton, & A. E. Norwood (Eds.), *Terrorism and disaster: Individual and community mental health interventions* (pp. 71–89). Cambridge, UK: Cambridge University Press.

Kenardy, J. (2000). The current status of psychological debriefing: It may do more harm than good. *British Medical Journal, 321,* 1032–1033.

Levant, R. F., Barbanel, L., & Delon, P. H. (2004). Psychology's response to terrorism. In F. M. Moghaddam & A. J. Marsella (Eds.), *Understanding terrorism: Psychosocial roots, consequences and interventions* (pp. 265–282). Washington, DC: American Psychological Association.

Myers, D. (1994). *Disaster response and recovery: A handbook for mental health professionals* (DHHS Publication No. [SMA] 94-3010). Monterey, CA: U.S. Department of Health and Human Services.

National Institute of Mental Health. (2002). *Mental health and mass violence: Evidence based early intervention for victims/survivors of mass violence: A workshop to reach consensus on best practice* (Vol. 109). Washington, DC: U.S. Government Printing Office.

Norris, F. H. (2002). Psychosocial consequences of disasters. *PTSD Research Quarterly, 13,* 1–7.

Norris, F. H., Murphy, A. D., Baker, C. K., & Perulla, J. L. (2003). Severity, training and duration of reactions to trauma in the population: An example from Mexico. *Biological Psychiatry, 53,* 769–778.

Ørner, R. J., & Schnyder, U. (2003). Progress made towards reconstructing early intervention after trauma: emergent themes. In R. J. Ørner & U. Schnyder (Eds.), *Reconstructing early intervention after trauma innovations in the care of survivors* (pp. 249–279). Oxford, UK: Oxford University Press.

Pfefferbaum, B., North, C. S., Flynn, B. W., Norris, F. H., & DeMartino, R. (2002). Disaster mental health services following the 1995 Oklahoma City bombing: Modifying approaches to address terrorism. *CNS Spectrums, 7,* 575–579.

Raphael, B. (1977). Preventative intervention with the recently bereaved. *Archives of General Psychiatry, 34,* 1450-1454.

Raphael, B. (1986). Psychosocial care. In B. Raphael (Ed.), *When disaster strikes: How individuals and communities cope with catastrophe* (pp. 245–290). New York: Basic Books.

Raphael, B., & Wilson, J. (2000). *Psychological debriefing: Theory, practice, and evidence.* Cambridge, UK: Cambridge University Press.

Robb, N. (1999). After Swissair 111, the helpers needed help. *Canadian Medical Association Journal, 160,* 394.

Rose, S., Bisson, J., & Wessley, S. (2003). A systematic review of single psychological interventions ("debriefing") following trauma: Updating the Cochrane review and implications for good practice. In R. J. Ørner & U. Schnyder

(Eds.), *Reconstructing early intervention after trauma innovations in the care of survivors* (pp. 24–39). Oxford, UK: Oxford University Press.

Shalev, A. Y., & Ursano, R. J. Mapping the multidimensional picture of acute responses to traumatic stress. In R. J. Ørner & U. Schnyder (Eds.), *Reconstructing early intervention after trauma innovations in the care of survivors* (pp. 118–129). Oxford, UK: Oxford University Press.

Watson, P. J., Friedman, M. J., Gibson, L. E., Ruzek, J. I., Norris, F. H., & Ritchie, E. C. (2003). Early intervention for trauma-related problems. In R. J. Ursano & J. E. Norwood (Eds.), *Trauma and disaster responses and management* (pp. 97–124). Washington, DC: American Psychiatric Publishing.

Wright, K. M., & Bartone, P. T. Community responses to disaster: The plane crash. In R. J. Ursano, J. Robert, B. G. McCaughey, & C. S. Fullerton (Eds.), *Individual and community responses to trauma and disaster: The structure of human chaos* (267–284). Cambridge, UK: Cambridge University Press.

CHAPTER 8

The Immediate Response to Disaster

Guidelines for Adult Psychological First Aid

BRUCE H. YOUNG

Nearly every survivor of mass violence or disaster experiences stress-related reactions in the immediate aftermath. Most recover. Nonetheless, in a communitywide disaster, the subset of survivors (11–15%) who develop posttraumatic stress disorder (PTSD) or other adverse mental health outcomes may number tens of thousands (Galea et al., 2002; Green & Solomon, 1995; McFarlane, 1995; Norris, 1992; Rubonis & Bickman, 1991).

As Chapters 8, 9, and 11 (this volume) demonstrate, preparedness and the systemic response to the mental health needs of survivors raise complex issues. Here the focus is on the issues specific to adult Psychological First Aid, one component of emergency public health services in the immediate response to disaster.

WHAT IS PSYCHOLOGICAL FIRST AID?

Psychological First Aid (PFA) is defined here as the use of pragmatic-oriented interventions delivered during the immediate-impact phase (first 4 weeks) to individuals who are experiencing acute stress reactions or who appear at risk for being unable to regain sufficient functional equilibrium by themselves, with the intent of aiding adaptive coping and problem solving. PFA is meant to be embedded in a systemic response involving mental health, public health, medical, and emergency response systems and federal, state, local, and nonprofit agencies (including non-mental health agencies such as law enforcement, fire and rescue, school systems, social services, etc.). Finally, PFA happens in the context of community intervention (publicly disseminated information about risk, resources, and care of self and family; memorials, VIP visits, etc.) and community-level surveillance/ assessment related to service needs.

Though PFA has not been empirically tested, it was endorsed by an international expert panel following mass violence or disaster because it is composed of empirically defensible interventions unlikely to be harmful when used in a conservative and culturally sensitive way related to the formulation of problems and ways of coping (see Watson, 2004). It is considered "safe" because it does not focus on emotional processing or detailed trauma narratives, is not meant to be "mandatory," and should be only used with individuals who meet certain criteria (National Institute of Mental Health, 2002).

The origins of PFA are tied to crisis intervention (Lindemann, 1944; Shneidman, Farberow, & Litman 1970) and the early disaster work of Raphael (1977) and Farberow (1978). In the late 1980s, critical incident stress debriefing (CISD), a protocol originally developed to mitigate stress response among emergency personnel (Mitchell, 1983), was increasingly used with victims of communitywide disasters. By the end of the 1990s, disaster mental health services were seen by many new to the field (planners, policymakers, and responders) as synonymous with debriefing (see Deahl, 2000)—despite a growing literature on PFA and principles of disaster mental health care (American Red Cross, 1991, 1995; DeWolfe, 2000; Farberow, 1978; Hartsough, 1985; Lystad, 1985; Myers, 1994; Raphael, 1986; Weaver, 1995; Young, Ford, Ruzek, Friedman, & Gusman, 1998) and the initial empirical evidence indicating that debriefing in general has no demonstrable preventive effect (Bisson & Deahl, 1994; Charlton & Thompson, 1996; Foa & Meadows, 1997; Gist, 1996; Kenardy & Carr, 1996; Rose, Bisson, & Wesseley, 2001).

Several recent reviews concluded that CISD cannot prevent long-term psychological sequelae, or it may worsen the outcomes of some individuals. Ørner, Kent, Pfefferbaum, Raphael, and Watson (Chapter 7, this volume) review this literature in detail.

WHO IS IN NEED OF PSYCHOLOGICAL FIRST AID?

If nearly all survivors experience acute stress reactions and most recover on their own, who is in need of PFA? Broadly speaking, two conceptual domains may be used for determining which survivors might benefit: individuals who exhibit extreme acute stress reactions (see Table 8.1) and those with notable risk factors linked to adverse mental health outcomes (see Table 8.2).

Assessment of risk factors may be used to monitor "high-risk individuals" and target the postdisaster factors that can be ameliorated. Risk assessment should enable disaster mental health (DMH) workers to avoid "overhelping" or denying the survivor the self-efficacy to mobilize existing resources (Gilbert & Silvera, 1996).

How do DMH workers engage survivors to gather sufficient information to determine if risk factors are present and if PFA is warranted? Young (2002) suggests guidelines for engaging survivors in settings in which survivors generally congregate (i.e., outreach) and conversing informally to assess risk. Survivors have imminent practical concerns and rapport is best established with topics related to present worries. While establishing rapport, talking about immediate concerns begins the assessment.

Postdisaster risk factor assessment of resource loss and immediate needs may help DMH workers assist in negotiating resources for survivors, a high-priority task in the immediate aftermath. It is also an opportunity to assess survivors' beliefs in their capacity to cope with the resulting losses and demands. The belief that one can manage demands related to the disaster has been shown to predict good psychological outcomes (e.g., Benight, Ironson, et al., 1999; Benight, Swift, Sanger, Smith, & Zeppelin, 1999). A survivor's response to the question "Do you believe you can cope with _____?" can help workers weigh the need for more in-depth services. The assessment process necessarily involves timing questions. Questions about perceived capacities to cope are clearly reasonable at

---

TABLE 8.1. Extreme Acute Stress Reactions

These reactions include:

- Extreme anxiety resulting in basic functional impairment.
- Dissociative symptoms include survivors experiencing pronounced:
  - Detachment.
  - Derealization.
  - Depersonalization.
  - Dreamlike interpretation of their surroundings.
- Prolonged, intense, and uncontrollable, distressful emotions (objectively or subjectively perceived.
- Prolonged inability to sleep or eat, or neglect of other basic self-care needs.
- Extreme cognitive impairment to include:
  - Confusion.
  - Poor concentration.
  - Poor decision making.

TABLE 8.2. Risk Factors Associated with Postdisaster Adverse Mental Health Outcomes

These factors include:

Predisaster factors

- *Female gender* (Caldera, Palma, Penayo, & Kulgren, 2001; Goenjian et al., 1995; Norris, Kaniasty, Conrad, Inman, & Murphy, 2002).
- *Age in the years of 40–60* (Gleser, Green, & Winget, 1981; Thompson, Norris, & Hanacek, 1993).
- *Ethnic-minority-group membership* (Palinkas, Petterson, Russell, & Downs, 1993; Perilla, Norris, & Lavisso, 2002).
- *Poverty or low socioeconomic status* (Dew & Bromet, 1993; Hanson, Kilpatrick, Freedy, & Saunders, 1995; Phifer, 1990).
- *Presence of exposed children in the home* (Bromet et al., 2000; Havenaar et al., 1997; Solomon, Bravo, Rubio-Stipec, & Canino, 1993).
- *Psychiatric history* (Dew & Bromet, 1993; Lonigan, Shannon, Taylor, Finch, & Sallee, 1994; North et al., 1999).

Within-disaster factors

- *Bereavement* (Green, Grace, & Gleser, 1985; Green et al., 1994; Murphy, 1984).
- *Injury* (Briere & Elliot, 2000; Norris & Uhl, 1993; Shariat, Mallonee, Kruger, Farmer, & North, 1999).
- *Severity of exposure* (Bravo, Rubio-Stipec, Canino, Woodbury, & Ribera, 1990; Palinkas, Petterson, Russell, & Downs, 1993; Pynoos et al., 1993).
- *Peritraumatic reactions, including panic* (Chung, Werrett, Farmer, Easthope, & Chung, 2000; Fullerton, Ursano, Tzu-Cheg, & Bharitya, 1999; Koopman, Classen, & Spiegel, 1996; McFarlane, 1989; Weisaeth, 1989).
- *Horror* (Clearly & Houts, 1984).
- *Life threat* (Bland et al., 1997; Briere & Elliot, 2000; Norris & Uhl, 1993).

Postdisaster factors

- *Resource deterioration* (Arata, Picou, Johnson, & McNally, 2000; Freedy, Shaw, Jarrell, & Masters, 1992; Smith & Freedy, 2000).
- *Relocation or displacement* (Najarian, Goenjian, Pelcovitz, Mandel, & Najarian, 2001; Norris & Uhl, 1993; Riad & Norris, 1996).
- *Social support deterioration* (Bland et al., 1997; Smith & Freedy, 2000).
- *Marital distress* (Norris & Uhl, 1993).
- *Loss of home/property and financial loss* (Bland, Leary, Farinaro, & Trevisan, 1996; Briere & Elliot, 2000; North et al., 1999).
- *Decline in perceived social support* (Kaniasty & Norris, 1993; Kaniasty, Norris, & Murrell, 1990; Solomon, Bravo, Rubio-Stipec, & Canino, 1993).
- *Alienation and mistrust* (Baum, Gatchel, & Schaeffer, 1983; Dohrenwend, 1983).
- *Avoidance coping* (Clearly & Houts, 1984; Maes et al., 1998; North et al., 1999).

In addition, other risk factors have been noted (McNally, Bryant, & Ehlers, 2003) including:

- Negative perceptions of other people's responses.
- Negative perceptions of symptoms.
- Exaggeration of future probability of trauma.
- Catastrophic attributions of responsibility.
- Secondary stressors.

postdisaster day 14 but may or may not be reasonable or informative at day 3 because of wide-ranging circumstances, personal characteristics, and history of survivors. Workers should take a case-by-case approach.

Asking survivors to talk about their "within"-disaster experience may be accomplished through inquiries about whereabouts (exposure), separation from family, bereavement, and displacement. Soliciting detail or any enhanced narrative related to exposure is unwarranted. Such narration outside multiple-session treatment could potentially harm (Bisson, 2003; Shalev, 2000).

Assessing predisaster risk factors may be accomplished via presenting brief educational points about risk related to previous traumatization and psychopathology, rather than through direct questions about chronic stress or psychiatric history. For example, a DMH worker might say:

> "We know from research and from talking with many survivors, that people with major health or financial concerns before a disaster, or who have had to cope with depression, anxiety, schizophrenia, or substance abuse are more often vulnerable after an event like this. The same is true for people previously traumatized. If this is your situation, you may need to take extra care or want to talk longer with a mental health professional when time permits."

If rapport is established, clinical judgment can decide whether to ask such questions:

> "What kind of stress were you dealing with before all this happened?"
> "Have you ever been through anything traumatic before?"

As part of any engagement or assessment process, workers should try to identify sources of strength and past successful coping.

OBJECTIVES AND INTERVENTIONS OF PFA

The principal objective of PFA can be stated as aiding the adaptive coping and problem-solving processes of survivors who appear at risk for being unable to regain sufficient functional equilibrium on their own. Problems may be related to safety and security, extreme acute stress reactions (see Table 8.1), and associated risk factors (see Table 8.2). Correspondingly, the primary objectives of PFA include establishing safety, reducing extreme acute stress-related reactions, and connecting survivors to resources that are restorative and better address respective problems through more in-depth services. Even in cases in which individuals are in need of PFA, not all interventions corresponding to the objectives are required. The following algorithm is a guide regarding the need for interventions:

1. If necessary, first help to establish safety and provide basic support.
2. If necessary, seek to reduce extreme acute stress-related reactions via:
   a. Interventions for specific traumatic stressors.
   b. Arousal reduction interventions.
3. If necessary, connect survivors to restorative resources via:
   a. Active help with problem solving.
   b. Referral.

Establishing Safety

Physical care is psychological care. DMH workers are not in the role of meeting survivors' physical needs, but if "first on-scene" as many were on 9/11, workers may give direction to areas away from danger, toxic and harsh elements, and exposure to further traumatic stimuli. Safe areas may vary from neighborhood to neighborhood. Common locations include designated shelters, information centers, emergency rooms, churches, schools, community centers, hotels, and medical clinics. Providing water, food, warmth, and respite gives basic support; it also can reassure survivors of altruism. Other interventions may be intrusive if the survivor is exhausted, hungry, and cold (Holloway & Fullerton, 1994; Raphael & Newman, 2000).

Reducing Extreme Acute Stress Reactions

Goal two of PFA is reducing extreme acute stress reactions from emotional, cognitive, physiological, or behavioral effects. There are at least two approaches to conceptualizing PFA to reduce severe stress: (1) describing interventions that address specific disaster-related stressors and (2) describing a "toolkit" of interventions to reduce severe disaster-related stress. Both conceptual approaches are used here. Whichever approach is used, all interventions require cross-cultural competency and the ability to exhibit empathy, genuineness, and positive regard for others.

Interventions for Specific Disaster-Related Stressors

Sudden Unexpected Bereavement. Violent death of a loved one has been linked with PTSD (Breslau et al., 1998). When working with the bereaved in the acute phases, workers must respect individual timing (e.g., avoidance may be a way to cope with grief).

TABLE 8.3. Conversational Guidelines for Working with the Bereaved

Possible things to say

"I am sorry that he/she is gone."
"I can't imagine what you are going through."

Suggestions:

Mention the name of the deceased during conversations.
Acknowledge the degree of distress and painful emotion that
    the survivor is willing to express.

Things *not* to say

"You should be glad the deceased passed quickly."
"She's/he's in his or her resting place now."
"I know how you feel."
"It is God's will."
"It was his or her time to go."
"Let's change the subject."
"It was probably for the best given what happened."
"You are strong enough to deal with this."

Providing support to individuals who suffer the death of a loved one is one of the more challenging aspects of DMH work. Weaver (2000) suggests that "less is more"; it is less what one says and more how one listens; it is knowing when to remain silent and when to intervene. Workers may encourage the bereaved to talk with other bereaved survivors, to identify their resilience, including past successful coping, support and spirituality, or help with understanding that bereavement from traumatic loss might be a different process than nontraumatic bereavement. Workers can expect to experience their own helplessness and must recognize that their presence alone can be valuable. Table 8.3 lists conversational guidelines for working with the bereaved (Weaver, 2000).

Exposure to Traumatic Stimuli. Extreme acute distress can come from witnessing grotesque death, dead bodies, strong smells, and frightening sounds, including those from dying, injured, or upset survivors. Protecting survivors from such exposure can reduce distress. For example, one may suggest to emergency medical staff at a triage site to keep the ambulatory minor injured apart from the seriously injured, or advise a shelter or family assistance center manager to limit television event coverage and keep young children away from viewing areas. Educating survivors about coping with external (e.g., disturbing media coverage) and internal (i.e., thoughts, emotions) traumatic memory triggers may help.

Resource Loss. The loss of critical resources can cause severe distress (see postdisaster risk factors, Table 8.2); interventions to prevent psychosocial resource loss may reduce long-term effects (Smith & Freedy, 2000). Interventions for resource loss may address pragmatic needs, the stress caused by such losses, or the connection to restorative resources.

Reexperiencing. A third possible cause of acute stress reactions is distressing intrusive thoughts. Survivors may directly complain about being unable to stop thinking about or visualizing some terrible aspect of the event, or a DMH worker may discover a frequent form of "reexperiencing." One way to disrupt the flow of intrusive thoughts is to guide a survivor's attention to the present (see Table 8.4; Young, 2002).

Cognitive Appraisal. Acute distress may relate to the survivors' cognitive appraisal of the event and their capacities to cope (Benight, Ironson, et al., 1999; Benight, Swift, et al., 1999). Workers may encounter survivors who have quickly developed cognitive distortions related to fear, helplessness, guilt, anger, and rage. Such beliefs can "unnecessarily" maintain a sense of threat and increase distress. DMH workers may have a chance to use brief cognitive restructuring or reframing to counter such distortions (see Table 8.5; Young, 2002).

TABLE 8.4. Example of Helping a Survivor Cope with Intrusive Thoughts

"[Person's name], I hear how you keep thinking about _____ [aspect of event] over and over again . . . and I can understand why this happens and how hard it is to not think about it. I also see how distressing it is for you to keep repeating _____ in your mind. If it is okay with you, I would like to help you get a break from _____. Is it okay with you?"

Gently suggest an activity that helps to orient the survivor to the present moment while asking him or her to describe the activity (e.g., walking, washing face and hands, deep breathing, and eating); alternatively, give the person something to hold or to touch, (e.g., a pen, a purse, a book, clothing, a chair) and ask him or her to describe what each feels like. Redirect attention to the experience of the activity to disrupt the flow of intrusive thoughts or distressing anxiety.

If the intrusive imagery is experienced as a "flashback," that is, a reliving of the traumatic experience, become even more directive, adding: "We are sitting in _____ [name of site], it is _____ [date, day of week, and time]. Please tell me where we are, today's date, and day . . . and what time it is."

If appropriate to the culture, consider asking the person to exchange reasonable eye contact.

TABLE 8.5. Example of a 2-Minute Version of Reframing

Theme: Guilt and shame

Negative thought or distortions
1. "I was a coward. Because of me, other people died."
2. "I should this have gotten over this by now."

Reframes
1. "I can only imagine how frightening that was and can hear that you are now doubting yourself. It's clear that your actions saved you from further injury. Many factors beyond your control resulted in the deaths that occurred and it's unfair to you to take any blame in this."
2. "I hear that you feel inpatient with yourself. It takes time get through something like this. I know for a fact, that many other survivors are at the same place that you are right now."

Theme: Helplessness and fear

Negative thought or distortion
1. "I was helpless then; I won't be able to cope with future events either."
2. "I just can't believe I felt so afraid. It's unacceptable to experience that degree of fear."

Reframes
1. "I hear you say that you believe you felt helpless and how distressful that was. Even when you believed you were helpless, it was your actions that saved your life . . . you helped yourself . . . and it appears that you continue to help yourself . . . this is coping with events as they unfold."
2. "A lot of people I've listened to said they were more afraid than anytime before in their life. Fear is natural and it helped you to survive. Gradually you can ease out of it."

Theme: Anger and trust

Negative thoughts or distortion
1. "Those jerks, or for that matter, most people just can't be trusted to help. I'm not interested in filing the relief forms. They tell me one thing one day and another the next. Everything's breaking down."

Reframe
1. "I can hear how angry you are—who wouldn't be? . . . and I hear how hard it is to bear so much loss . . . and that you feel let down by those who you thought would help you and your family. I would like to ask you to consider for a moment, even though you are very angry, that most likely there are people who can and will help you and there are people who neither can or won't. And that you and your family would probably benefit more if you were to reconsider filing the forms necessary to replace the furniture you lost. You can still be angry *and* fill out the forms that will help you."

As with other cognitive reframing techniques, care must be given to validation of the affective component (*feelings* of helplessness, fear, grief, rage, etc.); addressing cognitions without reference to their potential exaggerated effect; recognizing that such cognitions are not unrealistic; and timing (e.g., such intervention is less likely than the other components of PFA in the first 72 hours postevent).

Arousal Reduction Interventions

A "toolkit" of interventions can reduce stress-related reactions.

Relaxation Procedures. If stress reactions involve extreme anxiety; marked cognitive impairment; or uncontrollable, prolonged, or intense, distress, instructing survivors on relaxation procedures (conscious/slow breathing; progressive muscle relaxation; visualization; meditation, etc.) may reduce these reactions. In rare cases, all forms of relaxation procedures may exacerbate anxiety, intrusive images, or dissociative states (Everly & Lating, 2002); clinical judgment and preparation of the individual for possible increase in anxiety are recommended.

Young and colleagues (1998) advise that while suggesting relaxation procedures to survivors, it is important to address any related concerns—for example, beliefs that one cannot relax amid continuing stress; fears that relaxing will compromise their coping; fears of being overwhelmed by intense memories or emotions; or negative past experiences with such procedures. DMH workers must know different relaxation techniques to allow for offering survivors various options and how to instruct survivors quickly. A 30-second version of conscious/slow breathing might involve gently saying: "Everyone feels overwhelmed now, how about we take a few slow breaths"—followed by a demonstration and practice of slow diaphragmatic breathing. If time allows, longer versions can be utilized (see Young, Ruzek, & Ford, 1999, pp. 171–172).

Education Techniques. Education can help to "normalize" experiences; provide information about stress reactions, stress management strategies, and resources; and create a sense of control and efficacy. Most postdisaster education is informal, occurring during brief conversations with survivors. Table 8.6 lists educational talking points (Young, 2002). Talking points are meant to be specific to each survivor; one need not cover all details. It is important to summarize key points, provide written materials, and offer a follow-up contact (if warranted and feasible).

DMH workers should use judgment regarding whether and when to present information. Care must be given to avoid introducing a "modeling"

TABLE 8.6. Educational Talking Points

Well-known traumatic stressors

Life-threatening exposure, (duration, intensity, frequency), loss of loved ones, resource loss (property, financial, social support, etc.).

Common stress reactions and their course

Emotional: Anger, anhedonia, emotional numbing, fear, grief, guilt, shame, feelings of rejection, feelings of distrust.

Cognitive: Confusion, difficult concentration, disorientation, indecisiveness, intrusive thoughts, memory loss, self-blame and negative appraisal, shattered beliefs and assumptions, shortened attention span.

Physical: Body aches, change in appetite, change in libido, diarrhea, difficult sleep, fatigue, hyperventilation, nausea, racing heartbeat, startle, tension, tremor.

Behavioral: Increased conflict with others, increase use of controlling behaviors, withdrawal from social support and social activity, substance abuse (if predisposed).

Risk factors associated with adverse mental health outcomes

See predisaster, within-disaster, and postdisaster variables associated with adaptation to trauma (Table 8.2).

Self-care and stress management strategies

Positive coping: Exercise, eating well, receiving and giving social support, relaxation techniques, etc.

Negative coping: Substance abuse, workaholism, social withdrawal, phobic avoidance of reminders of event.

Benefits of self-awareness: Emotional experience, mindfulness, and selected self-disclosure.

Parenting/support guidelines: How to monitor children other family members' reactions; how to support children and other family members.

Characteristics of recovery: Guidance about general course of individual and community recovery.

Information about available resources.

When and where to seek additional help.

---

effect by suggesting symptoms (Shalev et al., 2003); some survivors in acute stages of recovery may not be receptive to education efforts.

The effectiveness of postdisaster education has not been evaluated, and recent evidence suggests that self-help instructions (fact sheets) alone may delay recovery in some survivors (Ehlers et al., 2003). Single-session education is not the best behavioral change procedure, and probably will not prevent PTSD in those at highest risk (Ehlers et al., 2003).

Cognitive Reframing Techniques. As mentioned, the subtle, supportive, and judicious use of cognitive reframing techniques may serve as a preliminary effort to help counter the potential negative affects of cognitive distortions. Though cognitive-behavioral treatment has demonstrated efficacy when used with trauma survivors (see, Foa, Keane, & Friedman, 2000), there is no study of the use of brief cognitive reframing techniques with disaster survivors.

Psychopharmacology. Use of psychopharmacological interventions may mitigate psychological stresses that are extremely distressful to survivors. Most individuals affected by disasters and mass trauma are resilient; long-term negative psychological sequelae are often minimal and long-term use of psychiatric medications is unnecessary.

Assessing for the indication of medication usage necessarily involves inquiring about past and current medical history: prior psychotropic use, drug allergies, contraindications to psychotropic use, as well as the survivor's ability to comply with medication regimen, and the potential for substance abuse. Effort should be made to ensure documented follow-up so that survivors can be monitored for the efficacy of the medication, potential side effects, or referrals to higher level of care if necessary.

Imipramine in low-doses shows significant reduction in acute stress disorder symptoms (Robert, Blakeney, Villarreal, Rosenberg, & Meyer, 1999). Propanolol administered in the first 6–12 hours shows a later reduction in conditioned response to trauma stimuli (Pitman et al., 2002). Risperidone administered 5 days posttrauma can decrease sleep disturbance, nightmares, flashbacks, and hyperarousal (Stanovic, James, & Van Devere, 2001). There is no evidence of a PTSD protective benefit, and some possibility of a negative affect with benzodiazepines (Friedman, 2000).

Connecting Survivors to Restorative Resources

The third goal of PFA is to direct survivors to additional resources. Survivors already in safe areas may still need being told where to receive information or services (e.g., medical care, shelter, relief and family assistance services, and information centers). In nonemergencies, therapeutic intervention generally seeks to develop empowerment and support independence while avoiding reinforcement of helplessness and self-defeating dependence. When survivors are so overwhelmed by losses, confusion, anxiety, grief, helplessness, guilt, and so on, that normal functioning is impaired, taking a more active role to ensure linkage or connection to resources may be appropriate. Caveat: Survivors' sense of control and self-efficacy are important and clinical judgment must be used to avoid acting on something that survivors themselves can act on, or creating situations where survivors are left thinking they had no say about the matters. Workers can always begin to identify and remind survivors of their existing coping skills and resources in their current social network.

Active Help with Problem Solving

Active help with problem solving includes helping survivors to obtain food, liquid, and clothing and to replace or obtain new medications; arranging transportation to a shelter, emergency mental health services clinic, or relief and information centers; helping connect to social support (family, significant others, friends); making phone calls on survivors' behalf when appropriate; linking survivors to information providers; advocating on their behalf; and referring them to more intensive financial, practical, or mental health services.

When and How to Refer to Mental Health Services

In the first 14 days, the decision to make a referral to more in-depth mental health services is complicated. During the immediate aftermath, workers often have only limited contact with survivors and may lack sufficient information to determine whether acute stress reactions will resolve without intensive services. Second, in the first 2 weeks to 1 month, community mental health resources may be overwhelmed or extremely limited (i.e., only emergency rooms available).

Because it can be expected that these resources will be limited, those needing referral can be sorted into two groups: (1) survivors needing immediate crisis intervention and (2) survivors at risk for long-term adverse mental health problems. Survivors needing crisis intervention are those experiencing suicidal ideation, symptoms of psychosis, and seemingly unremitting panic reactions, or those who no longer have the capacity for basic self-care (e.g., nourishment, hygiene, and rest). Crisis intervention would most likely resemble routine procedures under ordinary conditions. In catastrophes involving severe widespread damage where community resources become unknown, intervention involving hospital or police authorities may best ensure a survivor's safety.

In the second group, the unavailability of resources often requires that individuals be informed about "warning signs" (e.g., what to monitor and when to self-refer once more extensive disaster-related mental health resources are in operation) (Table 8.7).

Several procedural steps should be considered to increase compliance with seeking additional help. First, the option of receiving more in-depth services and what might be expected of such services is explained. If necessary, negative reactions (e.g., perceived stigma and perceptions of counseling) are explored: the stigma of disaster-related counseling might be

TABLE 8.7. Advising Survivors When to Seek Treatment: Persistent Stress Reactions and "Warning Signs"

Persistent stress reactions

- Phobic avoidance of reminders.
- Inordinate grief (dissonant with cultural values).
- Frequent episodes of intense inappropriate anger.
- Severe sleep disruption or frequent nightmares.
- Severe unremitting anxiety.
- Symptoms of clinical depression.
- Significant impaired problem-solving ability.
- Severely distressing intrusive thoughts.

Warning signs

- Abuse of alcohol/drugs.
- Significant social isolation.
- Spiritual/existential despair.
- Significant social isolation.
- Inability to work.
- Suicidal ideation.

reduced if it is described as an opportunity to receive practical support, information, and help with problem solving. Compliance may increase with written referral information and help with scheduling an appointment.

SUMMARY

The components of PFA described previously are endorsed by expert consensus as empirically defensible interventions unlikely to cause harm. When incorporated into a systematic disaster response system, they are expected to offer a critical mental health response in the first month following catastrophe. Interventions included in PFA have not been tested empirically and research is needed to determine if they are sufficient to prevent adverse mental health outcomes. Research is further needed to clarify the timeline for offering different elements of PFA, whether other components should be added, and which circumstances call for the use of specific components.

The field is currently progressing along several lines that should assist with more effective delivery: encouraging collaboration between mental health public health agencies, strategies, and interventions (Institute of Medicine, 2003); innovative delivery strategies (i.e., Internet and email); development of intervention manuals and videotaped vignettes (National Center for PTSD, Center for Mental Health Services [CMHS]; National

Child Traumatic Stress Network); development of more efficient assessment procedures and algorithms to identify individuals at high risk for progressing to chronic posttraumatic problems (Brewin, Rose, & Andrews, 2003); and adapting early interventions for ethnocultural populations (CMHS). Advances in psychobiology and genetics also may promise keys to identify and improve acute response to trauma (Charney, 2004). It is anticipated that these developments will contribute to a more comprehensive strategy for preventive mental and behavioral health following disasters, reducing recovery time and morbidity in survivors.

ACKNOWLEDGMENTS

I would like to acknowledge Anthony Ng, MD, for his contribution to the section on "Psychopharmacology" and to Patricia J. Watson, PhD, for her summary of current initiatives related to PFA.

REFERENCES

American Red Cross. (1991). *Disaster services regulations and procedures: Disaster mental health services* (ARC3050M). Washington, DC: Author.

American Red Cross. (1995). *Disaster mental health services I.* Washington, DC: Author.

Arata, C. M., Picou, J. S., Johnson, G. D., & McNally, T. S. (2000). Coping with technological disaster: An application of the conservation of resources model to Exxon Valdez oil spill. *Journal of Traumatic Stress, 11*, 23–39.

Baum, A., Gatchel, R., & Schaeffer, M. (1983). Emotional, behavioral and physiological effects at Three Mile Island. *Journal of Consulting and Clinical Psychology, 51*, 565–572.

Benight, C. C., Ironson, G., Klebe, K., Carver, C. S., Wynings, C. G., Burnett, K., et al. (1999). Conservation of resources and coping self-efficacy predicting distress following a natural disaster: A causal model analysis where the environment meets the mind. *Anxiety, Stress, and Coping, 12*, 107–126.

Benight, C. C., Swift, E., Sanger, J., Smith, A., & Zeppelin, D. (1999). Coping self-efficacy as a mediator of distress following a natural disaster. *Journal of Applied Social Psychology, 29*, 2443–2464.

Bisson, J. I. (2003). Single-session early psychological interventions following traumatic events. *Clinical Psychology Review, 23*, 481–499.

Bisson, J. I., & Deahl, M. P. (1994). Psychological debriefing and prevention of post-traumatic stress: More research is needed. *British Journal of Psychiatry, 165*, 717–720.

Bland, S. H., O'Leary, E. S., Farinaro, E., Jossa, F., Krogh, V., Violanti, J. M., et. al. (1997). Social network disturbances and psychological distress following Earthquake evacuation. *Journal of Nervous and Mental Disease, 185*, 188–194.

Bland, S. H., O'Leary, E. S., Farinaro, E., & Trevisan, M. (1996). Long-term psychological effects of natural disasters. *Psychosomatic Medicine, 58*, 18–24.

Bravo, M., Rubio-Stipec, M., Canino, G. J., Woodbury, M. A., & Ribera, J. C. (1990). The psychological sequelae of disaster stress prospectively and retrospectively evaluated. *American Journal of Community Psychology, 18*, 661–680.

Breslau, N., Kessler, R. C., Chilcoat, H. D., Schultz, L. R., Davis, G. C., & Andreski, P. (1998). Trauma and posttraumatic stress disorder in the community: The 1996 Detroit Area Survey of Trauma. *Archives of General Psychiatry, 55*, 626–631.

Brewin, C., Rose, S., & Andrews, B. (2003). Screening to identify individuals at risk after exposure to trauma. In R. Orner & U. Schnyder (Eds.), *Reconstructing early intervention after trauma: Innovations in the care of survivors* (pp. 130–142). Oxford: Oxford University Press.

Briere, J., & Elliot, D. (2000). Prevalence, characteristics, and long-term sequelae of natural disaster exposure in the general population. *Journal of Traumatic Stress, 13*, 661–679.

Bromet, E. J., Goldgaber, D., Carlson, G., Panina, N., Golovakha, E., Gluzman, S. F., et al. (2000). Children's well-being 11 years after the Chernobyl catastrophe. *Archives of General Psychiatry, 57*, 563–571.

Caldera, T., Palma, L., Penayo, U., & Kulgren, G. (2001). Psychological impact of the Hurricane Mitch in Nicaragua in a one year perspective. *Social Psychiatry and Psychiatric Epidemiology, 36*, 108–114.

Charlton, P. F., & Thompson, J. A. (1996). Ways of coping with psychological distress after trauma. *British Journal of Clinical Psychology, 35*, 517–530.

Charney, D. S. (2004). Psychobiological mechanisms of resilience and vulnerability: Implications for successful adaptation to extreme stress. *American Journal of Psychiatry, 162*, 195–216.

Chung, M.C., Werrett, J., Farmer, S., Easthope, Y., & Chung, C. (2000). Responses to traumatic stress among community residents exposed to a train collision. *Stress Medicine, 16*, 17–25.

Clearly, P. D., & Houts, P. S. (1984). The psychological impact of the Three Mile Island incident. *Journal of Human Stress, 10*, 28–34.

Deahl, M. P. (2000). Psychological debriefing: Controversy and challenge. *Australian and New Zealand Journal of Psychiatry, 34*, 929–939.

Dew, M. A., & Bromet, E. J. (1993). Predictors of temporal patterns of psychiatric distress during 10 years following the nuclear accident at Three Mile Island. *Social Psychiatry and Psychiatric Epidemiology, 28*, 49–55.

DeWolfe, D. J. (2000). *Training manual for mental health and human service workers in major disasters* (2nd ed.) (DHHS Publication No. ADM 90-538). Rockville, MD: Substance Abuse and Mental Health Services Administration.

Dohrewend, B. P. (1983). Psychological implications of nuclear accidents: The case of Three Mile Island. *Bulletin of the New York Academy of Medicine, 59*, 1060–1076.

Ehlers, A., Clark, D. M., Hackmann, A., McManus, F., Fennell, M., Herbert, C., & Mayou, R. A. (2003). A randomized controlled trial of cognitive therapy, a self-help booklet, and repeated assessments as early interventions for posttraumatic stress disorder. *Archives of General Psychiatry, 60,* 1024–1032.

Everly, G. S., & Lating, J. M. (2002). Neuromuscular relaxation. In G. S. Everly & J. M. Lating (Eds.), *A clinical guide to the treatment of the human stress response* (2nd ed., pp. 225–239). New York: Kluwer/Plenum Press.

Farberow, N. L. (1978). *Field manual for human service workers in major disasters* (DHHS Publication No. ADM 78-537). Rockville, MD: National Institute of Mental Health.

Foa, E. B., & Meadows, E. A. (1997). Psychosocial treatments for posttraumatic stress disorder: A critical review. *Annual Review of Psychology, 48,* 935–938.

Foa, E. B., Keane, T. M., & Friedman, M. J. (2000). *Effective treatments for PTSD: Practice guidelines from the International Society of Traumatic Stress Studies.* New York: Guilford Press.

Freedy, J. R., Shaw, D., Jarrell, M., & Masters, C. (1992). Towards an understanding of the psychological impact of natural disasters: An application of the conservation resources stress model. *Journal of Traumatic Stress, 5,* 441–454.

Friedman, M. J. (2000). A guide to the literature on pharmacotherapy for PTSD. *PTSD Research Quarterly, 11,* 1–7.

Fullerton, C. S., Ursano, R. J., Tzu-Cheg, K., & Bharitya, V. R. (1999). Disaster-related bereavement: Acute symptoms and subsequent depression. *Aviation, Space, and Environmental Medicine, 70,* 902–909.

Galea, S., Resnick, H. S., Ahern, J., Gold, J., Bucuvalas, M. J., Kilpatrick, D. G., et al. (2002). Posttraumatic stress disorder in Manhattan, New York City, after the September 11th terrorist attacks. *Journal of Urban Health: Bulletin of the New York Academy of Medicine, 79,* 340–353.

Gilbert, D. T., & Silvera, D. H. (1996). Overhelping. *Journal of Personality and Social Psychology, 70,* 678–690.

Gist, R. (1996). Is CISD built on a foundation of sand? *Fire Chief, 40,* 38–42.

Gleser, G. C., Green, B. L., & Winget, C. N. (1981). *Prolonged psychological effects of disaster: A study of Buffalo Creek.* New York: Academic Press.

Goenjian, A., Pynoos, R., Steinberg, A., Najarian, L., Asarnow, J., Karayan, I., et al. (1995). Psychiatric comorbidity in children after the 1988 earthquake in Armenia. *Journal of the American Academy of Child and Adolescent Psychiatry, 34,* 1174–1184.

Green, B. L., Grace, M. C., & Gleser, G. (1985). Identifying survivors at risk: Long-term impairment following the Beverly Hills Supper Club fire. *Journal of Consulting and Clinical Psychology, 53,* 672–678.

Green, B. L., Grace, M. C., Vary, M. G., Kramer, T. L., Gleser, G. C., & Leonard, A. C. (1994). Children of disaster in the second decade: A 17 year follow-up of Buffalo Creek survivors. *Journal of the American Academy of Child and Adolescent Psychiatry, 33,* 71–79.

Green, B. L., & Solomon, S. D. (1995). The mental health impact of natural and technological disasters. In J. R. Freedy & S. E. Hobfoll (Eds.), *Traumatic stress: From theory to practice* (pp. 163–180). New York: Plenum Press.

Hanson, R. F., Kilpatrick, D. G., Freedy, J. R., & Saunders, B. E. (1995). Los Angeles County after the 1992 civil disturbances: Degree of exposure and impact on mental health. *Journal of Consulting and Clinical Psychology, 63,* 987–996.

Hartsough, D. M. (1985). Stress and mental health interventions in three major disasters. In D. M. Hartsough & D. G. Myers (Eds.), *Disaster work and mental health: Prevention and control of stress among workers* (pp. 1–44) (DHHS Publication No. ADM 85-1422). Rockville, MD: National Institute of Mental Health.

Havenaar, J. M., Rumyantzeva, G. M., van den Brink, W., Poelijoe, N., van den Bout, J., van Englelend, H., & Koeter, M. (1997). Long-term mental health effects of the Chernobyl disaster: An epidemiologic survey in two former Soviet regions. *American Journal of Psychiatry, 154,* 1605–1607.

Holloway, H. C., & Fullerton, C. S. (1994). The psychology of terror and its aftermath. In R. J. Ursano, B. G. McCaughey, & C. S. Fullerton (Eds.), *Individual and community responses to trauma and disaster: The structure of human chaos* (pp. 31–45). Cambridge, UK: Cambridge University Press.

Institute of Medicine Committee on Responding to the Psychological Consequences of Terrorism. (2003). *Preparing for the psychological consequences of terrorism: A public health strategy.* Washington, DC: National Academies Press.

Kaniasty, K., & Norris, F. H. (1993). A test of the support deterioration model in the context of natural disaster. *Journal of Personality and Social Psychology, 64,* 395–408.

Kaniasty, K., Norris, F. H., & Murrell, S. A. (1990). Perceived and received social support following natural disaster. *Journal of Applied Social Psychology, 20,* 85–114.

Kenardy, J. A., & Carr, V. (1996). Imbalance in the debriefing debate: what we don't know far outweighs what we do. *Bulletin of the Australian Psychological Society, 18,* 4–6.

Koopman, C., Classen, C., & Spiegel, D. (1996). Dissociative responses in the immediate aftermath of the Oakland/Berkeley firestorm. *Journal of Traumatic Stress, 9,* 521–540.

Lindemann, E. (1944). Symptomatology and management of acute grief. *American Journal of Psychiatry, 101,* 141–148.

Lonigan, C., Shannon, M., Taylor, C., Finch, A., & Sallee, F. (1994). Children exposed to disaster: II. Risk factors for the development of post-traumatic symptomology. *Journal of the American Academy of Child and Adolescent Psychiatry, 33,* 94–105.

Lystad, M. (Ed.). (1985). *Innovations in mental health services to disaster victims* (DHHS Publication No. ADM 85-1390). Rockville, MD: National Institute of Mental Health.

Maes, M., Delmeire, L., Schotte, C., Janca, A., Creten, T., Mylle, J., et al. (1998). Epidemiological and phenomenological aspects of post-traumatic stress disorder: DSM-II-R diagnosis and diagnostic criteria not validated. *Psychiatry Research, 81,* 179–193.

McFarlane, A. C. (1989). The aetiology of post-traumatic morbidity: predisposing, precipitating and perpetuating factors. *British Journal of Psychiatry, 154,* 221–228.

McFarlane, A. C. (1995). Stress and disaster. In S. E. Hobfoll & M. W. de Vries (Eds.), *Extreme stress and communities: Impact and intervention* (pp. 247–266). Dordrecht, The Netherlands: Kluwer.

McNally, R. J., Bryant, R. A., & Ehlers, A. (2003). Does early psychological intervention promote recovery from posttraumatic stress? *Psychological Science in the Public Interest, 4,* 45–79.

Mitchell, J. T. (1983, January). When disaster strikes: The critical incident stress debriefing process. *Journal of Emergency Services, 8,* 36–39.

Murphy, S. A. (1984). Stress levels and health status of victims of a natural disaster. *Research in Nursing and Health, 7,* 205–215.

Myers, D. G. (1994). *Disaster response and recovery: A handbook for mental health professionals* (DHHS Publication No. SMA 94-3010). Rockville, MD: National Institute of Mental Health.

Najarian, B., Goenjian, A., Pelcovitz, D., Mandel, F., & Najarian, B. (2001). The effect of relocation after a natural disaster. *Journal of Traumatic Stress, 14,* 511–526.

National Institute of Mental Health. (2002). *Mental health and mass violence— Evidence based early psychological intervention for victims/survivors of mass violence: A workshop to reach consensus on best practices* (NIH Publication No. 02-5138). Washington, DC: U.S. Government Printing Office.

Norris, F. H. (1992). Epidemiology of trauma: Frequency and impact of different potentially traumatic events on different demographic groups. *Journal of Consulting and Clinical Psychology, 60,* 409–418.

Norris, F. H., Kaniasty, D. Z., Conrad, M. L., Inman, G. L., & Murphy, A. D. (2002). Placing age differences in cultural context: A comparison of the effects of age on PTSD after disasters in the United States, Mexico, and Poland. *Journal of Clinical Geropsychology, 8,* 153–173.

Norris, F. H., & Uhl, G. A. (1993). Chronic stress as a mediator of acute stress: The case of Hurricane Hugo. *Journal of Applied Social Psychology, 23,* 1263–1284.

North, C. S., Nixon, S. J., Shariat, S., Mallonee, S., McMillen, J. C., Spitznagel, E. L., et al. (1999). Psychiatric disorders among survivors of the Oklahoma City bombing. *Journal of the American Medical Association, 282,* 755–762.

Palinkas, L. A., Petterson, J. S., Russell, J., & Downs, M. A. (1993). Community patterns of psychiatric disorders after the Exxon Valdez oil spill. *American Journal of Psychiatry, 150,* 1517–1523.

Perilla, J. L., Norris, F. H., & Lavisso, E. (2002). Ethnicity, culture, and disaster response: Identifying and explaining ethnic differences in PTSD six months after Hurricane Andrew. *Journal of Social and Clinical Psychology, 21,* 20–45.

Phifer, J. F. (1990). Psychological distress and somatic symptoms after natural disaster: Differential vulnerability among older adults. *Psychology and Aging, 5,* 412–420.

Pitman, R. K., Sanders, K. M., Zusman, R. M., Healy, A. R., Cheema, F., Lasko, N. B., et al. (2002). Pilot study of secondary prevention of post-traumatic stress disorder with Propranolol. *Biological Psychiatry, 51,* 89–92.

Pynoos, R., Goenjian, A., Tashjian, M., Karakashian, M., Manjikian, R.,

Manoukian, G., et al. (1993). Post-traumatic stress reactions in children after the 1988 Armenian earthquake. *British Journal of Psychiatry, 163*, 239–247.

Pynoos, R. S., & Nader, K. (1988). PFA and treatment approach to children exposed to community violence: Research implications. *Journal of Traumatic Stress, 1*, 445–473.

Raphael, B. (1977). The Granville train disaster: psychological needs and their management. *Medical Journal of Australia, 1*, 303–305.

Raphael, B. (1986). *When disaster strikes: How individuals and communities cope with catastrophe.* New York: Basic Books.

Raphael, B., & Newman, L. (2000). *Disaster mental health response handbook.* North Sydney, Australia: NSW Health.

Riad, J., & Norris, F. H. (1996). The influence of relocation on the environmental, social, and psychological stress experienced by disaster victims. *Environment and Behavior, 28*, 163–182.

Robert, R., Blakeney, P., Villarreal, C., Rosenberg, L., & Meyer, W. (1999). Imipramine treatment in pediatric burn patients with symptoms of acute stress disorder: A pilot study. *Journal American Academy Child and Adolescent Psychiatry, 38*, 873–882.

Rose, S., Bisson, J., & Wesseley, S. (2001). *Psychological debriefing for preventing posttraumatic stress disorder* (The Cochrane Library, Issue 3). Oxford, UK: Update Software.

Rubonis, A. V., & Bickman, L. (1991, May). Psychological impairment in the wake of disaster: The disaster–psychopathology relationship. *Psychological Bulletin, 109*, 384–399.

Shalev, A. Y. (2000). Stress management and debriefing: Historical concepts and present patterns. In B. Raphael & J. P. Wilson (Eds.), *Psychological debriefing* (pp. 17–31). Cambridge, UK: Cambridge University Press.

Shalev, A. Y., Adessky, R., Boker, R., Bargai, N., Cooper, R., Freedman, S., et al. (2003). Clinical intervention for survivors of prolonged adversities. In R. J. Ursano, C. S. Fullerton, & A. E. Norwood (Eds.), *Terrorism and disaster: Individual and community mental health interventions* (pp. 162–188). Cambridge, UK: Cambridge Press.

Shariat, S., Mallonee, S., Kruger, E., Farmer, K., & North, E. (1999). A prospective study of long-term health outcomes among Oklahoma City bombing survivors. *Journal of the Oklahoma State Medical Association, 92*, 178–186.

Shneidman, E. S., Farberow, N. L., & Litman, R. E. (Eds.). (1970). *The psychology of suicide.* New York: Science House.

Smith, B., & Freedy, J. R. (2000). Psychosocial resource loss as a mediator of the effects of flood exposure on psychological distress and physical symptoms. *Journal of Traumatic Stress, 13*, 349–357.

Solomon, S., Bravo, M., Rubio-Stipec, M., & Canino, G. (1993). Effect of family role on response to disaster. *Journal of Traumatic Stress, 6*, 255–269.

Stanovic, J. K., James, K. A., & Van Devere, C. A. (2001). The effectiveness of Risperidone on acute stress symptoms in adult burn patients: A preliminary retrospective pilot study. *Journal of Burn Care and Rehabilitation, 22*, 210–213.

Udwin, O., Boyle, S., Yule, W., Bolkton, D., & O'Ryan, D. (2000). Risk factors for long-term psychological effects of a disaster experienced in adolescence: Predictors of PTSD. *Journal of Child Psychology and Psychiatry, 41*, 969–979.

Watson, P. J. (2004). Behavioral health interventions following mass violence. *Traumatic Stresspoints, 18*(1).

Weaver, J. D. (1995). *Disasters: Mental health interventions.* Sarasota, FL: Professional Resource Press.

Weaver, J. D. (2000). Working with those who have experienced sudden loss of loved ones. *Internet Journal of Rescue and Disaster Medicine, 2*, 1–10. Retrieved June 9, 2004, from www.ispub.com/ostia/index.php?xmlFilePath=journals/ijrdm/vol2n1/loss1.xml

Weisaeth, L. (1989). The stressors and the post-traumatic stress syndrome after an industrial disaster. *Acta Psychiatrica Scandinavica, 80*(Suppl.), 25–37.

Young, B. H. (2002). Emergency outreach: Navigational and brief screening guidelines for working in large group settings following catastrophic events. *NCPTSD Clinical Quarterly, 11*, 1–6.

Young, B. H., Ford, J. D., Ruzek, J. I., Friedman, M. F., & Gusman, F. D. (1998). *Disaster mental health services: A guidebook for clinicians and administrators.* St. Louis, MO: Department of Veterans Affairs Employee Education System, National Media Center. Retrieved from www.ncptsd.va.gov/publications/disaster

Young, B. H., Ruzek, J. I., & Ford, J. D. (1999). Cognitive-behavioral group treatment for disaster-related PTSD. In B. H. Young & D. D. Blake (Eds.), *Group treatments for post-traumatic stress disorder* (pp. 149–200). Philadelphia: Taylor & Francis.

CHAPTER 9

Intermediate Interventions

RICHARD A. BRYANT and BRETT T. LITZ

Mental health interventions between 1 and 4 weeks after trauma exposure have a different goal and employ different strategies than responses that typically occur in the initial days after trauma exposure. In the context of mass violence, there are typically inadequate mental health resources to allocate to all people immediately affected by the event. Accordingly, some kind of preselection based on risk for chronicity is critical so that valuable and scarce resources are used effectively. With this goal as a priority, this chapter outlines the range of responses that occur in the initial month, discusses strategies to focus on people who require mental health assistance, reviews evidence-based interventions designed to reduce the risk of chronic posttraumatic difficulties, and discusses strategies for managing stress reactions in the military.

THE COURSE OF PSYCHOLOGICAL RESPONSES

The initial month after trauma exposure is typically characterized by considerable levels of distress (for a review, see Bryant, 2003). Despite the commonality of initial stress reactions, there is marked remission in most of these people in the following weeks and months. For example, whereas 94% of rape victims displayed symptoms of posttraumatic stress disorder (PTSD) 2 weeks posttrauma, this rate dropped to 47% eleven weeks later (Rothbaum, Foa, Riggs, Murdock, & Walsh, 1992). In terms of nonsexual assault, 70% of women and 50% of men display PTSD at an average of

155

19 days after an assault; the rate of PTSD at 4-month follow-up dropped to 21% for women and zero for men (Riggs, Rothbaum, & Foa, 1995). Similarly, half of a sample meeting criteria for PTSD shortly after a motor vehicle accident had remitted by 6 months and two-thirds had remitted by 1-year posttrauma (Blanchard et al., 1996). In terms of victims of mass violence, surveys of New Yorkers affected by the terrorist attacks on the World Trade Center reported similar patterns. Whereas 7.5% of residents reported PTSD within 5–8 weeks after the attacks (Galea et al., 2002), the rate dropped to 1.7% of people living south of Canal Street 4 months later (Galea, Boscarino, Resnick, & Vlahov, in press).

WHOM DO WE TREAT?

Considering that the majority of people appear to adapt in the months after trauma exposure, where should we focus our treatment resources? Much attention has focused in recent years on identifying acutely traumatized people who will subsequently develop PTSD and related disorders. One of the major developments has been the introduction of the acute stress disorder (ASD) diagnosis. In 1994, the fourth edition of the *Diagnostic and Statistical Manual of Mental Disorders* (DSM-IV; American Psychiatric Association, 1994) introduced the ASD diagnosis to describe stress reactions in the initial month after a trauma. One goal of this diagnosis was to discriminate between recent trauma survivors who are experiencing transient stress reactions and those who are suffering reactions that will persist into long-term PTSD (Koopman, Classen, Cardeña, & Spiegel, 1995). DSM-IV stipulates that ASD can occur after a fearful response to experiencing or witnessing a threatening event (Cluster A). The requisite symptoms to meet criteria for ASD include three dissociative symptoms (Cluster B), one reexperiencing symptom (Cluster C), marked avoidance (Cluster D), marked anxiety or increased arousal (Cluster E), and evidence of significant distress or impairment (Cluster F). The disturbance must last for a minimum of 2 days and a maximum of 4 weeks (Cluster G) after which time a diagnosis of PTSD should be considered.

The primary difference between the criteria for ASD and PTSD is the time frame and the former's emphasis on dissociative reactions to the trauma. ASD refers to symptoms manifested during the period from 2 days to 4 weeks posttrauma, whereas PTSD can only be diagnosed from 4 weeks. The diagnosis of ASD requires that the individual has at least three of the following: (1) a subjective sense of numbing or detachment, (2) reduced awareness of one's surroundings, (3) derealization, (4) depersonalization, or (5) dissociative amnesia. The extent to which ASD does accurately identify people who will develop PTSD has been studied across 12 prospective studies (Brewin, Andrews, Rose, & Kirk, 1999; Bryant & Harvey, 1998; Creamer, O'Donnell, & Pattison, 2004; Difede et al., 2002; Harvey & Bryant 1998, 1999, 2000; Holeva, Tarrier, & Wells, 2001; Kangas, Henry, & Bryant, 2005; Murray, Ehlers, & Mayou, 2002; Schnyder, Moergeli, Klaghofer, & Buddeberg, 2001; Staab, Grieger, Fullerton, & Ursano, 1996). In general, approximately three-quarters of trauma survivors who display ASD subsequently develop PTSD.

These studies suggest that the ASD diagnosis is performing reasonably well in predicting people who will develop PTSD. However, when one evaluates the proportion of people who eventually developed PTSD and who initially displayed ASD, the utility of the ASD diagnosis is questionable. Across the majority of studies, the minority of people who eventually developed PTSD initially met criteria for ASD. This pattern suggests that whereas the majority of people who develop ASD are high risk for developing subsequent PTSD, there are many other people who will develop PTSD who do not initially meet ASD criteria. It appears that the major reason for ASD not identifying people at risk for chronic PTSD is the requirement that they display acute dissociation (Harvey & Bryant, 1999). These data suggest that whereas the ASD diagnosis may be useful in identifying recently trauma-exposed individuals who develop PTSD, one should not require dissociative responses in the determination of high risk. Consistent with this approach, some studies have indicated that overall symptom severity several weeks after exposure is associated with subsequent PTSD (Harvey & Bryant, 1998; Koren, Arnon, & Klein, 1999; Murray et al., 2002). There is also evidence of a range of other factors that may predict subsequent PTSD, including initial depression (Shalev et al., 1998), catastrophic appraisals of the trauma and one's capacity to cope with it (Ehlers, Mayou, & Bryant, 1998), functional impairment (Norris, Murphy, Baker, & Perilla, 2003), taking excessive precautions (Dunmore, Clark, & Ehlers, 2001), and dissociative responses (Koopman, Classen, & Spiegel, 1994).

WHEN SHOULD WE ASSESS PEOPLE FOR EARLY INTERVENTION?

One of the first questions to be asked is when should we try to identify people who will require mental health interventions. Although the ASD diagnosis specifies that one can make a diagnosis 2 days after trauma exposure, there is no evidence to support the utility of such an early identification. The sooner one makes an identification of high risk, the more likely one will incorrectly classify a transient stress reaction as a case of high risk. For example, ASD is more than twice as accurate in predicting subsequent PTSD if it assessed 4 weeks after trauma exposure compared to 1 week after trauma exposure (Murray et al., 2002). Clinicians need to remember that there is rapid diminishment in stress reactions in the initial weeks after trauma (Solomon, Laor, & McFarlane, 1996), and thus one should delay assessment if possible to optimize accurate identification and cost-effective use of resources. It should be noted that early screening that occurs only once includes the possibility that delayed-onset cases of PTSD may not be detected, and that people can develop problems at later times, especially if there are subsequent stressors impeding adequate recovery.

ASSESSMENT OF ASD

Despite the limitations of the ASD diagnosis, there are currently three measures of ASD available that may be useful for early identification of people who are high risk for PTSD. The first measure to be developed was the Stanford Acute Stress Reaction Questionnaire (SASRQ). The current version of the SASRQ (Cardeña, Koopman, Classen, Waelde, & Spiegel, 2000) is a self-report inventory that encompasses each of the ASD symptoms. Each item asks respondents to indicate the frequency of each symptom on a 6-point Likert scale (from 0 = "not experienced" to 5 = "very often experienced") that can occur during and immediately following a trauma. The SASRQ possesses high internal consistency (Cronbach's alpha = .90 and .91 for dissociative and anxiety symptoms, respectively) and concurrent validity with scores on the Impact of Event Scale ($r = .52 - .69$; Koopman et al., 1994). The Acute Stress Disorder Interview (ASDI; Bryant, Harvey, Dang, & Sackville, 1998) is a structured clinical interview that is based on DSM-IV criteria. The ASDI possesses good internal consistency ($r = .90$), test–retest reliability ($r = .88$), sensitivity (91%), and specificity (93%) relative to independent clinician diagnosis of ASD. The ASDI contains 19 dichotomously scored items that relate to the dissociative (Cluster B, 5 items), reexperiencing (Cluster C, 4 items), avoidance (Cluster D, 4 items), and arousal (Cluster E, 6 items) symptoms of ASD. Summing the affirmative responses to each symptom provides a total score indicative of acute stress severity (range 1 to 19). The Acute Stress Disorder Scale (ASDS; Bryant, Moulds, & Guthrie, 2000) is a self-report inventory that is based on the same items described in the ASDI. Each item on the ASDS is scored on a 5-point scale that reflects degrees of severity. This measure has been shown to have good predictive capacity in identifying people who subsequent develop PTSD (Bryant et al., 2000).

Each of the ASD measures suffers from the same validity problems associated with the ASD diagnosis. If the dissociative symptom requirement is adhered to, many high-risk individuals will be neglected. Although the ASD measures appear useful as a gross screen for the early identification of those at risk, clinicians should focus more on overall severity of symptom presentation in the weeks after trauma exposure than any prescribed constellation of symptoms.

EARLY INTERVENTION FOR PTSD

There have been attempts in recent years to prevent chronic PTSD by focusing on people who are at risk. There is very strong evidence for the efficacy of cognitive-behavioral therapy (CBT) for chronic PTSD (Foa & Meadows, 1997; Harvey, Bryant, & Tarrier, 2003). It is understandable that recent attempts to prevent chronic PTSD have adapted these proven interventions in the intermediate phase after trauma exposure.

Clinicians have attempted to prevent PTSD by early provision of CBT. Foa, Hearst-Ikeda, and Perry (1995) provided a brief cognitive-behavioral treatment to sexual and nonsexual assault victims shortly after the assault. This study compared CBT (including exposure, anxiety management, *in vivo* exposure, and cognitive restructuring) with matched participants who had received repeated assessments. Each participant received four treatment sessions and then received assessment by blind assessors at 2 months posttreatment and 5 months follow-up. Whereas 10% of the CBT group met criteria for PTSD at 2 months, 70% of the control group met criteria; there were no differences between groups at 5 months, although the CBT group was less depressed. This pattern suggests that CBT accelerated recovery relative to the rate of natural remission. Inferences from this study were limited, however, by the lack of random assignment. This team conducted a subsequent study of assault survivors who met criteria for PTSD in the initial weeks after the trauma (mean: 21 days), in which participants were randomly allocated to four weekly 2-hour sessions of CBT (n = 31), repeated assessment (n = 30), or supportive counseling (n = 29) (Foa, Zoellner, & Feeny, 2002). Surprisingly, this study found that participants in the CBT and repeated assessment conditions enjoyed comparable levels of improvement. At follow-up (approximately 9 months after treatment), comparable proportions of participants in each group had PTSD (CBT: 32%; repeated assessment: 30%; supportive counseling: 29%).

A problem with early-intervention studies is that it is difficult to disentangle the gains resulting from the treatment intervention and natural remission (Brewin, 2001). One approach that has been adopted in recent years is to provide secondary prevention interventions only to trauma survivors who are high risk for developing PTSD. Although the current evidence suggests that the ASD diagnosis does not identify all people who will develop PTSD, there is sufficient convergent evidence that it is a good indicator of risk for chronic PTSD. Focusing treatment efforts on people with

ASD is also a stricter test of any early-intervention strategy because it is less likely that symptom reduction is a function of natural remission.

In the initial study of this approach, Bryant, Harvey, Dang, Sackville, and Basten (1998) randomly allocated motor vehicle accident or nonsexual assault survivors with ASD to either CBT or supportive counseling. Both interventions consisted of five 1½-hour weekly individual therapy sessions. CBT included education about posttraumatic reactions, relaxation training, cognitive restructuring, and imaginal and *in vivo* exposure to the traumatic event. Supportive counseling condition included trauma education, general problem-solving skills training, and nondirective support. At 6-month follow-up, there were fewer participants in the CBT group (20%) who met diagnostic criteria for PTSD compared to supportive counseling control participants (67%). In a subsequent study that dismantled the components of CBT, 45 civilian trauma survivors with ASD were randomly allocated to five sessions of (1) CBT (prolonged exposure, cognitive therapy, anxiety management), (2) prolonged exposure combined with cognitive therapy, or (3) supportive counseling (Bryant, Sackville, Dang, Moulds, & Guthrie (1999). This study found that at 6 months follow-up, PTSD was observed in approximately 20% of both active treatment groups compared to 67% of those receiving supportive counseling. A 4-year follow-up of these studies has indicated that treatment gains are maintaining 4 years after treatment (Bryant, Moulds, & Nixon, 2003).

A third study attempted to enhance treatment effects of CBT by preceding imaginal exposure with hypnosis. This study randomly allocated civilian trauma survivors (*n* = 89) with ASD to CBT, CBT + hypnosis, or supportive counseling (Bryant, Moulds, Guthrie, & Nixon, 2005). The hypnosis component was provided immediately prior to imaginal exposure in an attempt to facilitate emotional processing of the trauma memories. In terms of treatment completers, more participants in the supportive counseling condition (57%) met PTSD criteria at 6-month follow-up than those in the CBT (21%) or CBT + hypnosis (22%) condition. Interestingly, participants in the CBT + hypnosis condition reported greater reduction of reexperiencing symptoms at posttreatment than those in the CBT condition. This finding suggests that hypnosis may facilitate treatment gains in ASD participants.

Finally, a recent study provided CBT to a sample of participants with ASD (*n* = 24) who sustained mild traumatic brain injury following motor vehicle accidents (Bryant, Moulds, Guthrie, & Nixon, 2003). This study investigated the efficacy of CBT in people who lost consciousness during the trauma as result of their traumatic injury. Consistent with the previous studies, fewer participants receiving CBT (8%) met criteria for PTSD at 6-month follow-up than those receiving supportive counseling (58%).

There is also evidence indicating the efficacy of CBT provided between 1 and 3 months after trauma exposure (Echeburua, de Corral, Sarasua, & Zubizarreta, 1996; Ehlers et al., 2003; Öst, Paunovic, & Gillow, 2002). This time frame overlaps, to a degree, with the intermediate period discussed in this chapter. These treatment studies have typically employed more treatment sessions but have also pointed to the efficacy of CBT in this period following trauma.

The components that typically constitute CBT for PTSD include psychoeducation, anxiety management, cognitive restructuring, and exposure. Psychoeducation includes education about the common reactions to a traumatic event, the cognitive and behavioral mechanisms that mediate core PTSD reactions, and a rationale for the treatment.

Anxiety management techniques provide individuals with coping skills to manage their fear, reduce arousal, and assist management of distressing activities and trauma reminders. Anxiety management approaches often include stress inoculation training that follows Meichenbaum's program of psychoeducation, relaxation skills, breathing retraining, thought stopping, and self-talk (Meichenbaum, 1975).

Cognitive Therapy

Cognitive restructuring is based on models that emphasize the importance of appraisals in the etiology and maintenance of PTSD (Ehlers & Clark, 2000). Cognitive restructuring involves teaching individuals to identify and evaluate the evidence for negative automatic thoughts, as well as helping patients to evaluate their beliefs about the trauma, the self, the world, and the future (Beck, 1976). For example, a person recently exposed to trauma may complain to a clinician that he believes he can never feel safe again. This belief will contribute to considerable pessimism and hopelessness and should be a focus of cognitive therapy. Following is an example of an interaction employing cognitive therapy to help the person shift this thought:

CLIENT: I can never go to New York City again.

THERAPIST: Why not?

CLIENT: Because I feel I can never feel safe again there.

THERAPIST: On a scale of 0–100, how strongly do you believe that you can never feel safe there again?

CLIENT: About 90. What happened to me was so bad and so unexpected that I can never feel safe again. I mean if New York can be attacked, then we are not safe anywhere.

THERAPIST: Let's see how realistic that thought is. Let's work out what the chances are of you being hurt in a terrorist attack in New York City. Now, how often has New York been attacked by terrorists?

CLIENT: I guess only the once.

THERAPIST: How often have you been to New York City?

CLIENT: Thousands of times.

THERAPIST: Now how many buildings are there in New York City?

CLIENT: I don't know. Hundreds, I guess.

THERAPIST: So what's the chance of you being in a building that will get attacked?

CLIENT: I guess if I can only be in one building and there's hundreds of them, the actual chance of me being in the one attacked is pretty small. But it doesn't feel like a small chance.

THERAPIST: I can appreciate that. But let's try to work out what is realistic thinking. Now, you are saying that you have been to the city thousands of times, that the city has only been attacked once, and the chances of you being in one of the hundreds of buildings in the city if it was attacked is pretty small. Now as you keep all these things in your mind, how likely do you think it is that you will be hurt in a terrorist attack in New York City?

CLIENT: Put that way, I guess it is not likely.

THERAPIST: On scale of 0–100, how likely do you think it is?

CLIENT: I guess only about 40.

THERAPIST: Good. Notice how you think differently about how scared you are when you consider the evidence a bit more realistically. I don't expect you to be able to believe these other thoughts so soon but the more we can practice testing our thoughts against the evidence that's really there, the more you will be able to believe in them because they line up with the reality that you experience every day.

There are several points to note in conducting cognitive therapy in the intermediate period after trauma exposure. First, clinicians need to recognize that catastrophic thoughts expressed by recently trauma-exposed people tend to be based on events that were very threatening and recent. Accordingly, clinicians should acknowledge that these thoughts are understandable in the circumstances, and they should not expect clients to shift their beliefs rapidly. Second, cognitive therapy is not positive thinking and should not aim to eradicate all negative appraisals. In the wake of trauma, many responses are appropriately negative (such as guilt, anger, and worry), and the goal of cognitive therapy is to appraise these responses in a realistic manner. Third, it is important to recognize that there may be subsequent stressors following the initial trauma, and cognitive therapy needs to avoid the mistake of communicating to the client that no further negative events will occur.

Finally, in the context of bioterrorism, the threat from biological agents can be ambiguous. For example, whereas concern about anthrax may be appropriate if there is genuine evidence of its presence, a preoccupation and persistent worry about anthrax may be deemed excessive. In these cases, cognitive therapy needs to help the client weigh the evidence to determine the distinction between adaptive concern and behavior and excessive rumination and maladaptive behavior.

Prolonged Exposure

There is much evidence in treating chronic PTSD that this strategy is effective in reducing an array of PTSD symptoms (Bryant & Friedman, 2001; Foa & Meadows, 1997). Prolonged imaginal exposure requires the individual to vividly imagine the trauma for prolonged periods. The goal of this technique is to achieve a state of reduced distress when the individual is thinking about the trauma experience. The individual typically provides a narrative of his or her traumatic experience in a way that emphasizes all relevant details, including sensory cues and affective responses. Individuals are typically instructed to vividly relive the trauma experience by having their eyes closed and recounting the experience in the first person and in the present tense. Therapists usually require the individual to focus on "hot spots," which are those sections of the narrative that are most distressing because these involve experiences that require therapeutic focus.

A variant of imaginal exposure involve requiring clients to repeatedly write down detailed descriptions of the experience (Resick & Schnicke, 1993). This exercise usually occurs for at least 50 minutes, and is usually supplemented by daily homework exercises. For example, a survivor of the New York City terrorist attack may be required to provide a narrative from the moment she heard the explosion and then provide vivid details of all the events that occurred until she was finally safe in hospital. This narrative may only require 15 minutes in its initial account, and thus the therapist would require the client to repeat the narrative three times. The client may skirt over a scene where she panicked when she was temporarily lost in a darkened room and believed that she would never get out. The therapist would subsequently require the client to revisit that scene and ask her to direct attention to that scene because it has special relevance to her. The therapist would ask the client to rate her distress (usually using a 100-point scale, from 0 = "not at all distressed," to 100 = "extremely distressed") every 10 minutes to index how she is coping with the exercise.

Most exposure treatments supplement imaginal exposure with *in vivo* exposure that involves graded exposure to the feared trauma-related stimuli. This procedure involves establishing a hierarchy of situations in which the individual is fearful and is avoiding. The therapist then requires the client to enter these situations, initially beginning with the lowest-ranked situation on the hierarchy. When the individual is able to experience a reduction of distress (usually a 50% reduction), the individual can leave the situation. Each situation is repeated until it is mastered, and then one attempts the next situation on the hierarchy. For example, the survivor of the 9/11 attacks, may have the following steps on a hierarchy: (1) to enter a tall building on the ground floor, (2) to walk up the stairs to the second floor with a friend, (3) to walk up the stairs to the second floor alone, (4) to take the elevator with a friend to the second floor, and (5) to take the elevator alone to the second floor. After a number of intervening steps, the client may finally attempt to take the elevator to the top floor by herself. It is important after conducting exposure exercises that the therapist encourages the client to participate in cognitive therapy of thoughts that arose during the exposure. Typically, exposure will lead to many beliefs that require considerable cognitive work because they are central to catastrophic appraisals about the trauma response.

Eye Movement Desensitization and Reprocessing

Eye movement desensitization and reprocessing (EMDR) is a variant of CBT in that it involves elements of exposure and cognitive therapy. It differs from the traditional delivery of CBT in that it requires the individual to focus his or her attention on a traumatic memory, and then the therapist elicits rapid horizontal eye movements by asking the client to visually follow the therapist's moving finger. The therapist then engages in attempting to integrate more adaptive thoughts and appraisals of the experience. A recent review of 17 randomized controlled trials of the effectiveness of EMDR concluded that eye movements do not appear to be necessary for improvement, and the effects observed suggest nonspecific effects or the effect of exposure alone (see Cahill, Carrigan, & Frueh, 1999; Lohr, Lilienfeld, Tolin, & Herbert, 1999). In comparing CBT to EMDR, the better-controlled studies have found that CBT is more effective than EMDR (Devilly & Spence, 1999; McNally, 1999). In any case, there are no studies pointing to the efficacy of EMDR in the initial month after trauma exposure. Accordingly, it is advisable to not employ EMDR in the intermediate stage because of the lack of supporting evidence for its application in this timeframe.

PRECAUTIONS REGARDING INTERMEDIATE INTERVENTIONS

This chapter points to a number of recommendations for managing stress reactions in the intermediate period after trauma exposure. Figure 9.1 presents an outline of suggested steps in the month after trauma. It is important to recognize that active early intervention is not indicated for all trauma survivors who display marked stress reactions, particularly following mass violence, which engenders significant chaos, potential multiple sources of trauma, and potentially significant secondary stressors. It is suggested that some acute presentations warrant exercising caution because these signs may suggest that these individuals may have an adverse reaction to intervention. These precautions include:

- Heightened anxiety, and particularly pretrauma anxiety states that may be exacerbated by exposure-based therapy.
- Severe dissociative reactions, which indicate that the individual is not capable of successfully regulating strong emotional reactions arising through active therapy.
- Substance dependence or severe substance abuse because active therapy may exacerbate the substance use.
- Ongoing stressors or threats because these people may not be able to manage the demands of therapy because of competing demands.
- Unresolved prior trauma because these past issues may arise during the therapy of the recent event, and it may be difficult to address these earlier traumas in the context of the recent stress.
- Significant suicide threat, in which case the individual requires psychiatric review and probably antidepressant medication.

A proportion of individuals assessed in the intermediate period will require referral because they have presented with problems that require specific interventions. Anybody presenting with marked suicidal impulses, psychotic or borderline tendencies, or substance dependence should be referred to appropriate specialist agencies. The issues pertaining to referral, and to the utility of pharmacological interventions, are outlined by Ørner, Kent, Pfefferbaum, Raphael, and Watson (Chapter 7, this volume). Ad-

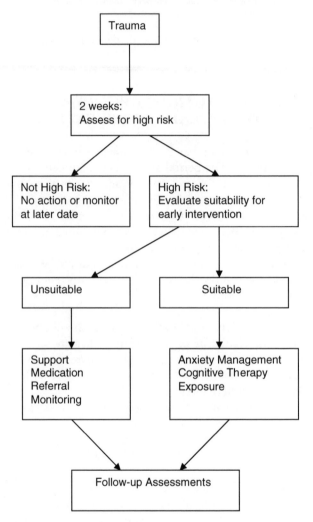

FIGURE 9.1. Flow chart for managing intermediate interventions.

vances in pharmacological interventions for ASD have not progressed at the same rate as they have for CBT. It is reasonable to conclude that the biological mechanisms involved in stress reactions in the intermediate phase are similar, although possibly not identical, to those that occur in more persistent phases after trauma exposure. Accordingly, it is probable that pharmacological interventions outlined by Raphael and Wooding (Chapter 10, this volume) on long-term interventions may be applicable to the intermediate phase.

APPLYING CBT FOLLOWING MASS VIOLENCE

It is important to note that all the research conducted on intermediate interventions has focused on survivors of discrete traumatic events that have affected individuals or small numbers of people. At the present time, there is no research on CBT in the context of mass violence. Several factors may limit the application of CBT in the intermediate period after mass violence. First, very few agencies have the resources to provide CBT in the initial month after mass violence. Considering the minimum level of expertise required to deliver CBT, it is difficult to utilize sufficient numbers of therapists to treat hundreds, let alone thousands, of affected people. Second, it is very common following mass violence for affected people to be dealing with an array of ongoing stressors. Physical injury, dislocation, medical investigations, financial loss, or other disturbances may be placing excessive demands on people. In these situations, many people may not be able to focus adequately on an intensive program, such as CBT, because they are preoccupied with these other stressors.

Under these circumstances, mental health practitioners may want to employ some sort of supportive counseling until the individual is capable of engaging in a trauma-focused cognitive-behavioral intervention. Stressors must be somewhat stabilized, and there should be some indication of successful coping with secondary adversities, so that the individual has the energy and motivation to complete CBT treatment. The expected outcome of supportive counseling is better coping, as expressed by improved task performance, better interpersonal interactions, controllable emotion, and sustained self-esteem. Supportive counseling following mass violence should be designed to reduce excessive, uncontrollable distress; identify coping strategies; facilitate social connectedness; and provide pragmatic resources. For instance, solution-focused methods of crisis counseling assist survivors in identifying and utilizing their strengths in the recovery process by helping them define concerns, imagine and set goals, identify strategies to achieve the goals, and develop an action plan (Madakasira & O'Brien, 1987).

In this context, it is worth noting that treatment studies of ASD that have employed supportive counseling have found it to be somewhat beneficial (although not as beneficial as CBT; Bryant, Harvey, Dang, Sackville, et al., 1998; Bryant et al., 1999). It is also worth noting that CBT of more chronic PTSD appears to be as effective as treatment of ASD, and thus it is appropriate to delay active treatment for months if there are insufficient resources or excessive demands on trauma survivors. In the meantime, supportive counseling can be a useful means to manage and monitor the distressed individual.

One example often employed following federally declared disasters in the United States is the FEMA-funded crisis counseling program. The goals of the crisis counseling program are to help an individual reduce distress, restore functioning, prevent chronic dysfunction and distress, and provide comfort and support. The key concepts of crisis counseling are (1) active listening, which helps to build rapport; this is at the heart of the work; (2) validation of responses, feelings, and reactions, whatever they may be; (3) education that some serious distress responses are an expectable and understandable reaction to an abnormal event, and it is very likely that many other individuals are experiencing the same types of distress responses; (4) education about coping, helping to draw on the individual's strengths and the coping skills that have worked for them in the past; (5) providing knowledge about when to self- or other-refer if symptoms become unmanageable; and (6) planning and helping move an individual toward the next steps in recovery. Plans are drawn out as to what they are going to do each day about practical issues and daily stressors. Although this program has not been empirically tested, it is based on crisis intervention models that have shown success in other populations (Madakasira & O'Brien, 1987), and plans are underway for a program evaluation toolkit and guidance so that effectiveness can be tested. It is critical that this line of evaluation be conducted so that multiple models of intervention are tested and verified for different populations and situations.

Prior to implementing an intervention program, the goals of intervening should be clearly determined (i.e., who we are providing services for, what we are doing, who will be conducting the intervention, and what outcomes we want to see). The experience of the person who was traumatized needs to be taken into account to maximize acceptability of screening and engagement for further follow-up. Developmental and cultural issues must be addressed, and intervention should be integrated into the natural helping network. The intervention program has to be practical, achievable, and implementable at the program level and should be part of the framework for a system of care (including public health community interventions, outreach, individual intervention services that range in intensity, and community events). It should include elements of strengthening existing strengths and resources, as well as ameliorating symptomatic response. Resources in the community must be able to meet the goals of the program. For instance, clinicians should be trained in the most empirically supported trauma interventions so that they will be available for the percentage of individuals who will most benefit from this modality.

Since the terrorist attacks in 2001, there has also been significant interest in delivering CBT through means that make these strategies available to whole communities. One way that has potential promise is through the World Wide Web. Internet-based therapies have proven to be effective in a range of problems (Carlbring, Westling, Ljungstrand, Ekselius, & Andersson, 2001), and there is initial evidence that this technology can be applied to assisting survivors of trauma (Litz, Williams, Wang, Bryant, & Engel, 2004; Lange, van de Ven, Schrieken, Bredeweg, & Emmelkamp, 2000). As these treatment programs become more available, the use of the Internet may facilitate dissemination of CBT techniques to survivors of mass violence. Not only does this approach bypass problems caused by limited resources involving traditional one-to-one therapy, it also provides anonymity for people who may be reluctant to approach mental health services.

FUTURE DIRECTIONS

Although there are some promising developments in early intervention after trauma, it needs to recognized that these interventions do not necessarily prevent subsequent PTSD. There is evidence that a significant proportion of participants do drop out of treatment. For example, 20% of participants in some studies dropped out of early intervention programs Bryant and colleagues (1999, 2005). Although exposure appears to be well tolerated in more chronic PTSD, it seems that exposure in the initial month may be less well managed by some individuals. Accordingly, clinicians may need to adopt a flexible approach in the initial month to ensure that they provide individuals with interventions that are tolerated. All clinicians should ensure that all interventions they apply are empirically defensible and that they err on the side of caution. Perhaps the most important lesson to be learned about interventions in the intermediate period is that it is not essential to provide early intervention in this period to all people. All the interventions described in this chapter can be equally well employed many months after the trauma. The major goal is to ensure that all people psychologically affected by trauma do not suffer persistent effects, and thus those individuals who may not be able to use therapy effectively in the intermediate period may benefit enormously at some later time.

REFERENCES

American Psychiatric Association. (1994). *Diagnostic and statistical manual of mental disorders* (4th ed.). Washington, DC: Author.

Beck, A. T. (1976). *Cognitive therapy and the emotional disorders.* New York: International Universities Press.

Blanchard, E. B., Hickling, E. J., Barton, K. A., Taylor, A. E., Loos, W. R., & Jones-Alexander, J. (1996). One-year prospective follow-up of motor vehicle accident victims. *Behaviour Research and Therapy, 34,* 775–786.

Brewin, C. R. (2001). Cognitive and emotional reactions to traumatic events: Implications for short-term intervention. *Advances in Mind–Body Medicine, 17,* 160–196.

Brewin, C. R., Andrews, B., Rose, S., & Kirk, M. (1999). Acute stress disorder and posttraumatic stress disorder in victims of violent crime. *American Journal of Psychiatry, 156,* 360–366.

Bryant, R. A. (2003). Early predictors of posttraumatic stress disorder. *Biological Psychiatry, 53,* 789–795.

Bryant, R. A., & Friedman, M. J. (2001). Medication and non-medication treatments of posttraumatic stress disorder. *Current Opinions in Psychiatry, 14,* 119–123.

Bryant, R. A., & Harvey, A. G. (1998). Relationship of acute stress disorder and posttraumatic stress disorder following mild traumatic brain injury. *American Journal of Psychiatry, 155,* 625–629.

Bryant, R. A., Harvey, A. G., Dang, S. T., & Sackville, T. (1998). Assessing acute stress disorder: Psychometric properties of a structured clinical interview. *Psychological Assessment, 10,* 215–220.

Bryant, R. A., Harvey, A. G., Dang, S. T., Sackville, T., & Basten, C. (1998). Treatment of acute stress disorder: A comparison of cognitive behavior therapy and supportive counseling. *Journal of Consulting and Clinical Psychology, 66,* 862–866.

Bryant, R. A., Moulds, M. L., & Guthrie, R. (2000). Acute stress disorder scale: A self-report measure of acute stress disorder. *Psychological Assessment, 12,* 61–68.

Bryant, R. A., Moulds, M. L., Guthrie, R. M., & Nixon, R. D. (2003). Treating acute stress disorder following mild traumatic brain injury. *American Journal of Psychiatry, 160,* 585–587.

Bryant, R. A., Moulds, M. L., Guthrie, R. M., & Nixon, R. D. (2005). The additive benefit of hypnosis and cognitive-behavioral therapy in treating acute stress disorder. *Journal of Consulting and Clinical Psychology, 73,* 334–340.

Bryant, R. A., Moulds, M. L., & Nixon, R. D. (2003). Cognitive behaviour therapy of acute stress disorder: A four-year follow-up. *Behaviour Research and Therapy, 41,* 489–494.

Bryant, R. A., Sackville, T., Dang, S. T., Moulds, M. L., & Guthrie, R. (1999). Treating acute stress disorder: An evaluation of cognitive behavior therapy and counseling techniques. *American Journal of Psychiatry, 156,* 1780–1786.

Cahill, S. P., Carrigan, M. H., & Frueh, B. C. (1999). Does EMDR work? And if so, why?: A critical review of controlled outcome and dismantling research. *Journal of Anxiety Disorders, 13,* 5–33.

Cardeña, E., Koopman, C., Classen, C. C., Waelde, L. C., & Spiegel, D. (2000). Psychometric properties of the Stanford Acute Stress Reaction Questionnaire (SASRQ): A valid and reliable measure of acute stress. *Journal of Traumatic Stress, 13,* 719–734.

Carlbring, P., Westling, B. E., Ljungstrand, P., Ekselius, L., & Andersson, G. (2001). Treatment of panic disorder via the Internet: A randomized trial of a self-help program. *Behavior Therapy, 32,* 751–764.

Creamer, M. C., O'Donnell, M. L., & Pattison, P. (2004). The relationship between acute stress disorder and posttraumatic stress disorder in severely injured trauma survivors. *Behaviour Research and Therapy, 42,* 315–328.

Deahl, M. P., Srinivasan, M., Jones, N., Thomas, J., Neblett, C., & Jolly, A. (2000). Preventing psychological trauma in soldiers: The role of operational stress training and psychological debriefing. *British Journal of Medical Psychology, 73,* 77–85.

Devilly, G., & Spence, S. H. (1999). The relative efficacy and treatment distress of EMDR and a cognitive-behavior trauma treatment protocol in the amelioration of posttraumatic stress disorder. *Journal of Anxiety Disorders, 13,* 131–157.

Difede, J., Ptacek, J. T., Roberts, J. G., Barocas, D., Rives, W., Apfeldorf, W. J., et al. (2002). Acute stress disorder after burn injury: A predictor of posttraumatic stress disorder. *Psychosomatic Medicine, 64,* 826–834.

Dunmore, E., Clark, D. M., & Ehlers, A. (2001). A prospective investigation of the role of cognitive factors in persistent posttraumatic stress disorder (PTSD) after physical or sexual assault. *Behaviour Research and Therapy, 39,* 1063–1084.

Echeburua, E., de Corral, P., Sarasua, B., & Zubizarreta, I. (1996). Treatment of acute posttraumatic stress disorder in rape victims: An experimental study. *Journal of Anxiety Disorders, 10,* 185–199.

Ehlers, A., & Clark, D. (2000). A cognitive model of posttraumatic stress disorder. *Behaviour Research and Therap. 38,* 319–345.

Ehlers, A., Clark, D. M., Hackmann, A., McManus, F., Fennell, M., Herbert, C., & Mayou, R. (2003). A randomized controlled trial of cognitive therapy, a self-help booklet, and repeated assessments as early interventions for posttraumatic stress disorder. *Archives of General Psychiatry, 60,* 1024–1032.

Ehlers, A., Mayou, R. A., & Bryant, B. (1998). Psychological predictors of chronic PTSD after motor vehicle accidents. *Journal of Abnormal Psychology, 107,* 508–519.

Foa, E. B., Hearst-Ikeda, D., & Perry, K. J. (1995). Evaluation of a brief cognitive behavioral program for the prevention of chronic PTSD in recent assault victims. *Journal of Consulting and Clinical Psychology, 63,* 948–955.

Foa, E. B., & Meadows, E. A. (1997). Psychosocial treatments for posttraumatic stress disorder: A critical review. *Annual Review of Psychology, 48,* 449–480.

Foa, E. B., Zoellner, L. A., & Feeny, N. C. (2002). *An evaluation of three brief programs for facilitating recovery.* Manuscript submitted for publication.

Galea, S., Ahern, J., Resnick, H. S., Kilpatrick, D. G., Bucuvalas, M. J., Gold, J., et al. (2002). Psychological sequelae of the September 11 terrorist attacks in New York City. *New England Journal of Medicine, 346,* 982–987.

Galea, S., Boscarino, J., Resnick, H., & Vlahov, D. (in press). Mental health in New York City after the September 11 terrorist attacks: Results from two population surveys. In R. W. Manderscheid & M. J. Henderson (Eds.), *Mental health, United States, 2001.* Washington, DC: Superintendent of Documents, U.S. Government Printing Office.

Harvey, A. G., & Bryant, R. A. (1998). Relationship of acute stress disorder and posttraumatic stress disorder following motor vehicle accidents. *Journal of Consulting and Clinical Psychology, 66,* 507–512.

Harvey, A. G., & Bryant, R. A. (1999). A two-year prospective evaluation of the relationship between acute stress disorder and posttraumatic stress disorder. *Journal of Consulting and Clinical Psychology, 67,* 985–988.

Harvey, A. G., Bryant, R. A., & Tarrier, N. (2003). Cognitive behaviour therapy of posttraumatic stress disorder. *Clinical Psychology Review, 23,* 501–522.

Harvey, A. G., & Bryant, R. A. (2000). A two-year prospective evaluation of the relationship between acute stress disorder and posttraumatic stress disorder following mild traumatic brain injury. *American Journal of Psychiatry, 157,* 626–628.

Holeva, V., Tarrier, N., & Wells, A. (2001). Prevalence and predictors of acute stress disorder and PTSD following road traffic accidents: Thought control strategies and social support. *Behavior Therapy, 32,* 65–83.

Kangas, M., Henry, J. L., & Bryant, R. A. (2005). The relationship between acute stress disorder and posttraumatic stress disorder following cancer. *Journal of Consulting and Clinical Psychology, 73,* 360–364.

King, D. W., King, L. A., Foy, D. W., Keane, T. M., & Fairbank, J. A. (1999). Posttraumatic stress disorder in a national sample of female and male Vietnam veterans: Risk factors, war-zone stressors, and resilience-recovery variables. *Journal of Abnormal Psychology, 108,* 164–170.

Koopman, C., Classen, C. C., Cardeña, E., & Spiegel, D. (1995). When disaster strikes, acute stress disorder may follow. *Journal of Traumatic Stress, 8,* 29–46.

Koopman, C., Classen, C., & Spiegel, D. (1994). Predictors of posttraumatic stress symptoms among survivors of the Oakland/Berkeley, California firestorm. *American Journal of Psychiatry, 151,* 888–894.

Koren, D., Arnon, I., & Klein, E. (1999). Acute stress responses and posttraumatic stress disorder in traffic accident victims: A one-year prospective, follow-up study. *American Journal of Psychiatry, 156,* 367–373.

Lange, A., van de Ven, J.-P. Q. R., Schrieken, B. A. L., Bredeweg, B., & Emmelkamp, P. M. G. (2000). Internet-mediated, protocol-driven treatment of psychological dysfunction. *Journal of Telemedicine and Telecare, 6,* 15–21.

Litz, B. T., Gray, M. J., Bryant, R. A., & Adler, A. B. (2002). Early intervention for trauma: Current status and future directions. *Clinical Psychology: Science and Practice, 9,* 112–134.

Litz, B. T., Williams, L., Wang, J., Bryant, R. A., & Engel, C. C. (2004). The development of an Internet-based program to deliver therapist-assisted self-help behavioral treatment for traumatic stress. *Professional Psychology: Science and Practice, 35,* 628–634.

Lohr, J. M., Lilienfeld, S. O., Tolin, D. F., & Herbert, J. D. (1999). Eye movement desensitization and reprocessing: An analysis of specific versus nonspecific treatment factors. *Journal of Anxiety Disorders, 13,* 185–207.

Madakasira, S., & O'Brien, K. F. (1987). Acute posttraumatic stress disorder in victims of a natural disaster. *Journal of Nervous and Mental Disease, 175,* 286–290.

McNally, R. J. (1999). Research on eye movement desensitization and reprocessing as a treatment for PTSD. *PTSD Research Quarterly, 10,* 1–7.

Meichenbaum, D. (1975). Self-instructional methods. In F. H. Kanfer & A. P.

Goldstein (Eds.), *Helping people change* (pp. 357–391). New York: Pergamon Press.

Murray, J., Ehlers, A., & Mayou, R. A. (2002). Dissociation and post-traumatic stress disorder: Two prospective studies of road traffic accident survivors. *British Journal of Psychiatry, 180,* 363–368.

Norris, F. H., Murphy, A. D., Baker, C. K., & Perilla, J. L. (2003). Severity, timing, and duration of reactions to trauma in the population: An example from Mexico. *Biological Psychiatry, 53,* 767–778.

Öst, L.-G., Paunovic, N., & Gillow, E.-M. (2002). *Cognitive-behavior therapy in the prevention of chronic PTSD in crime victims.* Manuscript submitted for publication.

Resick, P. A., & Schnicke, M. K. (1993). *Cognitive processing therapy for rape victims: A treatment manual.* London: Sage.

Riggs, D. S., Rothbaum, B. O., & Foa, E. B. (1995). A prospective examination of symptoms of posttraumatic stress disorder in victims of non-sexual assault. *Journal of Interpersonal Violence, 10,* 201–214.

Rothbaum, B. O., Foa, E. B., Riggs, D. S., Murdock, T. B., & Walsh, W. (1992). A prospective examination of posttraumatic stress disorder in rape victims. *Journal of Traumatic Stress, 5,* 455–475.

Schnyder, U., Moergeli, H., Klaghofer, R., & Buddeberg, C. (2001). Incidence and prediction of posttraumatic stress disorder symptoms in severely injured accident victims. *American Journal of Psychiatry, 158,* 594–599.

Shalev, A. Y., Freedman, S. A., Peri, T., Brandes, D., Sahar, T., Orr, S. P., et al. (1998). Prospective study of posttraumatic stress disorder and depression following trauma. *American Journal of Psychiatry, 155,* 630–637.

Solomon, Z., Laror, N., & McFarlane, A. C. (1996). Acute posttraumatic reactions in soldiers and civilians. In B. A. van der Kolk, A. C. McFarlane, & L. Weisaeth (Eds.), *Traumatic stress: The effects of overwhelming experience on mind, body, and society* (pp. 102–114). New York: Guilford Press.

Staab, J. P., Grieger, T. A., Fullerton, C. S., & Ursano, R. J. (1996). Acute stress disorder, subsequent posttraumatic stress disorder and depression after a series of typhoons. *Anxiety, 2,* 219–225.

Longer-Term Mental Health Interventions for Adults Following Disasters and Mass Violence

BEVERLY RAPHAEL and SALLY WOODING

In humanitarian terms the focus of emergency response in circumstances of mass violence and disasters will always be to maximize survival, to "save" as many as possible from death and destruction, and to protect individuals and communities from further threat and the consequences of the event. Thus a critical priority in terms of response aims to deal with the emergency phase of threat, rescue, triage, and care for casualties, and progressively to hand over responsibilities to recovery organizations. There is a transition process from these early days and weeks to a longer-term focus beyond the first month.

CONTEXT FOR LONGER-TERM INTERVENTIONS

Social Context

The social context of longer-term intervention to deal with potential mental health outcomes needs to be considered before these interventions are dealt with in depth. There are changing and evolving social processes over time;

the initial "honeymoon" where there is intense affiliative behavior, convergence of support, and public acknowledgment of heroism and suffering. This phase may merge into angry protest and disillusionment and demoralization, then progressive recovery and renewal (Raphael, 1986). The interest of outside agencies is likely to be maximum during the early weeks, when media attention is high. Many promises are made in the initial period by those coming to the aid of affected groups; promises that resources will be provided to deal with the damage and destruction; that things will be "made right" again. Many of these promises arise from the goodwill of those coming to the aid of affected groups, and perhaps a deeper and unrecognized wish to undo the death and destruction and to return to the previous state.

The promises of this "honeymoon phase" may be unable to be kept, giving way to the phase of disillusionment. The realities of the extent of loss, of what cannot be replaced, what cannot be undone, the costs and the question of who will pay, and who is to blame all come into play. These social processes may lead to stresses in and of themselves that may complicate the psychological and social processes of recovery for those affected. Communities and social systems may be affected, particularly if there has been extensive destruction and death, and it may be difficult to reconstitute "normal" community structures for homes, work, school, and basic utilities. All these factors may lead to an adverse social context, with additional stressors, as well as the unfavorable environment. Among these losses and additional stresses are those related to resource depletion.

Disempowerment

A second major issue is the tendency for those affected, the "victims," to become further *disempowered by social responses* to them. First, others may converge and attempt to direct the recovery strategies of individuals or communities by telling them what do, as opposed to supporting an environment and strategies that can complement their own leadership and action. Affected communities will have the learning, personal growth, and mastery that come from their own experience of dealing with challenges generated by the event and can utilize help offered on their own terms. Another form of disempowerment may come from the "victim" status, which may bring rewards of attention, support, and resources. The victim role may be the most significant the person perceives him- or herself to have. Social processes may reinforce victim status when those offering assistance feel empowered and strong in relation to "weak" and "helpless" victims.

It is important to recognize these social expectations and to ensure that they do not further contribute to social and psychological morbidity. This may involve consulting with response agencies and leaders to encourage hopeful and positive expectations and the critical role of those affected as powerful agents in their own and their community's recovery.

Resources and Funding

A third major issue relates to *resources*. If it is agreed that additional resources will be needed to deal with the impact of the disaster or mass violence incident, the provision of these resources and their disbursement and utilization may be contentious. Disbursement of resources involves government and nongovernment organization funding grants, as well as specific funding pools donated by the public in response to the incident. Who is eligible, who controls the funds, what can they be used for, and with what expected outcomes? Funds for "rebuilding" damaged property may seem straightforward, but determining priorities, such as homes and workplaces, for affected populations, may be very difficult and further complicated by the differing patterns of insurance payout. These may be significant individual and community stressors—for instance, competition for resources may include requests for funerals of deceased, travel of relatives to the disaster site, provision of a memorial, and so forth. These may be seen as priorities by those bereaved, in contrast to the professional community's requests for funds for treatment of posttraumatic stress disorder (PTSD) or other psychological consequences among those traumatized by such a disaster or mass violence.

A key issue for mental health will be the level of resources that will be provided for prevention and treatment of adverse psychiatric outcomes. How may purchasing of services for those affected over the longer term be controlled or managed to ensure the provision of good practice in evidence-based care, with accredited providers, and how will the outcomes of such work be evaluated? A further consideration is that in some mental health care settings the capacity for any additional response to such events may be difficult when services are already overstretched, as is often true in remote or poverty-stricken environments.

A critical requirement will be the human resources that have the skills and expertise and are available to provide longer-term interventions. Preparation and training of such a workforce needs to build on existing capacities. There needs to be a capacity for mobilization, the setting of clear guidelines, and frameworks for the work to be done and for supervision and review. In addition, formats for documentation of systematic assessment and outcome monitoring need to be available and to be subsequently evaluated.

INTERVENTIONS AFTER THE FIRST MONTH

The following are key elements for response: defining populations in need of continuing or specific interventions; identifying and engaging the individuals and groups that have potentially been placed at risk or have developed a disorder; determining the methods of providing effective, acceptable, and implementable interventions; assessing and targeting such interventions for those with prioritized need; and monitoring these interventions and outcomes.

Defining Populations in Need of Continuing or Specific Interventions

Work by a wide range of researchers has highlighted the impacts of multiple stressors in the aftermath of mass violence and disaster (Norris, 2002). The effects are frequently prolonged and are highlighted by work such as that of North and colleagues (1999) following the Oklahoma bombing, Weisaeth (1985, 1989) and others.

By *1 month postincident* the impact of loss of human life, injury, and destruction of physical and social resources should be fairly clearly defined, depending on the nature of the episode. The cause has also usually been revealed, such as a planned terrorist attack, a "loner" acting for diverse reasons, or a predictable or unpredictable natural or man-made disaster. All these factors will have implications in terms of defining populations that may require mental health interventions. The intensity or quantitative exposure of different survivor populations will also need to be taken into consideration.

In addition, there are other *factors known to add to vulnerabilities* on the basis of available research, as shown in Table 10.1. First responders, emergency workers, and community leaders may also be vulnerable. Thus in planning the mental health interventions that may be necessary for the longer-term period beyond 1 month, the first stage of planning a prospective intervention strategy would include defining the following populations, in terms of both numbers of those potentially exposed and where they may be found.

- *Those most severely exposed* are at risk of posttraumatic stress-related morbidity and may require clinical screening or assessment. Importantly, persisting dissociation, high levels of reexperiencing symptoms, numbness or avoidance, arousal, heightened and persistent rumination about the experience (Murray, Ehlers, & Mayou, 2002), and persisting acute stress disorder (Bryant & Harvey, 1997) at the first month and subsequently may all indicate heightened risk of chronic PTSD.

TABLE 10.1. Vulnerable Populations following Disaster or Mass Violence

Vulnerability factors	Affected populations
Disaster-related stressor exposures	
Severe life threat/death encounter	Those closest to incident whose lives were at risk, or who thought they might die. Those exposed to multiple, gruesome mutilating deaths, or deaths of children.
Bereavement as a result of disaster-related deaths	Those who lost a loved one in the disaster, especially where there are traumatic circumstances or remains difficult to identify.
Injury as a result of the incident	Those injured in significant ways with ongoing effects, such as disability, disfiguration, pain (e.g., loss of limbs or burns).
Resource loss and other losses including dislocation and relocation	Those who have lost homes, jobs, personal effects, finances, or other resources. Those separated from home, community, family, or social network.
Causation-related stressors (e.g., human malevolence)	Whole population, but especially those already directly affected or at further risk of harm.
Responder stressors	Those with formal or informal response roles who may be directly exposed to all of the above, indirectly exposed to all of the above, vicariously or through role-related stressors (e.g., perceived inadequacy of response).
Prolonged uncertainty, ongoing threat	Whole population.
Preexisting potential vulnerabilities	
Previous trauma exposure	Those who have had previous traumatic experiences, such as child abuse, refugees, etc.
Preexisting psychiatric disorder	Those with a range of preexisting or past disorders including depression, anxiety, psychosis, etc.
Preexisting physical disability	Those with extra needs or dependencies may be more vulnerable.
Sociodemographic factors	
Social disadvantage	Those with poorer economic resources, poorer neighborhoods.
Education	Those with low education levels.
Gender	Women are more likely to develop PTSD, according to many studies.
Older adults	Children and older adults are suggested to be more vulnerable.

Note. It should be emphasized that while all of the above have been shown to contribute to increased risk of adverse mental health outcomes in some studies, morbidity is not an inevitable consequence and a greater proportion of people and populations with such vulnerabilities will nevertheless be resilient.

• *The bereaved* are also likely to be at heightened risk of adverse outcomes. The deaths of children may be associated with a very adverse outcome for parents so bereaved (Singh & Raphael, 1981), but other sudden violent deaths have also been associated with poorer outcomes (Lundin, 1984). Whether bodies could be found and identified, whether those who were bereaved felt that they could say their good-byes, might add significantly to risk, as might the ability to follow religious or cultural requirements about burial. Such sudden deaths may also cut across prior ambivalent relationships with the deceased. In addition, those bereaved may have also been present and traumatized by the event, thus having traumatic grief, PTSD, and bereavement phenomena coexisting.

• *The injured* are at greater risk for adverse for adverse mental health problems (North et al., 1999). The nature and severity of injuries may allow an estimate of possible mental health impacts, building on data from nondisaster populations (e.g., from motor vehicle accidents, burn injuries, and assault injuries).

• *Those whose physical and social resources have been destroyed* may be vulnerable in complex ways. They face stressors such as dislocation from home and community and the loss and grief associated with this experience. Separation from family members, neighborhood, community, place of work, or school through dislocation and relocation has been shown to increase risk of morbidity, particularly if there are repeated moves. Social networks, which would normally mitigate the impact of adversity, may be destroyed or at the least disrupted, or so taken up with dealing with their own issues that they cannot assist. On the other hand, it is also possible that in some communities the shared adversity leads to strong bonding and effective actions. Causation-related stressors are those that may be a focus for ongoing rumination, with increased vulnerability to psychiatric morbidity. Human malevolence such as is involved in a terrorist attack is prominent in this way.

• *Helpers and emergency responders* such as police, fire, rescue, ambulance, health, and other formal first responders may be to some degree protected by their formal training and specific roles. Nevertheless, there is much to suggest that such groups may suffer mental health impacts in severe and extreme circumstances. They will require assessment, monitoring, and response and some longer-term follow-up as part of an occupational health and safety care system (Raphael & Wilson, 2000). Informal first responders may be particularly vulnerable because they lack the training and normal systems of support; thus some assessment should be made of these people and their longer-term needs.

• *Populations that have been previously traumatized* may require individual assessment and specific interventions to meet their complex needs. Indigenous or refugee populations may be particularly vulnerable. Those abused in childhood are more vulnerable to adverse mental health outcomes.

• While studies of the vulnerability of *those with a preexisting mental illness* in the face of disaster or mass violence are limited, data following the Three Mile Island nuclear leak demonstrate that this population may be at greater risk (Bromet, Parkinson, Shulberg, Dunn, & Gondek, 1982; Bromet, Shulberg, & Dunn, 1982; Dew, Bromet, Schulberg, Dunn, & Parkinson, 1987). Nevertheless, such preexisting vulnerability is a consistent finding in many studies and reviews (Norris, 2002, 2005). Another issue that may arise is the incorporation of the incident into delusional systems, for instance, believing that "terrorists" are pursuing you as victim.

• *Those with a preexisting physical disability* are at increased risk for other forms of trauma and their consequences, such as homelessness and increased hospitalizations (Mueser, Hiday, Goodman, & Valenti-Hein, 2003). In some cases the prominent diagnosis of disability may overshadow the existence of a comorbid disorder such as PTSD, for example.

• Among *other vulnerable groups* are those exposed to the *prolonged uncertainty* and *possible ongoing threat* that occur following a nuclear, biological, or chemical attack. Perceptions of the threat of actual exposure, no clear way of ensuring safety, and the hidden and possibly prolonged nature of this exposure may all cause heightened anxiety and depression at community and individual levels. This is well demonstrated in the work showing the impact of the Chernobyl nuclear disaster (Spivak, 1992; Viinamäki et al., 1995). Uncertainties may be heightened by political, societal, and particularly media response. It is well demonstrated by findings that excessive media exposure to repeated traumatic incidents (e.g., September 11) or other violent and traumatic events may heighten vulnerabilities in populations such as children (Krug, Dahlberg, Mercy, Zwi, & Lozano, 2002; Pfefferbaum et al., 2000).

Identifying and Engaging the Individuals or Groups That May Require Intervention

It has increasingly been recognized that those affected by disaster or mass violence may be reluctant or resistant in terms of recognizing their needs for mental health interventions, and engaging with those who can provide help. In terms of early intervention and emergency response there has frequently been a public expectation that "trauma counseling," "grief counseling," or "debriefing" will be almost automatically offered to all affected persons. Recent studies have made it clear that while outreach, support and information may be helpful, there has been no identified benefit and possibly a potential risk associated with universal provision of unsupported and unnecessary interventions for populations that may, on the whole, demonstrate resilience and recovery in the majority of instances (National Institute of Mental Health, 2001).

Identifying Those Who May Benefit from Longer-Term Interventions

Methods of *identifying* those who may need longer-term interventions may be through:

- Clear links and follow-up related to early- and intermediate-intervention strategies and follow-up of those identified in the emergency as likely to be in need or at heightened risk, for instance those with acute stress disorder or very severe exposure.
- Outreach alongside other recovery organizations.
- Lists of victims.
- People who spontaneously present to systems of postdisaster response or are referred by others.
- Help lines or other sources of information.
- People referred after presenting to primary care or elsewhere.
- People presenting to disaster identified or other mental health counseling and treatment services.
- People coincidentally, or driven by their experience, presenting to mental health services.
- Screening of specific or general populations of affected communities.

Key to effective follow-up is systematic documentation and recording so that those who may be in need can be contacted, their needs assessed, and their management and programs of care evaluated.

Engaging Populations

In planning a disaster response, provisions should be made to effectively engage populations through outreach, using paraprofessionals from similar backgrounds as well as key constituent leaders, and to introduce the concept of intervention in a way that is trusted and acceptable. Engaging populations affected by disaster or mass violence may be difficult for the following reasons:

- People may not identify their needs in terms of mental health.
- Practical and survival issues will have much greater priority.
- People may feel others have greater need.

- They may fear retraumatization and be relying on denial and avoidance either as current or longer-term defenses.
- They may choose other coping strategies.
- They may see accepting mental health intervention as indicating that they are weak and cannot cope and thus see this kind of intervention as stigmatizing.
- They may fear that interventions will require them to open up or "disclose" and that they will not be able to keep on going if they do so or will be overwhelmed.

There may be many other reasons, but one that is important and not well considered is that of the *skills and capacities of those who try to engage the disaster-affected populations* and offer specific programs (Lindy, Green, Grace, & Tichener, 1983). The different nature of this client population, the different skills, and the changed client/provider relationships when people do not identify themselves as having an illness for which they need help may well make engagement more difficult. Another factor that has been observed to interfere with such engagement in intervention for longer-term follow-up is the issue of *litigation*. People may focus on litigation in the search for meaning and justice, and therapies may be seen as interfering with this process or placing legal outcomes at risk.

Determining Interventions That May Be of Benefit and Their Implementation

Consensus on Interventions for Traumatized Populations and PTSD

A recent review of the treatment outcome literature has examined the efficacy of a range of interventions for PTSD (Gibson & Watson, 2003). In summary, this working group reported that cognitive-behavioral therapy (CBT), selective serotonin reuptake inhibitors (SSRIs), and eye movement desensitization and reprocessing (EMDR) were the interventions that have been subjected to the most empirical study. They concluded that "the strongest evidence supports the use of CBT packages (involving exposure, cognitive restructuring, and anxiety management), which have now been examined in multiple randomized controlled clinical trials" (p. 18; see Foa, Keane, & Friedman, 2000, for a more thorough discussion of these interventions).

In summary, there are a number of interventions in the longer term for *established PTSD* that have been shown to be effective, including CBT, as with survivors of sexual and other assault (Foa, Davidson, & Frances, 1999; Foa, Hearst-Ikeda, & Perry, 1995); motor vehicle accidents

(Blanchard et al., 2003; Bryant, Harvey, Dang, Sackville, & Basten, 1998); and a range of other traumatic events (Lange, van de Ven, Schrieken, & Emmelkamp, 2001; Marks, Lovell, Noshirvani, Livanou, & Thrasher, 1998; Tarrier et al., 1999). A number of other studies also support the value of behavioral/CBT components of intervention in reducing PTSD symptoms as well as certain pharmacological agents such as SSRIs (Brady et al., 2000; Davidson, Pearlstein, et al., 2001; Davidson, Rothbaum, van der Kolk, Sikes, & Farfel, 2001; see also Davidson, 2002). Fortunately, CBT techniques and SSRIs also have benefit for depressed populations, as comorbid depression is common.

In one of the studies of *CBT intervention for trauma effects following a terrorist incident,* Gillespie, Duffy, Hackmann, and Clark (2002), implemented a community-based CBT program with survivors (with chronic PTSD) of the Omagh bombing in Northern Ireland in 1998. The median interval between the bombing and treatment was 10 months with a median of eight treatment sessions (range < 5 to 20) administered by clinicians who had modest prior training in CBT. Treatment consisted of reliving the traumatic event via imaginal and sometimes direct exposure, which was then closely integrated with cognitive restructuring techniques. The researchers report "significant and substantial" improvement in PTSD symptoms. In line with other research findings, patients who were physically injured showed less improvement. Despite a number of significant methodological limitations, this study is encouraging as it addresses concerns raised about the generalizability of CBT implemented by experienced clinicians in laboratory settings as opposed to its use in a front-line, nonselective service (National Health Service staff with heavy caseloads and only brief training in CBT). Implementation in such a naturalistic setting suggests the potential feasibility and effectiveness of providing CBT interventions more broadly.

While this study suggests that CBT may be feasible, further quantification of the implementation of certain components of this approach is needed. Although these initiatives are promising they need to be carefully monitored in terms of their appropriateness for the delivery of interventions in these disaster contexts and their impact on longer-term mental health outcomes.

In situations of mass violence, creative implementation strategies may be necessary when face-to-face contact is not feasible. In a recent study of *Internet-driven therapy for treatment of posttraumatic stress and grief,* Lange and colleagues (2003) found that patients in the treatment condition improved significantly more than those in the wait-list control group. "Interapy" was 10 sessions (twice weekly for 5 weeks) of psychoeducation, screening, effect measures, and a protocol-driven treatment. Treatment was divided into three phases: "self-confrontation" (psychoeducation and exposure); cognitive reappraisal (restructuring and skills for positive coping);

and a "sharing and farewell ritual," which focused on use of social support networks and closure via a letter to themselves or someone who had been involved in the traumatic event. On most subscales, more than 50% showed reliable change and clinically significant improvement, with the highest percentages for depression and avoidance.

Although Web interventions are not always accessible for people who have been traumatized, educational and self-help strategies can be made readily available in such formats for many potential users during the postdisaster and mass violence aftermath. Whether or not it will be an effective preventive or therapeutic strategy remains to be empirically established (e.g., Kronik, Akhmerov, & Speckhard, 1999; Lange et al., 2001).

Key Elements for an Implementation Plan for Longer-Term Interventions Following Disaster

Implementing potentially effective interventions is a critical step that must be carried out with speed and clarity following a traumatic event. It requires agreement as to who the target populations for interventions will be, how these interventions will be delivered, and who will provide them. Who is trained and skilled to intervene and what sanctions they have are further issues. The outcomes sought, how they will be measured or evaluated, and the implications for ongoing or future mental health service delivery also need to be part of such implementation strategies.

Key elements for effective implementation include:

- *Identifying* affected populations and their numbers and level of exposure to estimate service need.
- *Developing*, in consultation with relevant community systems, agreed intervention programs and modalities including education, group and individual prevention, and therapy strategies and ensuring that providers are trained and prepared and that documentation, review, supervision, and support programs are in place.
- *Providing* educational, community, social, psychotherapeutic/psychological, and biological interventions as appropriate in terms of current evidence but ensuring that they are linked to understanding of cultural, language, and human diversity and the multiple and complex ways in which people adapt to life adversities.
- *Determining sites*, how intervention programs will be described and publicized, and how those who need them will be assisted in accessing and engaging with them.
- *Ensuring systematic assessment and documentation* procedures and protocols are in place.

- *Establishing processes for linkage* from early intervention to these longer-term programs.
- *Defining and specifying* prevention, early intervention, and treatment goals.
- *Ensuring expectations of recovery and positive outcomes* and building personal hopefulness and resilience are key aspects of intervention frameworks.
- *Identifying and providing for informational,* educational, and self-care components of intervention.
- *Building protocols and processes with other relevant systems* and agencies involved in the longer term, including primary care, non-government and community services, and welfare and other groups that may be part of the network of care clients will need to optimize their outcomes.
- *Identifying budget and resource availability* to support implementation of best-practice intervention in terms of assessed need and methods for determining priorities within resource availability.
- Building *links to advocacy and other self-help* and community groups as these develop and provide mental health input as appropriate.
- *Identifying key clinical issues* that may need to be dealt with (e.g., providing interventions as appropriate for the full range of reactions and disorders; balancing disaster stress with other life stressors; assisting in active and positive role identification; facilitating positive family and network dynamics; determining goals of interventions and criteria for return to routine systems of mental health care; and taking care of physical as well as mental health problems).
- Setting in place *mechanisms for program evaluation and reporting* so that what has been learned can further *inform* this program as well as future plans and responses.

Assessing and Targeting Interventions for Those with Prioritized Need

Interventions with Bereaved Populations

There is little evidence of benefit for formalized interventions in the earliest stages postbereavement, particularly the types of traumatic bereavement that occur as a result of disasters and mass violence. Nevertheless, there is a history of providing bereavement interventions, as with Lindemann's (1944) classic description of, and intervention with, acute grief after the Coconut Grove Nightclub fire and others (see Lindy et al., 1983).

For longer-term interventions, these initiatives provide some directions. In two randomized controlled trials of widows, Vachon, Lyall, Rogers, Freedman-Letofsky, and Freedman's (1980) widow-to-widow support provided stimulus for enhanced recovery for a general population of widows, and four to eight sessions of psychodynamically informed interventions aimed at facilitating normal grief and mourning had considerable benefits for health and health care utilization in widows considered higher risk because of perceived lack of social support, traumatic circumstances of death, a complex relationship with the deceased, and other concurrent crises (Raphael, 1977).

Treatments for *traumatic grief* are showing some promise. Pilot testing of a treatment protocol (16 sessions over 4 months) using a combination of interpersonal therapy for depression and CBT for PTSD resulted in significant improvement in grief symptoms and associated anxiety and depression (Shear et al., 2001). A randomized controlled trial of *group-based* psychoeducation and supportive intervention over 10 weeks with parents whose children had violent deaths indicated that those with high distress scores (problems) improved but other subjects were worse (Murphy, 1996). This may represent retraumatization in the group or greater expression of distress but highlights the *problems of universal groups for intervention* in such sensitive circumstances.

In a bereavement intervention specific to a disaster (e.g., a rail disaster in Australia; Singh & Raphael, 1981), when intervention was perceived as helpful it was associated with some improvement in outcomes, but this was not a major effect. In addition, seeing and being able to say good-bye to the dead person in the period immediately after the death was one intervention of benefit and was associated with better outcomes.

In contrast to complicated and traumatic grief constructs, which deal with the stress of the separation and loss as traumatic (Prigerson & Jacobs 2001), *traumatic bereavement* is the complex interplay of traumatic stress and bereavement phenomena over time when the circumstances of the death are violent and horrific (Pynoos, Frederick, et al., 1987; Pynoos, Nader, Frederick, Gonda, & Stuber, 1987; Raphael, Martinek, & Wooding, 2004). Traumatic bereavement requires both assessing and managing these complex reactive processes to prevent or treat adverse outcomes. This is a relatively new field and will require much further systematic investigation.

Finally, grief and traumatic stress reactions are not diseases, and the majority of those exposed, even in circumstances of disaster or mass violence, will be resilient and may even experience personal growth. Interventions should be targeted to those at heightened risk or already demonstrating adverse outcomes. Although there is some discussion regarding assessment and targeted treatment in this area (Raphael et al., 2004; Raphael & Wooding, 2004), further research is required.

Other Affected Populations

Chronic stressors in the longer-term recovery periods are multiple and fre-quently "wear down" populations experiencing them. After the devastation of a cyclone destroying an Australian city, a community leader commented that the acute stress was bad but was not so disabling as the multiple and chronic stressors of the recovery process. Family interventions, individual therapy, and community-based approaches may all be relevant but have not been studied systematically in this context, nor have there been adequate evaluation studies of the interventions that have been provided.

Emergency and recovery workers should also be assessed and sup-ported for mental health needs related to exposures and the secondary stressors of their work, both as members of the community and through occupational mental health programs. They should receive appropriate follow-up and earlier or later interventions as indicated previously in terms of their direct or indirect stressor exposures.

The impact of trauma and grief should also be considered in the assess-ment and management of people with preexisting psychiatric disorders who are affected by disaster or terrorism.

Monitoring Interventions and Outcomes

One of the major difficulties with a great deal of work in this field is that many of the interventions are provided by diverse groups, the interventions themselves may be relatively nonspecific and may not be systematically documented, and proximal and distal outcomes may not be measured. Much recent work has involved trials with disaster-affected populations at a later stage (e.g., Chemtob, Nakashima, & Carlson, 2002; Litz, 2004), but they do not deal with evaluation of the multiple interventions that may be provided. There is also the difficulty in carrying out randomized controlled trials, which may be both ethically and operationally problematic in the postdisaster period, or particularly in the aftermath of a terrorist incident where threat may be ongoing. Most reports, guidelines, comprehensive review papers, and books have a strong focus on cognitive-behavioral inter-ventions for PTSD (e.g., Shalev, Tuval-Mashiach, & Hadar, 2004; Walser et al., 2004). Other common consequences, such as traumatic bereavements, have recently come to attention, with systematic interventions being pro-vided and evaluated in some trials. The effects of and intervention with chronic long-term stress, human malevolence, mass violence, exacerbation of preexisting psychiatric disorders and vulnerabilities, and comorbid pathologies have little systematic attention.

A critical issue, as indicated previously and as identified by the World Health Organization's Assessment Instrument Mental Health Services—

Emergency (AIMS-E), is to have an information system that will provide a basis for identifying clients, documenting their risk and need, and describing the interventions provided and assessment of outcomes. Preexisting systems linked to other data sets, with protection of privacy, are thus a critical prerequisite to progressing this field.

Systematic population surveillance for mental health can demonstrate the overall impact of a mass event. Such surveillance can also provide the data both on those affected and those who received intervention, as well as on outcomes of both preventative and treatment programs.

Careful predisaster work can set up methodologies for research that can be carried out at the time of or following incidents and that can progressively contribute to knowledge in this field.

CONCLUSIONS

Understanding and responding to the social contexts of the postdisaster recovery period over the longer term will call on a range of mental health skills. Community consultations and work with community leaders and general health and mental health systems will be critical so that mental health interventions can have an appropriate and acknowledged place. The ongoing stressors facing traumatized, bereaved, and devastated communities may become very chronic, and disillusionment and anger may complicate the capacity to recover. Hopefulness and positive expectations are critical, as are tools for communities, families, and individuals to use in their own recovery. Supporting the return to "normal" and the functioning of social networks and institutions can greatly enhance the sense of safety and security and form structures that will facilitate resilience and opportunities for mastery. Support for families is critical as they may be torn apart by what has happened and may face many stressors as they struggle to overcome trauma and loss. Social rituals of reintegration and renewal, as well as memorialization, are part of the recovery process over the longer term and may be opportunities to further enhance mental health and well-being. Making meaning of what has happened is a significant issue in resolution of the experience, both for communities and for individuals. Giving "testimony" in accounts of what has happened may also be part of this. Specialized mental health intervention programs should be carefully planned to meet identified needs in terms of both preventing more adverse outcomes and treating established psychiatric morbidity. Populations of traumatized and/or bereaved adults and children may need to be assessed or screened.

Implementation of good-practice interventions can be informed by available evidence, but it is increasingly recognized that this is limited in terms of those exposed to mass violence or major disasters. Implementation of mental health interventions also needs to be integrated with other resource, support, and assistance programs. All interventions should, however, be informed by expectation of positive outcomes, hopefulness, and compassionate human response to those who have been affected by the catastrophe. Systematic assessment and documentation of problems and targeted interventions are important and form a basis for evaluation. Resourcing these implementation plans and programs will require careful management and clear relationships with systems of ongoing mental health care for more chronic disorders, either caused or exacerbated by the disaster. Most important, research and evaluation should be core requirements throughout—to extend knowledge and to better inform mental health response for future disaster, mass violence, and other inevitable life adversities.

REFERENCES

Blanchard, E. B., Hickling, E. J., Devineni, T., Veazey, C. H., Galovski, T. E., Mundy, E., et al. (2003). A controlled evaluation of cognitive behavioural therapy for posttraumatic stress in motor vehicle accident survivors. *Behaviour Research and Therapy, 41*, 79–96.

Brady, K., Pearlstein, T., Asnis, G. M., Baker, D., Rothbaum, B., Sikes, C. R., et al. (2000). Double-blind placebo-controlled study of the efficacy and safety of sertraline treatment of posttraumatic stress disorder. *Journal of the American Medical Association, 283*, 1837–1844.

Bromet, E. J., Parkinson, D. K., Shulberg, H. C., Dunn, L. O., & Gondek, P. C. (1982). Mental health of residents near the Three Mile Island nuclear reactor: A comparative study of selected groups. *Journal of Preventive Psychiatry, 1*, 225–276.

Bromet, E. J., Shulberg, H. C., & Dunn, L. O. (1982). Reactions of psychiatric patients to the Three Mile Island nuclear accident, *Archives of General Psychiatry, 39*, 725–730.

Bryant, R. A., & Harvey, A. G. (1997). Acute stress disorder: A critical review of diagnostic issues. *Clinical Psychology Review, 17*, 757–773.

Bryant, R. A., Harvey, A. G., Dang, S., Sackville, T., & Basten, C. (1998). Treatment of acute stress disorder: A comparison of cognitive-behavioral therapy and supportive counseling. *Journal of Consulting and Clinical Psychology, 66*, 862–866.

Chemtob, C. M., Nakashima, J., & Carlson, J. G. (2002). Brief treatment for elementary school children with disaster-related posttraumatic stress disorder: A field study. *Journal of Clinical Psychiatry, 58*(1), 99–112.

Davidson, J. R. T. (2002). Surviving disaster: What comes after the trauma? *British Journal of Psychiatry, 181*, 366–368.

Davidson, J. R. T., Pearlstein, T., Londborg, P., Brady, K. T., Rothbaum, B., Bell, J., et al. (2001). Efficacy of setraline in preventing relapse of posttraumatic stress disorder: Results of a 28-week double-blind, placebo-controlled study. *American Journal of Psychiatry, 158*, 1974–1981.

Davidson, J. R. T., Rothbaum, B., van der Kolk, B. A., Sikes, C. R., & Farfel, G. (2001). Multicenter, double-blind comparison of setraline and placebo in the treatment of posttraumatic stress disorder. *Archives of General Psychiatry, 58,* 485–492.

Dew, M. A., Bromet, E. J., Schulberg, H. C., Dunn, L. O., & Parkinson, D. K. (1987). Mental health effects of the Three Mile Island nuclear reactor restart. *American Journal of Psychiatry, 144,* 1074–1077.

Foa, E. B., Davidson, J. R. T., & Frances, A. (1999). The expert consensus guideline series: Treatment of posttraumatic stress disorder. *Journal of Clinical Psychiatry, 60,* 3–76.

Foa, E. B., Hearst-Ikeda, D., & Perry, K. J. (1995). Evaluation of a brief cognitive-behavioral program for the prevention of chronic PTSD in recent assault victims. *Journal of Consulting and Clinical Psychology, 63,* 948–955.

Foa, E. B., Keane, T. M., & Friedman, M. J. (2000). *Effective treatments for posttraumatic stress disorder: Practice guidelines from the International Society for Traumatic Stress Studies.* New York: Guilford Press.

Gibson, L., & Watson, P. (2003). *A review of the published empirical literature regarding early- and later-stage interventions for individuals exposed to traumatic stress.* Unpublished manuscript.

Gillespie, K., Duffy, M., Hackmann, A., & Clark, D. M. (2002). Community based cognitive therapy in the treatment of post-traumatic stress disorder following the Omagh bomb. *Behaviour Research and Therapy, 4,* 345–357.

Kronik, A. A., Akhmerov, R. A., & Speckhard, A. (1999). Trauma and disaster as life disrupters: A model of computer-assisted psychotherapy applied to adolescent victims of the Chernobyl disaster. *Professional Psychology: Research and Practice, 30,* 586–599.

Krug, E. G., Dahlberg, L. L., Mercy, J. A., Zwi, A., & Lozano, R. (2002, October). *World report on violence and health.* Geneva, Switzerland: World Health Organization.

Lange, A., Rietdijk, D., Hudcovicova, M., van de Ven, J. Q. R., Schrieken, B., & Emmelkamp, P. M. G. (2003). Interapy: A controlled randomized trial of the standardized treatment of posttraumatic stress through the Internet. *Journal of Consulting and Clinical Psychology, 71,* 901–909.

Lange, A., van de Ven, J., Schrieken, B., & Emmelkamp, P. M. G. (2001). Interapy: Treatment of posttraumatic stress through the Internet: A controlled trial. *Journal of Behavior Therapy and Experimental Psychiatry, 32,* 73–90.

Lindemann, E. (1944). Symptomatology and management of acute grief. *American Journal of Psychiatry, 101,* 141–148.

Lindy, J. D., Green, B. L., Grace, M., & Tichener, J. (1983). Psychotherapy with survivors of the Beverly Hills Supper Club fire. *American Journal of Psychotherapy, 37,* 593–610.

Litz, B. T. (Ed.). (2004). *Early intervention for trauma and traumatic loss.* New York: Guilford Press.

Lundin, T. (1984). Morbidity following sudden and unexpected bereavement. *British Journal of Psychiatry, 144,* 84–88.

Marks, I., Lovell, K., Noshirvani, H., Livanou, M., & Thrasher, S. (1998). Treatment of post-traumatic stress disorder by exposure and/or cognitive restructuring: A controlled study. *Archives of General Psychiatry, 55,* 317–325.

Mueser, K. T., Hiday, V. A., Goodman L. A., & Valenti-Hein, D. (2003). People with mental and physical disabilities. In B. L. Green, M. J. Friedman, J. de Jong, et al. (Eds.), *Trauma interventions in war and peace: Prevention, practice, and policy* (pp. 129–154). New York: Kluwer/Plenum.

Murphy, S. A. (1996). Parent bereavement stress and preventive intervention following the violent deaths of adolescent or young adult children. *Death Studies, 20,* 441–452.

Murray, J., Ehlers, A., & Mayou, R. A. (2002). Dissociation and post-traumatic stress disorder: Two prospective studies of road traffic accident survivors. *British Journal of Psychiatry, 180,* 363–368.

National Institute of Mental Health. (2001). *Mental health and mass violence: Evidence-based early psychological intervention for victims/survivors of mass violence. A workshop to reach consensus on best practices* (NIH Publication No. 02-5138). Washington, DC: U.S. Government Printing Office. Retrieved from www.nimh.nih.gov/research/massviolence.pdf

Norris, F. H. (2002). 60,000 disaster victims speak: Part I. An empirical review of the empirical literature, 1981–2001. *Psychiatry, 65,* 207–239.

Norris, F. H. (2005). *Range, magnitude and duration of the effects of disaster on mental health: Review update 2005.* White River Junction, VT: Research Education in Disaster Mental Health. Available at www.redmh.org/research/general/REDMH_effects.pdf

North, C. S., Nixon, S. J., Shariat, S., Mallonee, S., McMillen, J., Spitznagel, E. L., et al. (1999). Psychiatric disorders among survivors of the Oklahoma City bombing. *Journal of the American Medical Association, 282,* 755–762.

Pfefferbaum, B., Seale, T. W., McDonald, N. B., Brandt, E. N., Jr., Rainwater, S. M., Maynard, B. T., et al. (2000). Posttraumatic stress two years after the Oklahoma City bombing in youths geographically distant from the explosion. *Psychiatry, 63,* 358–370.

Prigerson, H. G., & Jacobs, S. C. (2001). Traumatic grief as a distinct disorder: A rationale, consensus criteria, and a preliminary empirical test. In M. S. Stroebe, W. Stroebe, R. O. Hansson, & H. Schut (Eds.), *New handbook of bereavement: Consequences, coping, and care* (pp. 613–645). Washington, DC: American Psychological Association Press.

Pynoos, R. S., Frederick, C., Nader, K., Arroyo, W., Steinberg, A., Eth, S., et al. (1987). Life threat and posttraumatic stress in school-age children. *Archives of General Psychiatry, 44,* 1057–1063.

Pynoos, R. S., Nader, K., Frederick, C., Gonda, L., & Stuber, M. (1987). Grief reactions in school age children following a sniper attack at school. *Israeli Journal of Psychiatry and Related Sciences, 24,* 53–63.

Raphael, B. (1977). Preventive intervention with the recently bereaved. *Archives of General Psychiatry, 34,* 1450–1454.

Raphael, B. (1986). *When disaster strikes.* New York: Basic Books.

Raphael, B., Martinek, N., & Wooding S. (2004). Assessing traumatic bereavement. In J. P. Wilson & T. M. Keane (Eds.), *Assessing psychological trauma and PTSD* (2nd ed., pp. 492–510). New York: Guilford Press.

Raphael, B., & Wilson, J. P. (Eds.). (2000). *Psychological debriefing: Theory, practice and evidence.* Cambridge, UK: Cambridge University Press.

Raphael, B., & Wooding, S. (2004, September 15–17). *Terrorist threat, mental health and the challenge of mental health promotion.* Paper presented at the Third World Conference, The Promotion of Mental Health and Prevention of Mental and Behavioral Disorders, Auckland, New Zealand.

Shalev, A. Y., Tuval-Mashiach, R., & Hadar, H. (2004). Posttraumatic stress disorder as a result of mass trauma. *Journal of Clinical Psychiatry, 65*(Suppl. 1), 4–10.

Shear, M. K., Frank, E., Foa, E., Cherry, C., Reynolds, C. F., Vander Bilt, J., et al. (2001). Traumatic grief treatment: A pilot study. *American Journal of Psychiatry, 158,* 1506–1508.

Singh, B., & Raphael, B. (1981). Post disaster morbidity of the bereaved: A possible role for preventive psychiatry. *Journal Nervous and Mental Disease, 169,* 203–212.

Spivak, L. I. (1992). Psychiatric aspects of the accident at Chernobyl nuclear power station. *European Journal of Psychiatry 6,* 207–212.

Tarrier, N., Pilgrim, H., Sommerfield, C., Faragher, B., Reynolds, M., Graham, E., et al. (1999). A randomized trial of cognitive therapy and imaginal exposure in the treatment of chronic post traumatic stress disorder. *Journal of Consulting and Clinical Psychology, 67,* 13–18.

Vachon, M. L., Lyall, W. A., Rogers, J., Freedman-Letofsky, K., & Freedman, S. J. (1980). A controlled study of self-help intervention for widows. *American Journal of Psychiatry, 137,* 1380–1384.

Viinamäki, H., Kumpusalo, E., Myllykangas, M., Salomaa, S., Kumpusalo, L., Kolmakov, S., et al. (1995). The Chernobyl accident and mental wellbeing—A population study. *Acta Psychiatrica Scandinavica, 91,* 396–401.

Walser, R. D., Ruzek, J. I., Naugle, A. E., Padesky, C., Ronell, D. M., & Ruggiero, K. (2004). Disaster and terrorism: Cognitive-behavioral interventions. *Prehospital and Disaster Medicine, 19*(1), 54–63.

Weisaeth, L. (1985). Post-traumatic stress disorder after an industrial disaster In. P. Pichot, R. Wolf, & K. Thau (Eds). *Psychiatry: The state of the art* (pp. 299–307). New York: Plenum Press.

Weisaeth, L. (1989). The stressors and the post-traumatic stress syndrome after an industrial disaster. *Acta Psychiatrica Scandinavica, 80,* 25–37.

CHAPTER 11

Consultation to Groups, Organizations, and Communities

JAMES E. MCCARROLL and ROBERT J. URSANO

Consultation by clinicians to operational groups, organizations, and communities helps people to determine and evaluate policies and procedures to reduce mortality and morbidity.

Since September 11, 2001, mental health consultation increasingly uses a public health model directed toward the prevention of and therapeutic intervention for psychological casualties in large-scale terrorist attacks as well as disasters (Butler, Panzer, & Goldfrank, 2003). This model uses a matrix to develop a system for interventions based on the individual or population affected, the agent, the physical and social environment, and the phases of the event (before, during, and after). The matrix encourages consultants to consider all characteristics of a terrorist attack or disaster and plan pre-event interventions to minimize postevent consequences. While current interest is in the large-scale public health consequences of terrorism and disaster, many principles of consultation are useful in both large-scale and more localized events such as a school, workplace, industrial or military accident site, or similar location.

Four standard epidemiological concepts can frame the characteristics of the event: agent, host, vector or vehicle, and environment. The agent is the violent act or threat, the host is the population of affected individuals, the vector or vehicle is the way the event was propagated (e.g., terrorist), and environment is the physical and social context surrounding the event.

TABLE 11.1. Community Needs for Psychological Health in Terrorism and Disaster

- Provision of basic services (e.g., food and shelter).
- Promotion of individual and community resilience.
- Surveillance for psychological consequences.
- Screening of psychological symptoms.
- Treatment for psychological trauma.
- Longer-term general needs (e.g., housing and financial assistance).
- Risk communication and information dissemination.
- Training service providers.
- Maintain capacity to manage increases in demand for mental health services.
- Case finding to locate individuals needing services.

Thus for the disease malaria, the population might be individuals in a swampy area, the vector is the mosquito, and the agent is the malarial parasite. Interventions can be made at any level, before, during, or after the infection. Similar perspectives can frame mental health consultations.

The consultant needs to assume that almost any organization or community is able to provide necessary disaster and terrorism support and core mental health services (see Table 11.1). Given the broad spectrum of consultation issues, this chapter focuses specifically on the mental health consultant and the consulting tasks; the information is largely practical.

HISTORY

One source of knowledge about how to conceptualize and perform psychiatric consultation to an organization grew out of war (McCarroll, Jaccard, & Radke, 1994). Army psychiatrists had experience with the treatment and management of psychiatric combat casualties in World War I (Salmon, 1929), World War II (Glass, 1947; Menninger, 1944), and Korea (Glass, 1955). As the understanding of how the stresses of military service and combat affected soldiers, the approaches of psychiatrists and other mental health professionals also evolved. Based on their findings from combat, psychiatrists felt they had proved that social–environmental circumstances were overriding determinants of behavior and the basis was set for wider application of preventive and consultative psychiatric services. Rioch (1955) wrote that during World War II, psychiatric concepts of prevention and treatment underwent pronounced changes, almost reversals. Appel (1966) wrote that prevention began where screening left off. The preventive measure that Rioch considered most important was the understanding of human relationships. The greatest defense against breakdown in combat, which can be considered a form of acute situational stress, was the development and reinforcement of group cohesiveness. One of the major lessons learned in World War II was that psychiatric disability correlated positively with external stress and was not limited to so-called intrapsychic determinants, as had been predicted. Although it may seem a long way between the experiences of psychiatrists and other mental health practitioners in war to consultation in the era of mass disasters and terrorism, many principals are the same. For example, organizational cohesion and social support are still important determinants of health and health behaviors (Berkman & Kawachi, 2000).

CURRENT ENVIRONMENT

Consultation is always *to someone*. It may be to an operational group (e.g., police or firefighters), a workplace (e.g., organization such as corporation, police, postal service, school, utility workers, and others), or a community (mayor or public official). Usually, the consultant directly addresses either the leadership of the group, organization, or community or its health official. Beneficiaries may be a local organization familiar to the consultant or at a distant location where the consultant is unknown. The major differences between these two include whether a relationship has already been established and whether continuity can be maintained following the initial visit, both more likely in local consultation. A consultant might be called to provide planning for training first responders, to assist supervisors in monitoring personnel for deterioration in performance and psychological symptoms, to evaluate performance in simulated disasters, to respond to questions by higher authority and from the media, and to deal quickly with situations that have mental health implications for individuals as well as specific groups. Thus, the range of consultative opportunities is broader than this chapter can envision, and is limited only by the vision of persons who may think of something helpful that has previously gone unnoticed or has not been corrected. Table 11.2 provides major topics to consider in planning and performing consultation.

PERFORMING THE CONSULTATION

Gaining Entry to the Organization

A consultation has to be requested and authorized by an appropriate authority. In almost all large-scale disasters, "consultants" flood the scene often without any authorization or support from higher authority. To be

TABLE 11.2. Major Consultation Tasks by Phase of Event in Disaster/Terrorism

Pre-event

- Obtain legitimacy with authority.
- Inventory resources.
- Develop and review disaster response plans for mental health response.
- Determine possible areas and levels of risk.
- Practice disaster drills.
- Establish networks of agencies, leaders, and key individuals.
- Prepare high-risk groups for likely traumatic events.
- Communicate contingency plans to all personnel.
- Promote individual and community resilience.

During event

- Communicate with authority, leaders, and key personnel.
- Educate leadership in risk communication.
- Determine locations, types, and extent of exposures.
- Decrease exposure of population to toxins/trauma and unnecessary risks.
- Triage behavioral problems.
- Establish work groups for rescue, repair, comfort, and other assistance operations.
- Advise leader on communication of information to the public.

Postevent

- Reconstruct history of event by leaders and personnel involved.
- Provide summary of responses event to the public.
- Acquaint mental health referral sources with information on event and likely responses of personnel.
- Provide referral for aftercare.
- Maintain long-term relationship with organization to follow natural developments.
- Assist leaders to obtain basic resources for personnel.
- Help reestablish normal working and living groups and conditions.

successful, the consultant has to obtain authorization for his or her services. However, this may not be easy. In seeking approval to assist the U.S. Navy after the terrorist bombing of the Pentagon on September 11, the Navy official who had the authority to grant the consultation team access to naval personnel asked the team leader what evidence the team had of its effectiveness and how the team could justify pulling personnel away from their duties to talk with team members (Grieger et al., 2003). The response from the team was that team members had received positive feedback in previous consultations, and they also agreed to limit the time with the sailors.

The consultant must also receive the cooperation of participants. Even though a higher authority has authorized the consultation, the participants may not fully participate. Acceptance is easiest when the consultant has personal and professional credentials that are credible to the organization's members, is known to the participants, has previously provided tangible assistance, is perceived as someone who can helpful, and is not conducting an investigation or pursuing a private agenda that would interfere with the consultation or assess blame.

Formulating the Initial Agreement and Clarifying the Question

Although the nature of the relationship between consultant and leadership of the organization is subject to change, without some sort of initial explicit contract between the parties, consultation is likely to fail. The consultation's goals may be somewhat general initially, but when the consultant approaches the tasks, the questions should be specific and the limits understood in terms of what can reasonably be expected and what cannot. The consultant's first task is to determine the primary questions to be addressed.

Forming a Consultation Team

The consultant may work alone or a consultation team may be necessary; the team should mirror to some degree the composition of the group to benefit from the consultation (hereafter known as "the participants"). There should be a similar mix of demography, culture, and work experience. The team can be expanded to include family members, military service members or veterans, and persons with special skills and from enough occupations to understand the nature of the problems.

Attire

It is important to consider the attire of the consultant and of the participants. This may seem trivial, but it deserves some thought before meeting the person who requested the consultation as well as the participants. A doctor who consults to disasters would not wear a white lab coat to the field. One might think twice before adopting the dress of those on the scene if this type of consultation is required. People may think casual attire disrespectful or that the consultant has the same type of job as they do, and credibility may suffer. It is usually helpful to talk to some participants about attire directly.

Understanding the Organization

If an organizational chart of the group, organization, or community and its parent organizations exists, it will provide valuable information prior to meeting the participants. It can also determine whether it is a useful representation of how the organization works or if an informal organization (which always exists) takes priority over formal structures and functions. Regardless of the formal structure, the consultant must attempt to become familiar with the set of informal subgroups to determine their influence on the operations of the larger organization.

Explaining the Purpose of the Consultation

The purpose of the consultation should be explained to everyone at every opportunity. Do not assume that participants have been told the purpose or that all agreed to the plan. Participants should be given the opportunity to ask questions and to opt out of participation, if possible. Generally, people may be required to attend meetings but not to disclose information. This discussion assumes that the consultant is not performing an investigation. Participants often believe they are being investigated or that securing critical resources depends on their answers or the results of the consultation, even when that is untrue. Usually investigations are separate, but the consultant can never ensure that this is the case. Suspicion by the participants is normal and should be expected. Such suspicion may be an inherent limitation that should be recognized. Assuming that the consultant is not to be used for investigative or resource allocation purposes, ways have to be developed to deal with the anxiety of those to whom you are consulting.

Talking with the Participants

A consultation usually begins with the head of the group, organization, or community. First questions are important because the answers provide the potential to go in many different directions. An understanding of each person's job and how that job fits together with others' is one place to start. Consultation, at least initially, requires the consultant to learn not to lecture. Certainly, there is an educational function for both parties, but the consultant should determine when each is appropriate because lecturing can easily be perceived (perhaps correctly) as "talking down."

Talk by the participants should be encouraged and supported. Participants, including the leadership, may tend to view themselves as passive recipients of the consultation process. It is essential that they participate actively. One framework proven useful in understanding the sequence of events after a disaster is to reconstruct it historically. Such a procedure was developed during wartime by the U.S. Army historian S. L. A. Marshall (Shalev, Peri, Rogel-Fuchs, Ursano, & Marlowe, 1996). Marshall's concepts and procedures have been adapted for use in understanding events by reconstructing a time line each person's participation and reactions to these events (Shalev, 2000).

Language

Knowing and using the language of the group is important. It is also important not to use terms familiar to group members if you are not sure of the meaning. It could lead to misunderstanding if both parties do not use the same terms in the same way. Do not assume that both persons, the one requesting the consultation and the one performing it, understand the question. Often, and this may be a particular risk between senior personnel, it is easy to assume that each knows what the other is talking about. When in doubt about meaning, clarify.

Terminating the Consultation

What happens at the end of the consultation depends on the type of consultation arrangement with the client. If it is a one-time consultation, the relationship usually ends at that point. If it is ongoing, the consultant will close out a particular question but continue the relationship established with the organization. At least three aspects need attention: the requestor, the participants, and the consultation team. There are also formal and informal aspects of termination. Formal aspects include filing a report, archiving notes, and arranging for follow-up work, if any. Informal aspects include attempting to inform the participants that the process is over and whatever findings can be given to them at that point. It is probably best if the organization provides feedback because it will have a broader view than just that of the consultant. At a minimum, the participants should be thanked for their cooperation.

Finally, if the members of the team do not regularly work together, they should be given an opportunity to say good-bye to each other and express their thoughts about the consultation efforts. In some instances, such as a particularly troubling event, a hostile group, or a long-term consultation where relationships have been established, a more formal opportunity to share perspectives and feelings may be advisable. This may also allow the team to discuss team recommendations, to try to resolve doubts and limits about the team's advice, and to improve the team's functioning in the event of such work in the future, either individually or in a group.

Report of the Consultation

Writing a report is a part of terminating the consultation. The report should serve the practical purpose of explaining what was done by whom, the recommendations, and the rationale for these. The success of the consultation may depend on the written report as verbal recommendations are likely to be forgotten or to be subject to faulty memory of all parties. It may be well for the consultant to defer a few days before writing and submitting the report until he or she has left the consultation site. Later reflection may provide additional perspective unavailable when people are tired and eager to leave. Thus, the report becomes a benchmark of the problems encountered by the organization at the time of the consultation and the plan for addressing them, particularly important if follow-up consultation is expected. The writing of this document should be carefully considered. The security of the document will be unknown, as few remain private. It should be considered a legal document that the consultant may have to defend publicly or see referenced in the media.

ADDITIONAL ISSUES IN CONSULTATION

Consulting to the Leader

Determining the key ingredients for consulting with the leader will vary depending on a host of factors such as the phase of time in which the consultant is involved, the nature and scope of the event, the experience of both the consultant and the consulted, and the demands on the leader and others. Bushnell (2002) gives an account of her experiences as the U.S. Ambassador to the Republic of Kenya in August 1998 when terrorists bombed the U.S. embassy. She warned that understanding how ordinary people react to extraordinary events is critical for leadership in this age. She also noted the importance of the three basic principles shown by Mayor Giuliani following the attack on the World Trade Centers in New York City on September 11: *visibility, empathy, and caring.*

   In the moments following the bombing of the embassy, Bushnell and her staff organized tasks for people. She noted that doing something—doing anything—provided a necessary comfort from feelings of helplessness and despair. Among her many other observations was the importance of the development of subgroups (e.g., those who had survived the bombing vs. those who came to the embassy to assist vs. persons assigned later to the embassy). The leader is also one of these subgroups and must balance a fine line between contributing as a member of such a group and retaining the leadership role for all persons.

The main lesson of Bushnell's experience is to learn to take care of people. She gives extensive examples of how she did this, including the need to re-create normalcy (even if it is an illusion), tolerate diminished results, use rituals to benefit from their healing powers, listen, and take care of oneself.

Community versus Person

One of the most important distinctions that the clinician must make is between clinical questions and organizational issues. This may be harder than it appears because the mental health provider is often approached about the welfare of an individual. When this happens, the next step is to assess whether it is a general problem that has surfaced in the presence of a single person or whether the problem is unique to that individual. Clinical training frequently neglects the work environment, which probably reflects a devaluing of the ways work contributes to health. Work may be seen as a stressor, not as something that maintains and sustains people, or it may be perceived as therapeutic.

Risks to the Consultant and Ethical Issues

The consultant should beware of believing too much in his or her own infallibility. There can be a tendency to make pronouncements not warranted by the data and the consultant may feel pressured to go beyond the data when there is insufficient information. A sense of humility on the consultant's part may make him or her less threatening to the participants. Likewise, one should not rely too much on previous experience. Every consultation problem should be treated as unique, one that deserves the same careful approach to understanding the problems.

Double Agency

"Double agency" is a dilemma for the consultant who works for the affected agency. It may limit the consultant's work but can also be valuable if he or she is familiar with the organization and its people. In restricted locations, such as overseas, there may be no alternative to consulting to one's own organization. As part of a military unit one usually develops bonds or emotional ties to the unit. On the positive side, because of this position, many informal mechanisms of consultation become available. However, it can be difficult to remember which role one is operating in: comrade or consultant.

Maintenance of the Consultative Role

There is an inherent danger of losing objectivity in the consultative process. One may become overinvolved with participants and enmeshed in the process, particularly when the consultant acts alone. When a consultative team is present, the team leader must check constantly with teammates as a type of reality check on the consultative process. When the consultant has developed a close relationship to a unit, he or she can be powerfully affected emotionally by losses. The consultant can also become a victim of the particular disasters or traumas of the unit to which he or she is trying to consult.

Confidentiality

Confidentiality to those who speak to a consultant may or may not exist in consultation and should not be promised except in rare circumstances. Promising confidentiality can often tie the hands of the consultant and may prevent valuable input from reaching the requestor. Still, discretion should be observed and private information with no bearing on the consultation question should be protected.

Special Issues

At the time of this writing, psychological responses to terrorism and disasters are still being developed (Ursano & Norwood, 2003). The mental health consultant is particularly important in this field as the public perception of danger and risk can often incapacitate the medical response systems (Ursano, Norwood, Fullerton, Holloway, & Hall, 2003). It has been shown that many more people believe they were exposed to a toxic agent than actually were (Stuart, Ursano, Fullerton, Norwood, & Murray, 2003). The communication of risk information is one of the most challenging tasks for leaders (Fullerton, Ursano, Norwood, & Holloway, 2003). Such information must be given to personnel within the organization and to the public. Communication of risk information to the public requires a working relationship with media personnel who will help translate complex scientific and medical information into messages helpful to the community.

The handling of the dead from disasters and terrorism can present special problems for groups, organizations, and communities (Ursano, McCarroll, & Fullerton, 2003). The major tasks are recovery, identification, storage and transportation of remains, and burial, but also the communication about the deaths to the families and the society, the removal and handling of personal effects, and the impact of the loss on all. Work with families and survivors can be a major task after such events.

SUMMARY

The task of consulting to an organization is not easy. Human needs have remained relatively similar over the years, but bioterrorism poses challenges previously unknown. People still have adjustment difficulties, although organizations still have difficult mission challenges and leadership and performance problems and must interact with a much wider variety of other organizations to do their job. In some situations, control has become more centralized and communication between organizations is a continual problem. Mental health practice has also changed. For psychiatry, the focus has gone toward biological treatment of the individual rather than community and group treatment.

Today, the consultant must have a broad range of skills. The consultant must know not only his or her own organization but also many others. Such skill development takes time and, more significant, the presence of a mentor who can teach younger people "the ropes" of consulting. Our impression is that most people who perform consultation successfully enjoy it and have a sense of having contributed something, as well as having obtained something special not ordinarily encountered in clinical or administrative life.

It should also be noted that while the mental health practitioner's task is normally to help a client achieve some kind of personal satisfaction, the consultation's emphasis tends to be more toward the group. Problem behaviors that arise from dissatisfaction are not always incapacitating. Many people suffer in war and disasters. The criterion of one's ability to perform his or her job should not necessarily include happiness at the task.

REFERENCES

Appel, J. W. (1966). Preventive psychiatry. In A. J. Glass & R. J. Bernice (Eds.), *Medical Department, United States Army: Neuropsychiatry in World War II: Vol. 1. Zone of the interior* (pp. 373–416). Washington, DC: U.S. Government Printing Office.

Berkman, L. F., & Kawachi, I. (2000). *Social epidemiology.* New York: Oxford University Press.

Bushnell, P. (2002). Leadership in the wake of disaster. In R. J. Ursano, C. S. Fullerton, & A. E. Norwood (Eds.), *Terrorism and disaster* (pp. 31–57). New York: Cambridge University Press.

Butler, A. S., Panzer, A. M., & Goldfrank, L. R. (Eds.). (2003). *Preparing for the psychological consequences of terrorism: A public health strategy.* Washington, DC: Institute of Medicine of the National Academies, National Academies Press.

Fullerton, C. S., Ursano, R. J., Norwood, A. E., & Holloway, H. C. (2003). Trauma, terrorism, and disaster. In R. J. Ursano, C. S. Fullerton, & A. E. Norwood (Eds.), *Terrorism and disaster* (pp. 1–20). New York: Cambridge University Press.

Glass, A. J. (1947). Effectiveness of forward neuropsychiatric treatment. *Bulletin of the U.S. Army Medical Department, 7,* 1034–1941.

Glass, A. J. (1955). Current problems in military psychiatry. *Journal of the American Medical Association,* 6–10.

Grieger, T. A., Bally, R. E., Lyszczarz, J. L. Kennedy, J. S., Griffeth, B. T., & Reeves, J. J. (2003). Individual and organizational interventions after terrorism: September 11 and the *USS Cole.* In R. J. Ursano, C. S. Fullerton, & A. E. Norwood (Eds.), *Terrorism and disaster* (pp. 71–92). New York: Cambridge University Press.

McCarroll, J. E., Jaccard, J. J., & Radke, A. Q. (1994) Psychiatric consultation to command. In F. D. Jones, L. R. Sparacino, V. A. Wilcox, & J. M. Rothberg (Eds.), *Military psychiatry: Preparing in peace for war.* Washington, DC: Office of the Army Surgeon General at TMM Publications, Borden Institute, Walter Reed Army Medical Center.

Menninger, W. C. (1944). Psychiatry and the Army. *Psychiatry: Journal of the Biology and Pathology of Interpersonal Relations, 7,* 175–181.

Rioch, D. M. (1955). Problems of preventive psychiatry in war. *Psychopathology of childhood* (Vol. 10, pp. 146–165). New York: Grune & Stratton.

Salmon, T. W. (1929). The care and treatment of mental diseases and war neurosis ("shell shock") in the British Army. In P. Bailey, F. E. Williams, & P. O Komora (Eds.), *The medical department of the United States Army in the World War: Vol X. Neuropsychiatry* (pp. 497–523). Washington, DC: Government Printing Office.

Shalev, A. Y. (2000). Stress management and debriefing: Historical concepts and present patterns. In J. P. Wilson & B. Raphael (Eds.), *Psychological debriefing: Theory, practice, and evidence* (pp. 17–31). Cambridge, UK: Cambridge University Press.

Shalev, A. Y., Peri, T., Rogel-Fuchs, Y., Ursano, R. J., & Marlowe, D. H. (1996). Historical group debriefing following exposure to combat stress. *Military Medicine, 163,* 494–498.

Stuart, J. A., Ursano, R. J., Fullerton, C. S., Norwood, A. E., & Murray, K. (2003). Belief in exposure to terrorist agents: Reported exposure to nerve or mustard gas by Gulf War veterans. *Journal of Nervous and Mental Disease, 171,* 431–436.

Ursano, R. J., McCarroll, J. E., & Fullerton, C. S. (2003). Traumatic death in terrorism and disasters: The effects on posttraumatic stress and behavior. In R. J. Ursano, C. S. Fullerton, & A. E. Norwood (Eds.), *Terrorism and disaster* (pp. 308–340). New York: Cambridge University Press.

Ursano, R. J., & Norwood, A. E. (Eds.). (2003). *Trauma and disaster responses and management*. Washington, DC: American Psychiatric Publishing.

Ursano, R. J., Norwood, A. E., Fullerton, C. S., Holloway, H. C., & Hall, M. (2003). Terrorism with weapons of mass destruction: Chemical, biological, nuclear, radiological, and explosive agents. In R. J. Ursano & A. E. Norwood (Eds.), *Trauma and disaster responses and management* (pp. 125–154). Arlington, VA: American Psychiatric Publishing.

CHAPTER 12

On a Road Paved with Good Intentions, You Still Need a Compass

Monitoring and Evaluating Disaster Mental Health Services

CRAIG S. ROSEN, HELENA E. YOUNG, and FRAN H. NORRIS

WHY EVALUATE DISASTER MENTAL HEALTH PROGRAMS?

Crisis mental health services, by their nature, are delivered in a chaotic, rapidly evolving environment in which decisions need to be made quickly, on the basis on limited information. The prejudice is toward action, not deliberation. As a result of this necessary bias, program activities may be implemented inefficiently, interventions may have unintended consequences, or the program may operate on a set of false assumptions about the best means of ameliorating acute stress symptoms or the nature of effective service delivery—particularly when the clinical and logistical knowledge base is drawn largely from impressions of previous disasters rather than empirical data. Racing down the road of good intentions, one can still end up in a ditch.

Contributions of Program Evaluation

This chapter aims to provide a brief guide to conducting or understanding program evaluations in the aftermath of disaster. Program evaluation refers to systematic efforts to collect, analyze, and interpret information about the execution or effectiveness of interventions (Shadish, Cook, & Leviton, 1991). During the crisis, there may be little interest in collecting systematic information on how the program is working. This shortcoming makes it difficult to monitor program progress, provides few data with which to later evaluate program achievements, and hampers sharing of innovations. Without systematic evaluation, programs have limited means of crystalizing what they discovered from experience in a way that can be communicated to other people planning responses to future events.

Beyond helping specific programs document their work, program evaluation is a promising strategy for increasing the knowledge base that guides program policy. Evaluation may identify key challenges that need to be addressed. For example, children are known to be a group at high risk for psychological problems following disasters. However, a recent review of crisis counseling grants funded by the Federal Emergency Management Agency (FEMA) and administered by the Center for Mental Health Services (CMHS) over a 5-year period indicated that children were consistently underserved by most crisis counseling programs (Norris et al., 2005). This finding might inform policy innovations such as negotiating advance agreements to allow delivery of disaster mental health services through the schools as part of predisaster planning.

Evaluation can also identify variations in effectiveness across programs. We found that some crisis counseling programs reached over four times as many consumers as did other programs with a similar level of funding (Norris et al., 2005). However, inconsistencies in evaluation methods and data quality across programs precluded our pinpointing the specific community or program design elements that contributed to some programs having more successful outreach. By collecting data more systematically and consistently across future programs, we may be able to make better judgments about program-level factors that influence service delivery.

In addition, empirical knowledge about best practices is still very limited. Unsound counseling practices may be perpetuated, while innovations and improvements are not disseminated. For example, in the past, many crisis counseling programs made frequent use of psychological debriefing, but recent research suggests that this practice typically has little benefit and can even exacerbate some survivors' symptoms (Litz & Gray, 2002; Rose, Bisson, & Wessely, 2003). By encouraging pilot testing of new innovations, such problems may be avoided in the future. This goal requires that programs have access to evaluation measures and strategies that they can use to test the outcomes of special initiatives.

In summary, whether the questions concern how to improve the reach of the service delivery system or how to improve the efficacy of the services themselves, program evaluation provides an empirical basis for the answers. Our proposed framework for future evaluation of disaster mental health services attempts to improve practice in a way that adheres to the goals and standards of program evaluation science.

Types of Program Evaluation

Evaluation has different purposes, and calls for different strategies, at different stages in the life of a program—from the earliest stages of its definition, or needs assessment, through its phases of development and organization, service delivery, and sustainability. One important distinction is between *process evaluations*, which focus on program processes, and *outcome evaluations,* which focus on a program's results (see Figure 12.1). Process evaluations often assume that we know what types of activities and services are potentially helpful and assess how they are implemented. Outcome evaluations assume that we do not in fact know whether various program processes are effective and directly assess their impact.

Distinctions are also made between *program monitoring* and *summative evaluation.* Both are systematic attempts to gather and analyze information on a program's performance, but their purposes and foci are somewhat different.

Program monitoring refers to data that are collected data throughout the life of a program to assess "in real time" whether service delivery processes are proceeding as planned. It is a management tool used to allow program administrators to make corrections as they go, to ensure that the project is proceeding (more or less) according to plan, and to enable midcourse corrections. Expanding on the driving metaphor of our chapter

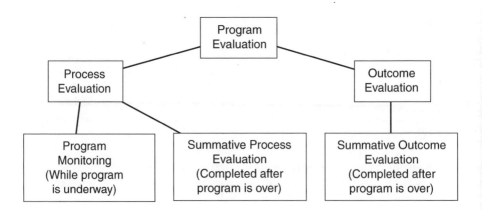

FIGURE 12.1. Types of program evaluations relevant to disaster mental health.

title, program monitoring can be thought of as looking through the windshield while driving to make sure that we are driving in the proper lane and checking the speedometer to make sure that we are going at the right speed. At its best, program monitoring is conceived of as a basic constituent of daily operations, not as an "add-on" activity conducted after the fact. Because it must be implemented quickly and efficiently, program monitoring typically focuses on easily measurable indicators that can be tracked over time, such as the number of treatment contacts or client satisfaction.

Summative evaluation is a more comprehensive review conducted to assess program processes and results. It may encompass a wider range of activities than does program monitoring. Like program monitoring, summative evaluation may consider how well a program is implemented, but it can also address more deep-seated questions about what makes a program effective. In the short course of most disaster mental health programs, the data that speak to these questions may not be on hand or fully analyzed until after a program is completed. These results may be more helpful for planning responses to *future* disasters than for modifying responses to the *current* crisis. A summative evaluation might not only consider implementation issues but also assess broader, policy-related questions such as objectives and strategies. Returning to our driving analogy, a summative evaluation might consider not only whether we were driving safely, but also whether the road we selected actually leads toward our desired destination *(policy objectives)* and whether it might have been wiser for us to fly rather than drive *(strategies)*.

STANDARDS OF A GOOD PROGRAM EVALUATION

Program evaluation standards provide a referent for decision making when trade-offs must be made in the evaluation process. Adherence to these benchmarks helps to produce an evenhanded assessment, one that is *useful, feasible* to accomplish, *ethical,* and technically *accurate.* (For more detail on these various points, the reader may consult Fleischman & Wood, 2002; Patton, 1978; Scriven, 1993; University of Kansas Work Group, 2004.)

Utility

Evaluations must answer questions of concern to the people who will be affected by, or have investment in, the evaluation results. To that end, these individuals ("stakeholders") must be identified, so that their needs can be addressed. Stakeholders include the persons involved in program operations, such as managers, team leaders, and crisis counselors. Stakeholders also include the people and communities that are served or affected by the program, such as consumers, potential consumers, neighborhood organizations and advocacy groups, and local political leadership. Funding and administrative agencies, such as FEMA and CMHS, are also stakeholders. Stakeholders will make different judgments about the utility of evaluations depending on what they believe to be important. For some stakeholders, adherence to empirically validated practice guidelines is most critical, whereas for other stakeholders, reaching out to the community may be most important. In part, the evaluator's job is to make these values explicit. Midcourse findings should be disclosed to the program sponsor so that results can be used in a timely way. Throughout, the evaluation should be conducted and reported in such a way to optimize its influence on stakeholder follow-through.

Feasibility

The practicality of an evaluation is reflected in the reasonableness of its scope, given available resources, and its political viability. Is the information gathered in such a way that interference with program process is minimized? Is the evaluation planned and conducted bearing in mind the different interests of the various stakeholders? Is the evaluation cost-effective (i.e., does it produce information sufficiently constructive so that the resource investment in the evaluation can be justified)?

Ethics

An ethical evaluation is conducted with regard for the rights and welfare of all involved parties. Formal agreements establish areas of accountability (deliverables, timelines, responsible parties) that can be renegotiated as appropriate. The rights of human participants must be protected, and ongoing consultations with participants should bear in mind their values and perspectives, so that neither the evaluation process nor the use of the data is viewed as threatening. A challenge for the evaluator is responding to the needs of a wide range of stakeholders while not becoming a sponsor of any one constituency. Conflicts of interest must be dealt with openly, to prevent compromise of the evaluation process and results.

Accuracy

The evaluation procedures should be described in enough detail so that they themselves can be monitored. Defensible sources of information lend integrity to results. Measures with empirically proven validity and reliability should be used to assess outcomes. Methodical data review minimizes error correction and missing information. Systematic examination of both quantitative (e.g., contact sheets, encounter logs, and questionnaires) and qualitative (coded narrative of interviews, focus groups) information provides a richness of source material, resulting in conclusions that can be justified.

CONDUCTING A PROGRAM EVALUATION

To achieve these attributes, effective program evaluation typically involves a sequence of integrated steps, summarized in Table 12.1. (For further detail, see Bickman, 1987; Lipsey, 1993; Mowbray, 1988; Rossi, Freeman, & Lipsey, 1999; University of Kansas Work Group, 2004; Weiss, 1997.)

TABLE 12.1. Steps in Conducting a Program Evaluation

Steps	Elements
1. Engage the stakeholders.	• Identify and enlist stakeholders. • Differentiate among immediate, intermediate, and long-term stakeholder concerns.
2. Describe how program works.	• Develop program logic model. • Define inputs, processes of care, outputs, and outcomes of care.
3. Focus questions and design.	• Articulate program questions. • Key the design to process vs. outcome assessments, tradeoffs between sound scientific method and pragmatism.
4. Gather credible evidence.	• Identify performance indicators and reliable information sources. • Outline logistics.
5. Justify conclusions.	• Elucidate methodology and present interpretations. • Attend to insider/outsider perspectives, considerations of timeliness versus accuracy, methodological and face validity, standards and values.
6. Share results, lessons learned.	• Obtain stakeholder feedback, follow-up comments and reactions. • Disseminate findings.

Step 1. Engaging Stakeholders

Without "buy-in" from key stakeholders, evaluations are unlikely to influence policy. Disaster mental health programs are conducted in partnership with agencies and individuals directly participating or interested in the evaluation process and its results, and thus any cooperative effort must consider the values held by those partners. Identification of stakeholders at the outset of an evaluation and encouragement of their involvement help to create a sense of ownership by ensuring that their perspectives are understood and that essential elements of the program are not being ignored, lending credibility to the process. Failure to engage stakeholders, on the other hand, may end in the discounting of findings, especially when conclusions contradict the policies of the program under study.

Evaluators must maintain equilibrium between scientific inquiry and the pragmatics of organizational imperatives and real-world constraints. Therefore, it is important to identify the primary client at the start of the process: Who will "own" the data, and who gets to put the "spin" on results? The evaluation is more likely to work well if it is designed to meet the needs of multiple parties.

When a program evaluation is planned in real time, particularly in a situation as emotionally charged as disaster recovery, evaluation may not be seen as a priority; instead, it may be viewed as arbitrary and burdensome, imposed by outsiders without a stake in serving survivors. For the evaluation process to proceed effectively, it must be seen as a relevant and worthwhile management tool that answers questions of concern to stakeholders and advances consumer care. Thus, a good deal of groundwork is required in order to obtain endorsement from stakeholder groups, across the spectrum of involved individuals.

What are the mechanics of stakeholder engagement in the evaluation process? We suggest that the evaluator start from the vantage of inquiring of the stakeholder representatives: "What will this evaluation do for you? What is it that you want to know? Who do you have to answer to? What does that mandating authority care about?" They should invite discussion about immediate, intermediate, and long-term concerns, with respect to both process and outcome issues. If a desired outcome of the evaluation process is to shape services delivery or impact policy, that agenda—detailing the types of policies the stakeholder is attempting to inform or influence—should be built into discussions about evaluation design and implementation at the start, and policy goals should be incorporated into the design. Allowing the stakeholders to review the first draft of findings may contribute to a sense of affiliation in the process.

Step 2. Describing How the Program Works

Program evaluation or program monitoring is much more likely to be useful and meaningful if it is grounded in an understanding of how a program operates: what resources it has, what it does, what it produces, and what societal benefits it is trying to achieve. This understanding is often termed a "program theory" or "logic model" (Weiss, 1997). Program theory can be thought of as the sequence of causal assumptions, as well as the beliefs and expectations underlying the processes of a program; these provide a rationale for the benefits that these processes are expected to produce. Program theory, however, is rarely articulated for social services programs, much less for those dealing in disaster mental health, which are usually designed around experience, practice knowledge, and intuition. One of the immediate benefits of an evaluation effort may be making explicit the assumptions on which the program is based. This enables evaluators, program staff, and sponsors not only to better assess *what* a program is achieving but also to better explore *why* a program is more or less successful in meeting its stated objectives.

A program logic model typically includes several elements—inputs, processes, outputs, and outcomes. Figure 12.2 presents an example model.

Inputs are the resources available to the program for use in achieving its goals. Some inputs are tangible resources: funding, program staff, office space, office supplies and other consumables, transportation, and so on. Others are less concrete but equally important: the skills and expertise of program staff, the relationships among staff and with local community leaders, and the delineation of responsibilities among the different agencies involved. Lack of one or more of these needed contributions can greatly limit an organization's ability to deliver services.

Given the unexpected nature of disasters, crisis counseling programs often are initiated *before* all the necessary inputs are in position. For example, service delivery may begin before there is a financial system in place for transferring funds, or a clear chain of command among agencies, and before working relationships have been established with key local community leaders. In these situations, one of the first tasks of the program is initiating the preparatory processes to obtain these needed inputs, such as working with state governments to set up a compatible fiscal accounting system and means of funds transfer, negotiating and delineating responsibilities with participating agencies, or soliciting the advocacy of local political leadership.

Activities or processes are the means used to bring about program objectives. Such processes might include outreach to affected people in the community, providing classes or community education on normal re-

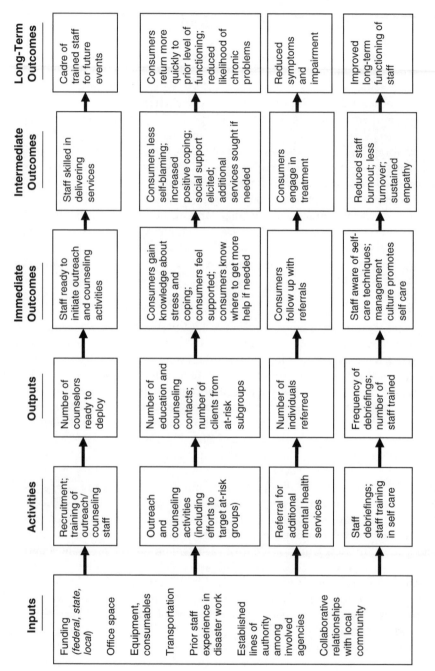

FIGURE 12.2. Example of a logic model for a crisis counseling program.

sponses to trauma, public relations efforts to increase community awareness of the agency's services, training secondary helpers in how to provide reassurance and support to facilitate recovery, providing brief individual or group counseling or more extensive intervention, or arranging treatment referrals for individuals with more severe mental health needs.

Outputs are the measurable units of product from a program's processes. Evaluations often focus on the outputs of the service delivery process, such as the numbers of outreach visits concluded, individuals in receipt of counseling, educational classes conducted, or individuals screened and referred for more extensive treatment. In some cases, evaluations conclude with the elucidation of outputs, which are used as a proxy for outcomes. In other cases, outcomes need to be measured directly in order to assess whether services are truly having an impact.

Outcomes are the societal benefits. While outputs assess "how much" was done, outcomes focus on "how much good" was done. Outcomes represent the least well specified, least understood, and least well measured arena in disaster mental health research. Currently, there exist limited solid empirical data on how much good disaster mental health interventions actually accomplish. Outcomes can be considered in the short (immediate), intermediate, and long term. *Immediate outcomes* are those that can be observed directly after completing an activity. *Intermediate outcomes* are those that derive from immediate outcomes such as alleviation of psychiatric symptoms, reduced substance use, or improved role functioning. *Long-term outcomes* may include posttraumatic growth, community cohesion, establishment of a disaster preparedness infrastructure, or community resilience in dealing with subsequent crises.

Step 3. Focusing the Evaluation Questions and Design

Evaluations are more likely to be successful if they are focused on particular issues or elements of concern. Focusing an evaluation requires articulating, "What is it we want to know?" The questions to be answered should then drive the evaluation design. Having a logic model can be useful in helping staff members decide which aspects of a program's operations should be evaluated. Historically, when disaster mental services are evaluated at all, they have typically focused on outputs: how many people got what types of services. Evaluations less commonly assess details of process: exactly what was done and how it was delivered. Aside from a few research studies, outcomes of disaster mental health services—indices of whether interventions actually improve the lives of consumers—have generally not been measured. Various questions might be advanced about a program by its staff, payors, or evaluators, and these will have implications for design.

The type of evaluation (process or outcome, monitoring or summative) to be conducted depends on the question to be answered.

Process evaluations (both program monitoring and summative process evaluations) can often be conducted with an observational design. The evaluator can monitor the number of outreach contacts completed each week to track changes over time or compare the number of outreach contacts achieved by teams that use different outreach strategies. Process evaluations and program monitoring may also involve benchmarking (i.e., comparing observations to some standard).

Outcome evaluations typically compare individuals who have and have not received an intervention along key variables. In the simplest case, consumers are compared with themselves before and after an intervention; this is called a preexperimental or pre–post design. Such a design may be adequate to assess an immediate outcome, such as knowledge gained from a workshop, which normally would not change with time. A pre–post design is typically inadequate for evaluating the effect of services on intermediate or long-term outcomes relating to symptoms, coping style, or role functioning because, for most trauma survivors, functioning normally improves over time. Evaluation of this sort usually requires some type of comparison group that did not receive the services to be assayed, the members of which are compared to program clients in a quasi-experimental or experimental design. The most valid test of an intervention is of course an experimental design in which receipt of an intervention is determined randomly. This methodology ensures that differences in outcomes are actually due to the intervention itself and not to self-selection on the part of certain types of clients who wish to obtain the service (e.g., psychologically minded clients may be more likely to request counseling). When experimental designs are not feasible to carry out, more limited conclusions can be drawn from quasi-experimental or naturalistic methods.

Step 4. Gathering Credible Evidence

The collection of data that lend believability to an evaluation requires identification of program performance indicators and reliable sources of information and workable logistics. Indicators are gauges that measure a program's dependent variables: They are the standards used to monitor or evaluate program success or outcome. Indicators are the program processes, outputs, or outcomes that need to be assessed in order to answer the evaluation question. It is the job of the evaluator to ensure that these criteria are defensible, and that the relative weight given to each criterion is justified. The evaluator needs to operationalize the concepts that address the outputs and outcomes of concern (e.g., number of clients receiving services, changes in consumer symptoms or behaviors, or changes in community conditions). For indicators of success to be meaningful, they must exhibit good construct validity (measure what they claim to be measuring). Sources of data include documents, observations of the program in action, structured self-report measures such as questionnaires, or the more open-ended testimony of people involved in program operations. Logistics are the pragmatic considerations of how data will be collected and how accuracy (validity and reliability) will be maximized. The logistics of evidence collection comprise the methods, timing, and physical infrastructure for gathering and managing information (e.g., instrument design, data collection procedures, and the training of personnel involved in data collection, coding, and data management, including routine error checking). Techniques used by evaluators must be in keeping with cultural norms and preferences and must ensure participant confidentiality.

Assessing changes in consumers' functioning presents the evaluator with a set of remarkable dilemmas: Assessing changes in functioning requires following people over time, but following people over time raises concerns about privacy. Tracking consumers' improvement over time requires knowing who they are and how to contact them. Measuring change over time requires that consumers agree to confidentiality ("We know who you are, but promise we won't tell anyone else") rather than anonymity ("Even *we* don't know who you are"). Standards for maintaining confidentiality in research are well established and could easily be adopted in disaster mental health evaluations; whether most consumers of crisis counseling would have adequate confidence in these procedures has yet to be determined. In addition, evaluating outcomes may require obtaining data from individuals who were not program clients. After a disaster, most people return to normal functioning with time. Demonstrating that an intervention produces better-than-normal-outcomes (or at least faster recovery) requires comparing the improvements shown by individuals who did and did not receive the intervention (or by those who received different ones).

Step 5. Justifying Conclusions

Evaluation is ultimately not about gathering data but about using data to draw conclusions. Is the program being implemented as planned? Is it effective in producing desired outputs and achieving desired outcomes? Which aspects of the program work well and which do not? A major question in program evaluation is who analyzes the data? Analysts internal to the organization have a deep understanding of its goals and procedures but may not be sufficiently independent to highlight problems with impunity. External evaluators, on the other hand, may lack sufficient understanding of program realities. One solution to this dilemma is a collaborative analytical process, drawing conclusions derived from both outsider and insider per-spectives.

In the program monitoring process, timeliness is as important as accu-racy. Data analysis will often be descriptive or visual (simple graphs) rather than statistical. In contrast, summative evaluations, which are conducted with less time pressure, and which may have more enduring effects on future policy, should involve more rigorous analytical techniques. Evalua-tions may require involvement of academic researchers or professional evaluators who can contribute appropriate technical expertise. A necessary but not sufficient requirement of evaluation is that the analysis and the con-clusions drawn from the data are methodologically sound. However, the analysis must also demonstrate face validity in the view of decision makers, for whom graphs and statistics may not be meaningful. Evaluators may find that their results are most credible if they use a combination of quanti-tative data, case-study findings, and compelling illustrative examples to shed light on the program.

Evaluations results are open to interpretation. A program may access a large number of clients but penetrate only a fraction of the total population at risk. Do stakeholders see this result as a glass "half empty" or "half full"? Evaluation results are more likely to be accepted as credible if the cri-teria for "success" are defined in advance and there is buy-in from stake-holders vis-à-vis reasonable standards for program achievement. Program results may also involve trade-offs in outcome: staffers who tirelessly throw themselves into their work may realize greater customer satisfaction but exhibit greater burnout. An innovative program may serve fewer clients but attain better results for those it serves. Different stakeholder groups may judge these exchanges differently.

Step 6. Sharing Evaluation Findings

Evaluations are only useful to the extent that their results are communi-cated effectively to people who have the power to improve programs. In program monitoring, program managers should regularly share results in staff meetings, quarterly updates, or even graphs posted on the wall. This feedback can then facilitate discussion on means to improve services. For example, noting that one outreach team dramatically increased its number of client contacts may promote sharing by field workers of an innovative outreach technique. Or, it might reveal that the team is counting cursory contacts as outreach visits, allowing the supervisor to give staffers feedback about ways to deepen their discussions with survivors. It is critical that monitoring results be shared in a climate that is supportive and curious ("What might these data be telling us?") rather than rigid and punitive.

Results of a summative evaluation may not be available until a program has been underway for some time, or after it is over. Even so, it is often extremely valuable to share preliminary results with program staff, sponsors, and other stakeholders (such as community leaders or a program's community advisors) prior to completing a final report. The occasion for commentary increases stakeholder buy-in to the results and provides opportunity for participants to identify important issues that the evaluator may have overlooked. Process evaluations may also generate information on good practices, innovative approaches, or common challenges, which can be shared with other programs through training materials, online discussion groups, or other venues. Some evaluations may produce results suitable for publication. Communication of evaluation findings are of course most likely to be effective if it employs simple nontechnical language, includes vivid examples, and conveys clear conclusions and recommendations.

CHALLENGES OF POSTDISASTER EVALUATIONS

Conducting program evaluation in the aftermath of disasters poses special challenges. For one thing, the kinds of mental health services delivered tend to evolve over time as the needs of the survivors change. They often must be adapted to address the distinctive ethnographic signature of the community, and providers in the field have a sense of "learning as they go." Therefore, evaluations cannot assume that services are being delivered based on a preordained, unchanging model. This makes it essential to continually (re)define and document the program services and delivery strategies in order to be able to evaluate what the program is actually doing at different points in time.

Evaluation results are impacted by the surrounding community context, which also evolves over time. For example, client satisfaction results may be higher during early phases of recovery than during later stages, when community services begin to be withdrawn and disillusionment sets in (see Athey, 1999; Lipsey, 1993). Longitudinal studies may be preferred to cross-sectional studies for this and other evaluation questions that may be phase-dependent.

Moreover, outreach programs may identify problems that existed prior to the disaster but that might otherwise have remained undiscovered (Athey, 1999). For example, a needs assessment survey conducted after September 11 confirmed that 64% of New York City schoolchildren had experienced other potentially traumatic events prior to the World Trade Center attack (Hoven et al., 2002). Evaluations must therefore be careful to differentiate increased detection of preexisting problems from those arising *de novo.*

An additional challenge in evaluating crisis counseling programs is that the need for assessment may not be apparent until it is too late to conduct a valid evaluation. Despite the increasing shift in the health care system toward greater accountability, standards are different in the wake of disaster. There is an ethic that disaster relief funds are more or less an entitlement of the affected community. Federal sponsors assume that something must be done and thus work with state agencies in a hurried and enthusiastic collaboration to establish programs and release funds. In the press to expedite service delivery, program managers may have limited interest in (or resources for) implementing an evaluation component that is not seen to have immediate benefit, even if it is useful in the long term. If an evaluation plan is not in place at the outbreak of a disaster event, then program assessment is likely not to occur. Demands for accountability and demonstrating effectiveness often are not heard until the initial crisis counseling grants are winding down and programs are seeking sustainability funding from other sources. By this point it is too late to put a strong evaluation effort in place. This leaves a program vulnerable to getting a grade after the fact, without knowing what the scoring criteria were.

DEVELOPING AN "EVALUATION CULTURE"

In this chapter, we have aimed to make the case that monitoring and evaluating disaster mental health programs can make critical contributions to improving services by enlarging the empirical knowledge base that informs disaster response. The tracking of activities and outputs in disaster mental health programs has been generally unsystematic; the tracking of outcomes has been virtually nonexistent. The question before us now is how to establish an evaluation infrastructure that will allow us to maximize learning in future crisis events. This requires laying groundwork in the various areas outlined below.

• *Build advance political support for evaluation.* Instilling an evaluation culture in disaster mental health requires creating an evaluation planning component in state emergency disaster preparedness programs. Embedded in this ethos would be a respect for quality management informed by empirical feedback, supported by sound recordkeeping and data collection, and the expectation of accountability. In conjunction with top-down support, it is equally important to establish a dialogue among key stakeholders involved in postdisaster recovery—at federal, state, and local levels—to set evaluation policy for future disaster events; this dialectic is needed to ensure that the evaluation mandate is feasible, relevant to real-world concerns, and not unduly burdensome. Sponsors of disaster mental health programs might consider convening an ongoing working group comprised of state disaster planners to share lessons learned and to give voice to their perceived evaluation needs.

• *Create a library of ready-to-use data collection, data management, and reporting tools.* We perceive a pressing need for a standardized data collection toolkit, to be used across disaster mental health programs countrywide, to record client contacts, client characteristics, and program activities. The toolkit should also include brief, reliable, and empirically validated measures of client symptoms and role functioning, both to evaluate program outcomes and to inform decisions about clinical intervention and referral. Together with common measures, the toolkit could include modular inserts pitched to the type of disaster event (e.g., a naturalistic event such as a flood or hurricane vs. an incident of mass violence). All these materials should include automated tools for data entry, scoring, analysis, and report generation from toolkit data.

• *Establish a cadre of technical assistance personnel.* Evaluation tools may be of little use without in-place technical support to assist programs in implementing, managing, and interpreting these tools and measures. Technical assistance will be needed to help program staff clarify evaluation questions and designs, to train local champions in techniques for eliciting buy-in for the evaluation process, to educate staff in the accurate use of toolkit materials, and to instruct managers in the use of program monitoring to inform administrative decisions. Provision of technical help may be especially important in less publicized disasters that do not attract assistance from academic researchers.

• *Initiate serious discourse about privacy protection in outcomes measurement.* Evaluating program outcomes is likely to require collecting data on individual consumers, contrary to the tradition in crisis counseling, for which few records are kept in deference to consumer concerns about stigma and privacy. Although some researchers have successfully resolved this problem in volunteer samples (North, Pfefferbaum, & Tucker, 2002), a broader discussion on the subject of reconciling data collection with the protection of consumer welfare is overdue (Jones, 2003). This exchange should bring together medical ethicists, evaluators, trauma researchers, crisis counseling staff, and consumer representatives.

• *Include funding for evaluation in disaster mental health assistance.* Conducting evaluations requires resources. Applications for disaster mental health services should request the financial and administrative support base needed to maintain monitoring and evaluation functions; grant-making authorities should provide support for such activities, including training in data collection, to avoid placing undue burden on service delivery operations.

Disaster mental health is in an extremely exciting stage of development. Most of the knowledge that guides crisis counseling services is based on anecdotal experience and conventional wisdom. Much of the empirical understanding we do have about the effectiveness of postcrisis interventions derives from more easily researched analog populations, such as motor vehicle accident victims. If the next generation of crisis mental health interventions is to be informed by empirical data from real disasters, that information cannot be obtained in the laboratory. We need to establish the necessary infrastructure to conduct meaningful program evaluation in the field, on the fly, as disaster mental health services are being delivered.

REFERENCES

Athey, J. (1999, November). *FEMA/CMHS Crisis Counseling Assistance and Training Program Work Group on Program Evaluation and Research*. Brookville, MD: Health Policy Resources Group.

Bickman, L. (1987). The functions of program theory. In L. Bickman (Ed.), *Using program theory in evaluation* (New Directions for Program Evaluation No. 33, pp. 5–18). San Francisco: Jossey-Bass.

Fleischman, A. R., & Wood, E. B. (2002). Ethical issues in research involving victims of terror. *Journal of Urban Health, 79,* 315–321.

Hoven, C. W., Duarte, C. S., Cohen, M. C., Lucas, C., Gregorian, N., Rosen, C. S., et al. (2002). *Effects of the World Trade Center attack on NYC public school students*. New York: New York City Board of Education.

Jones, G. E. (2003). Crisis intervention, crisis counseling, confidentiality, and privilege. *International Journal of Emergency Mental Health, 5,* 137–140.

Lipsey, M. W. (1993). *Theory as method: Small theories of treatments* (New Directions for Program Evaluation No. 57, pp. 5–38). San Francisco: Jossey-Bass.

Litz, B., & Gray, M. (2002). Early intervention for mass violence: What is the evidence, what should be done? *Cognitive and Behavioral Practice, 9,* 266–272.

Mowbray, C. T. (1988). Getting the system to respond to evaluation findings. In J. A. McLaughlin, L. J. Weber, R. W. Covert, & R. B. Ingle (Eds.), *Evaluation utilization* (New Directions for Program Evaluation No. 39. pp. 5–38). San Francisco: Jossey-Bass.

Norris, F. H., Rosen, C. S., Elrod, C. L., Young, H. E., Gibson, L. E., & Hamblen, J. L. (2005). *Retrospective 5-year evaluation of the crisis counseling assistance and training program*. White River Junction, VT: U.S. Department of Veterans Affairs, National Center for Posttraumatic Stress Disorder.

North, C. S., Pfefferbaum, B., & Tucker, P. (2002). Ethical and methodological issues in academic mental health research in populations affected by disasters:

The Oklahoma City experience relevant to September 11, 2001. *CNS Spectrum, 7,* 580–584.

Patton, M. Q. (1978). *Utilization-focused evaluation.* Beverly Hills, CA: Sage.

Rose, S., Bisson, J., & Wessely, S. (2003). A systematic review of single-session psychological intervention ("debriefing") following trauma. *Psychotherapy and Psychosomatics, 72,* 171–175.

Rossi, P. H., Freeman, H. E., & Lipsey, M. W. (1999). *Evaluation: A systematic approach* (6th ed.). Thousand Oaks, CA: Sage.

Scriven, M. (1993). *Hard won lessons in program evaluation* (New Directions in Program Evaluation No. 58). San Francisco: Jossey-Bass.

Shadish, W. R., Cook, T. D., & Leviton, L. C. (1991). *Foundations of program evaluation: Theories of practice.* Newbury Park, CA.: Sage.

University of Kansas Work Group on Health Promotion and Community Development. (2004). *Community toolbox* [Online]. Retrieved from www.ctb.ku.edu

Weiss, C. H. (1997). How can theory-based evaluation make greater headway? *Evaluation Review, 21,* 501–524.

P A R T   I V

SPECIFIC SITUATIONS AND POPULATIONS

CHAPTER 13

Interventions for Children and Adolescents Following Disasters

JUDITH A. COHEN, ANTHONY P. MANNARINO, LAURA E. GIBSON, STEPHEN J. COZZA, MELISSA J. BRYMER, and LAURA MURRAY

Children and adolescents are not immune from the ill effects of disasters and mass violence. Children respond not only to the traumatic nature of such situations but also to the emotional distress of their parents, teachers, and community leaders. Adult support is a strong protective factor for traumatized children (Pine & Cohen, 2002), and, conversely, community traumas that adversely affect adults can make at-risk children more vulnerable to potentially serious and long-lasting mental health problems. Children who lose loved ones in disasters may develop childhood traumatic grief, a condition in which trauma symptoms impinge upon the child's ability to negotiate the normal grieving process (Cohen, Mannarino, Greenberg, Padlo, & Shipley, 2002). Combined with the interruption of parental support that often accompanies a familial death, this condition may place children at even greater risk for ongoing emotional difficulties. It is therefore important to consider the special needs of children in the wake of community traumas.

This chapter reviews empirical treatment studies of children following disasters and mass violence, as well as the more extensive literature on treating children traumatized by interpersonal violence. It discusses the benefits and challenges of conducting widespread early screening of children following disasters and offers a synthesis of which children to treat, how to treat them, when such treatment should be offered, and how to optimally train community therapists to provide these treatments. Special attention is paid to children of emergency services and military members, and a case study of outreach efforts in New York following the World Trade Center bombing in 2001 is described. Future clinical and research needs are also addressed.

EMPIRICAL LITERATURE

Child Interventions Following Disasters

Few scientifically rigorous child treatment studies have been conducted in the early aftermath of disasters for a variety of reasons discussed elsewhere (Cohen, 2003). It is important to recognize that although most treatment studies for traumatized children focus on symptoms of posttraumatic stress disorder (PTSD), children respond to trauma with a wide variety of symptoms and may develop depressive, behavioral, substance use, or other anxiety problems in addition to or instead of PTSD. These children obviously also deserve clinical attention, but this multiplicity of symptoms complicates screening and treatment, both clinically and from a research standpoint. The following section attempts to briefly review and synthesize what is known about treating children following disaster or mass violence. Due to space limitations, this review only includes studies that used well-defined treatment interventions and reported the use of pre- to posttreatment changes on standardized assessment instruments.

The strongest conclusions can be drawn from studies that use a randomized controlled treatment (RCT) design. Unfortunately RCTs for disaster-exposed children are scarce. Field, Seligman, Scafidi, and Schanberg (1996) compared two sessions of massage therapy to an attention control condition provided to children within the first month after being exposed to a hurricane and found that children in the massage condition experienced greater reduction in depression and anxiety. PTSD was not measured, and the study had a number of methodological shortcomings. Another RCT conducted by Chemtob, Nakashima, and Carlson (2002) compared eye movement desensitization and reprocessing (EMDR) to a wait-list control condition, provided to children who continued to have PTSD 3 years after exposure to a hurricane. They demonstrated that three sessions of EMDR resulted in greater improvement in PTSD, anxiety, and depression. Another RCT by this group compared individual or group cognitive-behavioral interventions to a lagged treatment control group and demonstrated that the active treatment (whether provided in individual or group settings) resulted in greater improvement in PTSD symptoms (Chemtob, Nakashima, & Hamada, 2002). Hardin and colleagues (2002) compared group catastrophic stress intervention (CSI) (psychoeducation, art, and "visual imagery" interventions, which were provided three times a year over 3 years) to no treatment. Subjects were adolescents who had been exposed to a hurricane. The treatment group had less psychological distress at 12, 18, and 24 months than the no-treatment group; these differences were no longer present at 30 and 36 months. These studies are the only published RCTs for disaster-exposed children.

Non-RCT studies have also provided useful information with regard to potentially effective interventions following mass disasters. Goenjian and colleagues (1997) compared a combined trauma- and grief-focused cognitive-behavioral group and individual intervention to a no-treatment control group, for early adolescents exposed to a severe earthquake in Armenia. Two schools received the intervention, while two other schools served as controls. Although PTSD symptoms improved and depressive symptoms were unchanged in the treatment group, both PTSD and depressive symptoms worsened in the untreated group. Yule (1992) provided debriefing and an open cognitive-behavioral group treatment to 24 children who survived a ship's sinking. Compared to children at another school who did not receive early interventions, the treated children had lower scores on the Impact of Event Scale (IES) and fewer self-reported fears. Unfortunately, the psychological characteristics of children in the untreated school and the specific treatment interventions used were poorly defined in this study.

Several uncontrolled treatment studies have also been conducted for children following mass violence. Debriefing was provided to 26 children involved in a hostage-taking incident, half of whom had developed PTSD symptoms. After 7 months only four of these children had PTSD (Vila, Porche, & Mouren-Simeoni, 1999). The lack of a control group and the fact that several of these children also received individual therapy make it impossible to assess how much if any of this improvement was due to the debriefing intervention. Stallard and Law (1993) provided debriefing 5 months after a school bus crash, to seven children who had survived the crash. Group scores on the IES and on depression and anxiety decreased 3 months later, but the absence of a control group and other methodological limitations make it difficult to evaluate what caused this improvement.

Treatment studies for children who have lost loved ones in traumatic circumstances also provide important information, as disasters and mass violence may result in child bereavement and some of these children will develop childhood traumatic grief (CTG). There is growing consensus that children with this condition need mental health interventions that focus on both trauma and grief. The only RCT for traumatically bereaved children was conducted by Pfeffer, Jiang, Kakuma, Hwang, and Metsch (2002). This study compared group cognitive-behavioral interventions without exposure components to a no-treatment control condition provided to 102 children and adolescents who had lost a parent or sibling to suicide. The active treatment group experienced greater improvement in anxiety and depression but not in PTSD. In an uncontrolled pilot study, Salloum, Avery, and McClain (2001) provided group cognitive-behavioral therapy without an exposure component, to 45 inner-city minority adolescent survivors of homicide and demonstrated significant improvement in PTSD symptoms at the end of treatment. These two studies were limited by the fact that neither specifically measured CTG, and neither included exposure procedures.

Layne and colleagues (2001) provided a trauma- and grief-focused group cognitive-behavioral treatment intervention to 55 bereaved Bosnian adolescents 4 years after the civil war in that country. Approximately half of these students showed improvements in PTSD and grief symptoms, with 35% showing improvement in depression. Saltzman, Pynoos, Layne, Steinberg, and Aisenberg (2001) used this same treatment model to treat 26 young adolescents with community violence-related PTSD, 7 of whom had lost a loved one to homicide. PTSD symptoms improved significantly in this group as well. Cohen, Mannarino, and Knudsen (2003) provided individual CTG-focused cognitive-behavioral treatment (CBT) to 22 children and adolescents with CTG symptoms following the death of a parent or sibling. Parallel individual treatment was also provided to surviving parents or primary caretakers. This study demonstrated large effect sizes in improvements in CTG, PTSD, depression, behavior problems, and anxiety in the children, as well as significant improvement in parental PTSD and depressive symptoms. The lack of control groups in these treatment studies limits the conclusions that can be drawn about the effectiveness of the index treatments, but the studies suggest the value of conducting RCTs to further evaluate these combined trauma-and grief-focused interventions.

Child Interventions with Multiple Traumas

Our experience following the terrorist attacks of September 11, 2001, suggests that many children who develop significant PTSD symptoms in the wake of community disasters had experienced previous interpersonal trauma such as child abuse, domestic or community violence, or multiple losses of loved ones. Indeed, one of the most consistent risk factors for developing mental health problems following trauma exposure is a history of past trauma (Pine & Cohen, 2002). Thus it is relevant to also review the child treatment literature with regard to interpersonal trauma. Several studies have evaluated the efficacy of trauma-focused CBT (TF-CBT) for sexually abused children.

Deblinger, Lippmann, and Steer (1996) compared TF-CBT provided to children only, to parents only, or to both children and parents to standard community care and found that the two TF-CBT conditions in which children received treatment resulted in greater improvement in PTSD symptoms, whereas the two conditions in which TF-CBT was provided to parents resulted in greater improvements in children's depressive symptoms and in positive parenting practices. Cohen and Mannarino (1996) demonstrated that TF-CBT provided individually to preschoolers and their parents was superior to nondirective supportive therapy in reducing PTSD, internalizing, externalizing, and sexualized behavior symptoms. A parallel study with 8–14-year-old sexually abused children similarly found that TF-CBT resulted in greater improvement in depression and social competence in treatment completers at posttreatment (Cohen & Mannarino, 1998) and in PTSD and dissociation at the 12-month follow-up (Cohen, Mannarino, & Knudsen, 2005). These two studies also demonstrated that resolution of parental distress about the child's abuse and parental support were strong predictors of children's response to treatment.

In a multisite RCT for 229 sexually abused children, Cohen, Deblinger, Mannarino, and Steer (2004) found that TF-CBT was superior to child-centered supportive therapy in improving PTSD, depressive, anxiety, behavior, and shame symptoms in the children and in improving depression, abuse-related distress, parental support, and positive parenting practices in the parents of these children. Of note is the fact that this cohort of children had experienced multiple traumas: 70% had experienced the traumatic death or terminal illness of a loved one, 58% had experienced domestic violence, 26% had experienced physical abuse, 38% had experienced a serious accident, 17% had experienced community violence, and 13% had experienced a natural disaster or fire. The results of this study suggest that TF-CBT is effective in treating PTSD and other symptoms in multiply traumatized children.

Another study (King et al., 2000) likewise demonstrated that TF-CBT was superior to a wait-list control condition in improving PTSD and depression in sexually abused children, and that inclusion of parents in treatment resulted in less anxiety symptoms at the 3-month follow-up. Studies of children with PTSD from community violence have compared group TF-CBT interventions to wait-list control or lagged treatment conditions in school settings and have shown that these are effective in reducing PTSD and depressive symptoms (Kataoka et al., 2003; Stein et al., 2003). Other studies have suggested the potential benefit of psychodynamic treatment for sexually abused children (Trowell et al., 2002) and for young children exposed to domestic violence (Lieberman & van Horn, 1998). However, these studies have yet to be replicated.

Pharmacological interventions are increasingly used to treat childhood PTSD, despite the absence of RCTs, which have been difficult to conduct with children. Only one pharmacological RCT has been conducted for traumatized children (Robert et al., 1999), and this was conducted in acutely burned children, who may have unique physiological insults not generalizable to other children. This study demonstrated that the tricyclic antidepressant imipramine was superior to a sedating agent, chloral hydrate, in reducing PTSD symptoms. More and better-designed studies are needed before pharmacological interventions can be recommended for the treatment of childhood PTSD. In the meantime, medication selection should be guided by known effective treatments for comorbid psychiatric conditions, or for symptomatic relief of specific symptoms known to be related to certain neurotransmitter activity (Cohen, Perel, DeBellis, Friedman, & Putnam, 2002).

APPLYING THE LITERATURE: BEST PRACTICE FOLLOWING MASS VIOLENCE

The treatment literature offers the strongest support for TF-CBT and related CBT approaches for traumatized children. These treatments have consistently been shown to decrease PTSD symptoms in children traumatized by a variety of different types of traumas. Most of the empirically tested TF-CBT models have similar components, which are described briefly here. A detailed treatment manual is available to therapists (Cohen, Mannarino, & Deblinger, in press). The following sections outline the most common components of TF-CBT.

Psychoeducation about PTSD and other common reaction to traumatic events may help to normalize parents' and children's experience of their own distress. Knowing that their children's responses are predictable and often self-limited reassures parents about their own parenting abilities (i.e., "my child's symptoms don't mean I am a terrible parent") as well as their children's resilience. This in turn can help parents to be more reassuring and supportive of their children at a time when parental support is crucial for optimal child recovery. Psychoeducation can also include safety planning for the future.

Affective identification and modulation skills include exercises that assist children in identifying a wide range of different feelings, including those that they may view as "bad" feelings. Children are then encouraged to accept the validity of all feelings and to learn optimal ways of expressing feelings. Children also learn skills for tolerating negative emotional states and for self-soothing.

Stress management techniques include helping children find personally effective ways of using relaxation, focused breathing, and other mind–body integration skills; positive self-talk; and thought stopping.

The cognitive triad is introduced to children through increasing their awareness of the connections between thoughts, feelings, and behaviors. Children then practice using cognitive restructuring to minimize negative emotion with regard to everyday situations as well as those related to their traumatic experiences.

Exposure and contextualizing interventions are introduced once children have mastered the skills introduced in earlier TF-CBT components. Most commonly this involves creating the child's trauma narrative, in the form of a book, poem, series of drawings, or other creative formats whereby the child gradually describes increasing details about the traumatic event and his or her feelings, thoughts, and body reactions to it. As children include more details, they become more able to tolerate memories of the traumatic event, thereby desensitizing the child to trauma reminders and fitting the trauma into the larger context of the child's life.

Cognitive processing of the traumatic event assists the child in examining and correcting cognitive errors such as self-blame or learned helplessness related to the traumatic event. Often cognitive distortions are identified in children's trauma narratives rather than by directly asking children about their attributions and safety planning for the future.

Some of these models also include a *parental treatment component* and *joint parent–child treatment sessions* (Cohen, Mannarino, & Deblinger, 2003; Deblinger & Heflin, 1996). Parental interventions parallel the child components described previously. They include parenting skills, which enhance parents' feelings of effectiveness and their ability to address children's behavioral problems, which often increase at times of stress such as after a community trauma. Typically the parenting skills include the use of praise and positive attention, active ignoring, effective use of time out, and/or the use of contingency reinforcement programs. Joint parent–child sessions are usually included near the end of treatment and offer children an opportunity to share their trauma narratives with their parents and to openly discuss all aspects of the traumatic experience together as a family.

Combined trauma- and grief-focused models for CTG (Cohen & Mannarino, 2004; Layne, Saltzman, Savjak, & Pynoos, 1999) include all of the foregoing trauma-focused components and, in addition, provide interventions designed to assist children in negotiating the normal grieving process once their trauma symptoms have subsided in response to the trauma-focused portion of treatment. These include education about grief in the context of the child's cultural, religious, and family beliefs about death and the afterlife; acknowledging what has been lost with the death of the loved one (interactive experiences in the past as well as future experiences that now can never be shared); addressing unfinished business or ambivalent feelings toward the deceased; preserving positive memories; recommitting to present and future relationships with living people; and making meaning of the traumatic loss.

Treating CTG typically takes somewhat longer than treating children with PTSD and other trauma symptoms in the absence of bereavement. More research is needed to identify the optimal length of treatment for both situations. There are potential advantages to conducting such treatment in group settings, particularly in community traumas (where large numbers of affected children may be most easily treated in school settings and where children affected by a common trauma can derive support from their peers), as well as for providing treatment to individual children and families (to optimize participation of parents in treatment and minimize the potential for vicarious traumatization). In the absence of research that indicates the superiority of one over the other, TF-CBT should be offered in either or both settings, depending on what is most acceptable and accessible for families and providers.

Based on our current knowledge, clinicians interested in preparedness for possible future disasters would be well advised to familiarize themselves with one or more of these TF-CBT treatment approaches. Training and ongoing consultation in these treatments is available through the National Child Traumatic Stress Network (www.nctsnet.org) funded by the Substance Abuse and Mental Health Services Administration (SAMHSA) and through the SAMHSA Center for Substance Abuse Prevention Model Programs initiative (modelprograms.samhsa.gov). Training is also available online at www.musc.edu/tfcbt.

Timing and Developmental Issues

Although we have growing information about effective treatments for traumatized children, we have much less empirical data to guide decisions about the optimal timing of such treatment, or about the early trauma response and natural recovery process in children of different ages. It is crucial to consider optimal ways to help children in the immediate aftermath of community traumas, but conducting rigorous scientific studies for children in this time frame is very difficult. No immediate mental health interventions for children such as group debriefing have been evaluated in controlled studies. The only RCT demonstrating the benefit of immediate interventions provided relaxation in the form of massage therapy rather than trauma-focused psychotherapeutic interventions (Field et al., 1996). Thus the following discussion is based primarily on clinical considerations rather than research data.

Children use social referencing to help them assess the meaning and seriousness of external events. Very young children look primarily to their parents in this regard, while older children also depend on teachers and other trusted adults, as well as their peers, to contextualize events. When the parents of young children are free of significant emotional distress and offer these children age-appropriate reassurance and support, these children tend to adjust well following traumatic events (Laor, Wolmer, & Cohen, 2001). In contrast, lack of social support and the presence of parental psychopathology heighten children's risk for developing mental health problems following trauma exposure (Pine & Cohen, 2002). Thus it makes sense that in the acute aftermath of community-level traumas, attending to the practical and mental health needs of parents and other adults may mitigate potential problems in children. As with adults, providing safety; shelter; food; accurate, age-appropriate information; and social support should be immediate priorities for children.

Many parents, teachers, and other adults are unsure whether to tell children the truth about horrifying events and thus often say nothing, allowing children to get inaccurate information elsewhere or to "fill in the gaps" with their imaginations, which are often more horrifying than reality. Thus a rule of thumb is to provide age-appropriate information that helps children understand what is happening while providing all reasonable reassurance about their personal safety. (This is more difficult when adults are themselves receiving frightening, inaccurate, inconsistent, or no official information; the importance of keeping the public informed in disaster situations is addressed elsewhere in this volume.) Mental health professionals can be of assistance to children in this regard by posting information sheets for children and parents on public websites, as occurred soon after September 11 (e.g., www.forourkids.org; www.ncptsd.org).

Unless RCTs demonstrate otherwise, we believe that in the acute aftermath of a disaster or mass violence, providing the basic necessities, optimizing parental adjustment, and providing social support and age-appropriate information and reassurance should take precedence over providing immediate mental health treatment to children (except for those children with severe symptoms of psychiatric impairment, who as always should be provided with appropriate clinical interventions). This type of information and reassurance is described as psychological first aid (PFA). A manual for PFA is available through www.nctsnet.org. The potential risks of conducting immediate group debriefing for children include exposing them to the extreme emotional distress of peers, thereby leading them to assign more catastrophic meaning to the event than they otherwise would have; sensitizing them to trauma reminders without the opportunity for desensitization that occurs in longer interventions such as TF-CBT; and depriving them of other natural occurring support in their community (e.g., if normal social interactions with peers in school are more health-promoting than debriefing groups, running groups at recess may deprive children of normal opportunities for these interactions). At this time we have no evidence that the benefit of such treatment outweighs these potential risks.

Child Mental Health Screening

Another acute response to community trauma should be screening children for significant mental health difficulties and referring identified children for in-depth evaluation. Accurately identifying PTSD and other trauma-related symptoms is particularly challenging in younger children, who are less able to accurately report their own internal emotional states and whose distress symptoms are often nonspecific (Scheeringa, Peebles, Cook, & Zeanah, 2001). Younger age of onset of PTSD is also associated with more severe impairments in brain development (DeBellis et al., 1999). Unlike adults, children rarely seek treatment on their own for mental health problems. A child with trauma-related symptoms typically depends on a parent, teacher, or other adult to recognize that such problems exist and to bring the child to treatment, with this dependency being greater in younger children. In disaster and mass violence situations such adults are often personally traumatized and thus may be less able to recognize the relevance or severity of the child's distress and/or less emotionally able to provide adequate support to the child. For these reasons, younger children may be the most likely to be severely impacted by community traumas, and the least likely to be provided with trauma-related treatment. There are therefore compelling reasons to conduct widespread screenings to detect children with mental health problems in the acute aftermath of community traumas.

Fortunately, brief psychometrically sound instruments are available to screen children and adolescents for trauma exposure and PTSD symptoms. For example, the UCLA PTSD Index for DSM-IV includes developmentally appropriate versions for child, adolescent and parent reports of children's trauma exposure and symptoms (Pynoos, Rodriguez, Steinberg, Stuber, & Frederick, 1998); instruments, administration, and scoring instructions are available at www.nctsnet.org. Procedures have been established to facilitate ease of administration of such instruments in school settings (Chemtob, Nakashima, & Hamada, 2002), and several studies have demonstrated that early screening (i.e., within 2 months following trauma exposure) successfully identifies children at greatest risk for developing PTSD (Brent, Moritz, Bridge, Perper, & Canobbio, 1996; Yule & Udwin, 1991).

There are many barriers to conducting such screening. The most efficient setting for screening children is in schools, but school boards, school staff, and parents are typically very protective of their students, particularly in the aftermath of a disaster or other community trauma, and are often resistant to "outsiders" coming into their schools to ask children what may be perceived as upsetting or intrusive questions. The successful school-based mental health screening 6 weeks after the Oklahoma City bombing was highly unusual; more typical is the New York experience after September 11, 2001, where screening of a representative sample of children occurred 6 months later, and universal screening was not instituted (Pfefferbaum et al., 2003).

To overcome these obstacles, it is important for mental health professionals with expertise in treating traumatized children to establish proactive ongoing relationships with school and public health officials in their respective communities. Providing education to people in these positions about the availability and value of established screening instruments and procedures may reduce barriers to conducting such screening as an early response to disaster situations. At-risk children should then be offered more extensive evaluation and children with significant symptoms should receive appropriate evidence-based treatments (EBTs). Providing such treatment in community settings requires that EBTs be accessible and acceptable to community providers and affected families as discussed next.

Cultural Issues: Community Training and Acceptance of EBTs

Following the September 11, 2001, terrorist attacks on New York City, many federal, state, and local entities collaborated to provide training to community therapists with regard to EBTs for traumatized and traumatically bereaved children and adolescents. The fortuitous initial funding of the National Child Traumatic Stress Network (NCTSN) by SAMHSA in October 2001 facilitated the availability of expert trainers and the coordination of training among several New York academic and community programs. Two EBTs for traumatized children and adolescents were selected for dissemination among community treatment providers (Cohen et al., 2001; Layne et al., 1999), and a series of intensive trainings and ongoing consultation calls between community providers and trainers were conducted. These are ongoing as part of the Child and Adolescent Trauma Treatment Services (CATS) program, a nine-site consortium coordinated by Columbia University.

Despite the fact that both of the treatment models had been developed, used, and tested in culturally diverse populations and settings, these ongoing trainer–community therapist interactions resulted in the treatment manuals for both EBTs undergoing extensive revisions, to be optimally responsive to the cultural and community needs of providers and the families they have been treating. In part this was due to the extreme cultural diversity of New York, but it was also because these therapists were particularly committed to protecting their child clients from any treatment not relevant to their specific religious, ethnic, racial, language, and cultural communities. Thus we believe the following considerations were crucial to the adoption of EBTs by these child therapists and will have relevance to future efforts to disseminate EBTs to community child therapists:

1. *Acknowledge the centrality of the therapeutic relationship with the child.* In an effort to provide intensive skills-based training in the brief time available, we initially focused solely on specific TF-CBT treatment components, without discussing the importance of the relationship between the therapist and child. We thought therapists would take for granted that we viewed the therapeutic relationship as the heart of any effective treatment. We learned that an essential part of establishing our credibility was to verbalize this core belief that we shared as therapists (i.e., that establishing a trusting therapeutic relationship with the child and parents takes precedence over specific treatment interventions).

2. *Emphasize flexibility.* There is great variability among community child therapists with regard to their theoretical orientations, years of experience, and favored treatment approaches. While very junior therapists may be receptive to rigidly defined treatment manuals that offer step-by-step implementation instructions, most therapists view such manuals as "cookbook" approaches that ignore the importance of therapist judgment and creativity. We found it much more helpful to present EBTs as a collection of core treatment components that can and should be implemented flexibly, in ways that are sensitive to the individual child's developmental level, culture, community and family values, and the personal preferences.

3. *Emphasize commonalities; solicit therapist input.* We found that most community child therapists were already utilizing some TF-CBT components in their usual treatment, without identifying them as such. By soliciting therapists' suggestions for how they would address a specific issue, we were often able to point out that their favored methods were totally consistent with TF-CBT interventions, and that they were teaching us novel ideas of how to implement these. This encouraged therapists to view the trainings as collaborative learning experiences rather than as a series of didactic directives telling them how to change their practices. We found this to be particularly beneficial with regard to cultural issues. For example, instead of saying "this is how you do the trauma narrative," we would ask therapists of different cultures, "What do you think would work best to encourage a child from your culture to talk about what happened to him?" Therapists offered wonderfully creative and culturally sensitive ideas in this regard, all of which were consistent with the TF-CBT model. We found that this approach both made therapists more receptive to adopting and adapting the model and taught us innovative ways to implement it.

4. *Trainers should be child therapists.* When challenging questions arise during the training, therapists did not want to hear theoretical answers. They were looking for practical suggestions for what might work in difficult real-life therapeutic situations. There was no substitute for extensive clinical experience in this regard: describing similar children we had treated, what worked (and what didn't) was critical to convincing ther-

apists of our personal therapeutic credentials as well as the credibility of our model.

5. *Provide ongoing consultation.* The most common training format is a one time didactic lecture. We found that therapists who ran into difficulties in implementing the TF-CBT model were more likely to continue to use it if we were available on an ongoing basis to suggest alternative ways to address these difficulties. Otherwise they reverted to their previous, more familiar treatment practices. Our experience suggests that as consultation calls progressed, therapists became more affiliated with the model, reported more successes in implementing it, and eventually started to advocate for its use in discussions with other therapists. Although this is a time-consuming process, we believe it is an important and worthwhile investment to make in disseminating the use of EBTs for traumatized children

CHILDREN OF MILITARY
AND EMERGENCY SERVICES PROFESSIONALS

In addition to the peril that all children face when impacted by trauma or disaster, children of military and other uniformed parents (including firefighters, emergency rescuers, and other first responders) contend with the constant reality that their parents may be injured or killed within the line of duty. The September 11 terrorist attacks had a profound impact on children of emergency services workers. Thousands of children lost their firefighter or other uniformed services parents in these attacks. Exemplary collaboration with the firefighter community allowed one pair of investigators to establish an extensive screening and treatment program for these children; an extraordinary achievement of this collaboration was developing and conducting an RCT for CTG, which started providing randomly assigned treatment within 6 months of September 11 (Brown & Goodman, 2002). This experience highlighted the heightened vulnerability experienced by these children in disaster situations. Other than this cited report, studies related to these special populations of children are few and largely restricted to military children.

The experience of military children has been variably reported in the literature. Although some authors have referred to a possible noxious influence of growing up in a military family and have proposed a possible "military family syndrome" (Lagrone, 1978), such a conclusion does not appear empirically supportable. In a study comparing children of active duty, reserve and civilian parents Ryan-Wenger (2001) found no evidence suggesting higher levels of anxiety or other psychopathology in military children. In fact, there is some evidence that military children exhibit fewer behavioral and emotional symptoms than civilian counterparts (Jensen,

Xenakis, Wolf, & Bain, 1991). Nevertheless, military children must contend with certain unique and potentially corrosive challenges. As military members routinely deploy on missions around the world, they are often separated from their children for extended periods. Separations during peacetime can be challenging. Separations during wartime are likely to be even more troubling for children whose parents are assigned to places that may bring them into harm's way. In addition to separations, other experiences may prove to be traumatic. Military children may be confronted with the illness, serious injury, or death of a parent serving in the line of duty. In addition, the children of service members who return from traumatic military duty may be vicariously traumatized through parental exposure or may face unique challenges as they are impacted by parental psychopathology. These topic areas are summarized in the following paragraphs.

Several studies have looked at the impact of parental separation on military children during deployment. In a study examining the effects of father absence during routine (noncombat) military deployments, Jensen, Grogan, Xenakis, and Bain (1989) found a significantly higher level of anxiety and depression symptoms in children of the father-absent group, compared to the father-present control group. Interestingly, the authors found that these symptoms were largely influenced by the effect of maternal psychopathology and the presence of family stressors, suggesting the importance of parental response and family stability to the healthy adaptation of the child during deployments.

Studies that looked at the impact of wartime separations during Operation Desert Storm (ODS) found moderate effects of such deployments on children's symptom development. Rosen, Teitelbaum, and Westhuis (1993) found high rates of reported internalizing and externalizing symptoms in children of ODS deployed parents. However, few of these children demonstrated symptoms of severity that required treatment and those who did were more likely to have had a past history of mental health treatment. These findings suggest that prior psychopathology is a risk factor for the development of more serious emotional problems in children during parental deployment. In a comparison of children of ODS deployed parents and a control group of children whose parents deployed during the same time period but under routine (noncombat) circumstances, Kelley (1994) found that ODS children evidenced greater internalizing and externalizing symptoms and that their families reported less cohesiveness than those within the control group.

While collecting data on children in military families prior to ODS, Jensen, Martin, and Watanabe (1996) fortuitously captured the impact of wartime deployment on children in a prospective fashion by measuring children's symptoms both pre- (prior to knowledge of deployment) and mid-ODS deployment. The authors compared those children whose parents deployed with those whose parents did not deploy. They measured a modest effect of deployment on symptom development, particularly depression and, to a lesser degree, anxiety. However, as a group, the ODS children's symptoms did not reach pathological levels. Other important findings of this study were that boys and younger children demonstrated greater vulnerability, suggesting a need for greater monitoring in these groups.

Peebles-Kleiger and Kleiger (1994) argued that deployment during wartime should be considered a "catastrophic" stressor to children and families, in comparison to routine deployments during noncombat periods. While the merits of the authors' conclusion can be argued, some consideration of differences between deployment types seems justified. During wartime children are much more likely to be aware of the dangers that the deployed parent faces. Military communities often rally in support of deployed soldiers during wartime, generating more visible reminders of the importance and potential danger of the mission. In addition, children often have awareness of those service members in the community who are returning as injured or deceased, portending greater danger regarding their own parents. Another source of graphic and potentially disturbing information for children during wartime deployments is exposure to the media (which should be limited as appropriate according to developmental age).

The military component to which a child's parent is assigned (e.g., active, reserve, or National Guard) must also be factored into a child's experience of parental deployment. Active-duty service members and their families may have an advantage over reserve or National Guard families in their level of preparation and readiness for deployment. Having served greater amounts of activated time in service, active-duty families may be better inculcated into the military system. They are often better prepared psychologically for deployment, as many have experienced prior deployments. Another advantage to active-duty families of deployed service members is that they are more likely to have access to military support services than reserve or National Guard families. This is particularly true when the latter live in areas that are remote from military bases. Additional financial burdens may be present in the families of activated reservists or National Guardsmen since activation may mean the loss of salary from a civilian job that is higher paying than their military positions. All these factors can affect a family's, and consequently a child's, ability to effectively integrate a deployment experience.

Other potential traumas to military children have been researched little. Inferences largely need to be made based on findings in the general psychiatric literature. As an example, the death of a parent clearly puts a child at higher risk for developing a psychiatric disorder or other emotional or behavioral problems (Dowdney, 2000). However, no information is available that specifically examines the impact of such an event when the insult occurred as a result of war. It can be hypothesized that a war-related parental death is a unique and potentially graver experience for a child due to the inherent aggressive, combatant, and directed nature of the assault that caused it. This experience may be more psychologically complicated for the child than those cases studied in the literature and might indicate graver consequences. Further research is required in this area.

Anecdotally, some information is available related to the loss of a military parent during wartime. In the aftermath of the death of a service member, a family is likely to be significantly disrupted. Emotional responses may include sadness, guilt and/or regret, and rage, as well as other emotions. An important role for the family in helping a child to integrate such a loss is to contain and process these emotions in a constructive fashion. Often, military families are not assigned to areas close to extended family. They may choose to travel distantly to bury their loved ones, leaving a supportive military community behind. Children are often uprooted for funerals, leading to disruption in peer support, school schedules, and other activities. Surviving parents will understandably be distracted by the many preparations that are required, potentially affecting their ability to parent. Also, when a military service member dies the family typically loses access to military installation housing. Although some families may choose to remain within the vicinity of the military community, many families choose to relocate back to areas of extended family or lifelong friends. It remains unclear how all these events affect children within these families and how the consequences are different from those of nonmilitary children whose parents die.

Similarly, scientifically collected information about the impact of injury of military parents during wartime on children is lacking. However, analogous to the foregoing discussion, it is expected that this impact is more complex and potentially more compromising than that of children whose parents are injured in nonviolent settings. Anecdotally, injuries to a service member are likely to result in a flurry of urgent activity and anxiety, leading to potential disruption within the family. Often immediate information regarding the nature and severity of the injury is limited, and sometimes inaccurate, causing further increased anxiety in families. Typically, when notified of the injury the spouse makes arrangements to join the service member who is receiving medical attention.

Children may also join the injured parent or remain at home. In either case children are likely to face challenges. As the military treatment facility may be at considerable distance from the family's residence, children who remain at home are faced with the threatened loss of the injured parent, as well as the real absence of the nonmilitary parent, on whom they depend. Local friends, neighbors, or out-of-town family members may care for them in the absence of parents. Children's stability and comfort will depend largely on the nature of their existing relationships with the assigned care-givers and the latter's capability to provide emotional support, appropriate discipline, and nurturance in the absence of the parents.

Children who travel to be with their injured parents are uprooted for varying periods of time, losing the structured support of their home and school schedules. On occasion, entire families may temporarily uproot to be closer to the injured parent who is undergoing longer-term rehabilitation. Under such circumstances, children are sometimes reenrolled in local schools or entered into parent-run home-schooling programs. Of course, many of these scenarios result in disruptions of friendships, other social contacts, and routine structured activities. Many military treatment facilities are not equipped to provide extensive services to visiting children, so they may find few activities to engage their time. The presence of children can sometimes complicate the ability of nursing and other health care professionals to treat their patients. Effective efforts allow some accommodations for these younger family members so that they can be involved in activities while their injured parent heals.

Of special concern is the potential trauma of the child's exposure to the injured parent. As service members may return from combat with amputations, shrapnel injuries, burns, and other disfiguring wounds, their children should be adequately prepared for the level of injuries they will see. Personnel in military treatment facilities are likely to be preoccupied with the fast pace of caring for the war wounded. Certain professionals, such as child-life workers, pediatric staff, and mental health providers, can assist by highlighting the unique needs of these children to the hospital leadership and to other health care providers with whom the families interact.

Finally, service members may return from war exposure suffering from either identified or nonidentified psychiatric illnesses (depression, PTSD, substance use disorders). The impact of these disorders on family members (including children) can be profound and must be recognized. While the findings are not entirely consistent, a literature exists that suggests the transgenerational transmission of posttraumatic symptoms. The children of Vietnam veterans with PTSD are more likely to evidence symptoms similar to those of their fathers (Rosenheck & Nathan, 1985; Rosenheck & Thomson, 1986). Motta (1990) has also described that veterans suffering from war-induced symptoms may transmit maladaptive behaviors to their children. Other studies have measured problems in family functioning (reduced family cohesion, decreased interpersonal expressiveness, greater interpersonal conflict, and reduced problem-solving ability) of Vietnam veterans suffering from PTSD (Davidson & Mellor, 2001; Solomon, 1988; Solomon et al., 1992). Recent developments within the military have focused on the importance of identifying and addressing these longer-term consequences in military members and their families upon redeployment.

PRACTICE IMPLICATIONS

Disasters and Mass Violence

The foregoing information has several practical implications for how to address the needs of children and adolescents following disasters and mass violence:

1. Families, schools and communities should attempt to *maximize support and normalcy* in children's lives as quickly as possible after a disaster has occurred. Providing emotional support, community resources, and accurate information to parents (and offering appropriate mental health interventions to severely traumatized parents) will likely optimize children's responses to community traumas.

2. Children should be protected from well-meaning "grief therapists" and other mental health professionals who flock to the scene of disasters; help from children's natural support systems within their own community is usually more beneficial. Volunteers should focus their efforts on normalizing these systems of support through providing practical support (food, clothing, money, babysitting, transportation, etc.) and psychological first aid rather than acute mental health interventions to children.

3. Early mental health screening should be instituted through schools, and child mental health care providers in the community should receive intensive training in empirically supported assessment and treatment models as soon after the disaster as possible (ideally this training would be obtained proactively, before a disaster occurs). TF-CBT treatments have the strongest evidence of efficacy for children; but these are typically not provided until more than 1 month after the disaster has occurred. This timing may be ideal in order to allow children's natural recovery process to occur; some children who are initially symptomatic may be free of symptoms a month after the disaster has occurred. Such children probably do not need mental health treatment.

4. TF-CBT may be provided in group or individual formats, in schools, or in community mental health settings. These treatments typically are provided over 10–16 weeks and may include a parental treatment component. Trauma- and grief-focused CBT for CTG are typically provided over 16–20 weeks and have been manualized for individual and group settings. Training in these treatments are available through the NCTSN (www.nctsnet.org). Other treatments with some evidence of efficacy are described earlier; training in these approaches may be available through

their developers. Therapists should make efforts to track progress in therapy through the use of standardized instruments that assess PTSD and other trauma-related symptoms. Children with comorbid psychiatric disorders or with severe psychiatric symptoms may benefit from adjunctive psychopharmacological treatments or from other therapeutic interventions known to effectively treat the comorbid conditions.

Military Children

Although there is no evidence suggesting higher levels of anxiety or other psychopathology in military children, and some evidence that military children exhibit fewer behavioral and emotional symptoms than do civilian counterparts, certain precautionary and reactive strategies are recommended for particularly stressful circumstances:

1. During *separations* due to wartime, maternal psychopathology, prior child psychopathology, and family stressors should be monitored and addressed or alleviated as much as possible. Exposure to the media should be limited as appropriate for the child's developmental age. Extra support should be given to families of activated reservists or National Guardsmen. Friends and extended family should be educated to provide extra support to children whose parents are understandably distracted by the many preparations that are required.

2. During situations in which the child is confronted with the *illness, serious injury, or death of a parent* serving in the line of duty, family members should be educated in helping a child to integrate such a trauma or loss and to contain and process their emotions in a constructive fashion. As much as possible, care should be taken to maintain peer support, school schedules, and other activities. In the case of injuries, as soon as possible, accurate information regarding the nature and severity of the injury should be conveyed. If the spouse of the injured service member must leave the child at home while he or she flies to be with the service member, local friends, neighbors, or out-of-town family members should be educated in how to care for the children in the absence of parents. If children must travel to be with their injured family member, accommodations should be made for these younger family members so that they can be involved in activities while their injured parent heals.

If the service member returns from combat with amputations, shrapnel injuries, burns, and other disfiguring wounds, his or her children should be adequately prepared for the level of injuries they will see. Mental health providers can assist by highlighting the unique needs of these children to the hospital leadership and to other health care providers with whom the families interact.

3. In a situation in which a child of a service member who returns from traumatic military duty is at risk for being *vicariously traumatized through parental exposure or is impacted by parental psychopathology*, families should be educated to reduce the likelihood that the service member transmits maladaptive behaviors to his or her children and prepared for possible reduction in family cohesion, decreased interpersonal expressiveness, greater interpersonal conflict, and reduced problem-solving ability. These potential affects should be identified and addressed as early as possible to avoid longer-term consequences in military members and their families upon redeployment.

A PHASED APPROACH TO RESPONSE IN DIFFERENT SETTINGS

The following recommendations attempt to summarize school, family, and community responses that may optimize children's recovery from community trauma.

Immediate Aftermath (Hours to Days)

Schools

In the immediate aftermath of a community trauma, it is critical to reunite children with their parents or other known caretakers as quickly as possible. Schools should have emergency contact information for parents and alternative caretakers; children and parents should proactively agree on reunification plans in case of emergency. For example, if parents work far away from children's schools, neighbors or other relatives might be designated to pick up children in emergency situations. School personnel should be apprised of these plans so that children are only released to authorized adults. Schools also need lockdown, parent notification, and other emergency plans in place and these should be tested periodically through scheduled drills. While children are waiting to be reunified with parents, they should be provided with age-appropriate reliable information about the nature of the emergency, steps being taken to keep students safe, and plans for family notification and reunification. Teachers should keep televisions or radios turned off in classrooms, as repeated viewing of disaster scenes on television is correlated with increased severity of PTSD in children (Pfefferbaum et al., 1999). If schools resume in the days following the disaster, normal routines should be followed to whatever extent is practical. Information should be provided on a regular basis, but TVs should remain off at school.

Parents

Steps should be taken to provide essentials such as heat, electricity, water, shelter, and food to displaced children and families as soon as possible. Children are often able to adapt well to such circumstances if parents are able to encourage such behavior by framing the experience as an adventure rather than a terrifying event. Providing children with storybooks, crayons, stuffed animals, handheld computer games, and so on, and playing games, telling stories, or singing songs together with other children or as a family may also help children regain a sense of safety and normalcy, even under abnormal circumstances. If children spontaneously want to talk about what they have seen and heard during the disaster, parents and other adults should listen and provide reassurance. At this stage adults should probably not actively prompt children to recount their upsetting experiences. Parents and other adults should provide as much realistic reassurance as possible to children while avoiding lying or making unrealistic promises. It is important for parents to reassure children that they are doing fine and will be there to help and protect their children.

In the acute aftermath of a community disaster it is common for children to become clingy with adults; many children may want to sleep in their parents' beds during these times. This is understandable and acceptable under these circumstances and children will typically return to their own rooms within several days or weeks if there is no further trauma exposure. Parents should try to maintain routines in order to reassure children that life is returning to normal, but common sense may dictate that certain rules will need to be bent slightly for a time. Parents may access information about helping children after different types of community disasters on the Terrorism and Disaster page of the NCTSN website (www.nctsnet.org).

Communities / Mental Health Professionals

Children whose parents, siblings, or other loved ones are missing should be comforted and provided with as much information as is available. They should be reassured that adults will take care of them and attend to their safety until their parents are located. Information about disruptions in telephone service, public transportation, and so on, may be reassuring to children who might otherwise not understand why their parents have not called or come for them. Relatives, neighbors, or other known adults should be located as soon as possible to care for and comfort children whose parents are not available.

As noted previously, there is no evidence that providing mental health interventions to unscreened children this soon after a disaster is helpful. Community leaders, mental health professionals, or schools may consult with the NCTSN Terrorism and Disaster Branch for information on responding to the needs of children following community traumas (310-235-2633, or www.nctsnet.org).

Short-Term Response (First 4 Weeks)

Schools

Screening procedures should be initiated in collaboration with child trauma or mental health professionals, public health officials, and/or researchers. Child and parental consent procedures have been developed for this purpose, but individual schools may need to modify these procedures. School administrators should be involved in planning and implementing these procedures as early in the process as possible, to avoid delays in screening. Schools may consult with the NCTSN (310-235-2633) with regard to appropriate screening procedures, instruments, or scoring. Children who screen positive for trauma symptoms should be referred for more detailed assessment. Schools may have the capacity to conduct such assessments themselves or may need to refer children to community child mental health providers for such assessments. School counselors or psychologists should consider requesting training in trauma assessment and/or EBTs for traumatized children, if they have the capacity and interest in providing school-based assessments or treatments. Education should be provided to teachers, student assistance staff, and other staff who interact directly with students and parents, about the effects of trauma on children, and how to recognize and cope with the effects of vicarious and personal trauma. Providing psychoeducation about common reactions to trauma and general stress management techniques may be reassuring and helpful to some students at this point, but there is no evidence that providing more trauma-specific interventions to unscreened children in school is beneficial in the first month after a disaster.

Families

In the absence of further trauma, children usually start to return to normal routines in the weeks after a community trauma. Parents should be alert to significant changes in their children that seem to worsen or not resolve over time, and they should also seek help if they experience worsening of their personal trauma symptoms.

Communities / Mental Health Professionals

Communities should arrange training for mental health professionals in assessment and EBTs for traumatized children. Specifically, professional should receive intensive skills-based training in TF-CBT for children and adolescents, with ongoing phone consultation from experienced trainers. Web-based training is available as described above (www.musc.edu/tfcbt). Several groups provide such training through the NCTSN. If possible, communities should coordinate training such that trained treatment providers are available in different neighborhoods for ethnically diverse populations of children. If the community lost large numbers of children or adults in the disaster, it should also request training in EBTs for CTG. Funding for treatment and other services should be sought through the Federal Emergency Management Agency or other federal disaster assistance programs, as described elsewhere in this volume.

Ongoing Response (Beyond 1 Month)

Schools

Schools should continue screening procedures until all children have been screened and identified children have been referred for additional services. School-based treatments for children with PTSD may begin as soon as 1 month after the disaster, although typically these are not offered so soon. Typically, school-based TF-CBT treatments are provided in group formats and last 10–15 weeks. Training and ongoing consultation with experts should be arranged prior to offering such groups. Individual therapists should also be identified for referrals of children who do not wish to participate in or do not benefit from group interventions. Consideration should be given to offering psychoeducational or therapeutic interventions for parents. Teachers should be encouraged to consult with school mental health professionals about concerns they have regarding individual students.

Parents

Parents should encourage children to return to normal routines and reinstate usual rules and expectations for most children. Parents should be aware of common signs of childhood PTSD and bring children with these symptoms to a mental health professional for assessment. Parents should continue to seek professional help for their own stress-related symptoms.

Communities/Mental Health Professionals

Ongoing outreach efforts should continue in order to identify and provide services to children with multiple family problems, no insurance, or other social and economic barriers to service seeking. EBTs for traumatized children should continue to be publicly available for at least 1–2 years after the disaster has occurred.

CLINICAL VIGNETTE

Presenting Complaints

Allison is a 7-year-old female who was referred due to sleep and school problems that began immediately after September 11. Chief complaints included:

1. Constant nightmares "about ghosts and goblins," which resulted in limited sleep for both Allison and her parents.
2. Being "fearful of everything since then" and constantly clinging to her parents. For example, Allison would refuse to use the bathroom or even brush her teeth unless her mother was standing right next to her.
3. Bedwetting shortly after the WTC attack.
4. Throwing tantrums every time she needed to go on the subway; breaking into tears and screams.

Background

Mrs. X denied any difficulties prior to September 11 and stated that she did not pay any attention to these recent difficulties until a discussion with Allison's teacher, who reported a decrease in performance over the past year and occasional aggressive outbursts from Allison, such as biting her peers on the playground. Mr. and Mrs. X stated that they were not convinced Allison's difficulties had anything to do with the World Trade Center (WTC) attack but were encouraged to see someone by school staff. Allison indicated previous exposure to community violence in different areas of New York, primarily aggressive acts within the subway or gang-related incidents.

Mrs. X presented with high anxiety and admitted avoiding numerous things such as subways, elevators, any area filled with dust, and many parts of downtown Manhattan. She reported that her husband has become "increasingly aggressive" by yelling at home and getting into fights with tourists who were observing the WTC site.

Allison lived in Battery Park (a neighborhood very close to the WTC) with her mother, father, and older brother. On September 11, Allison had been dropped off at school by her mother, who ran back to Allison's school to pick her up after witnessing the planes crashing into the WTC. She arrived as the school began evacuating the children. Mrs. X and Allison ran together from the school amidst the crowds of frantic New Yorkers, many covered in dust. For some time, Mrs. X was carrying Allison so that Allison was directly facing the WTC towers. They moved from place to place in the city, attempting to escape the falling debris, fires, dust, and putrid smell. Mrs. X was not able to get in touch with her husband or her son until the next day.

The family survived the event but they were displaced for over 6 months in various hotels. Both Mr. and Mrs. X lost their jobs. Since the disaster, Mrs. X and Allison have been together on two subway rides that were stopped for over an hour in darkness due to unknown reasons.

Treatment

The treatment used was *Individual Trauma-Focused Cognitive Behavioral Therapy for Children and Parents* (Cohen et al., 2001). The following components were included:

1. Psychoeducation was communicated by playing a game listing all the scary things that could happen and reactions people may have. Through this, Allison's own reactions were normalized and validated.
2. Feeling identification was conveyed by drawing a person, identifying emotions she felt (such as "icky"), picking a color, and coloring where in her body she felt that. Stories were told and pictures drawn about different times the therapist and she felt different ways.
3. Deep "belly breathing" was taught for relaxation during which "rides" were given to stuffed animals, and competitions between therapist and Allison were engaged in. All these skills were taught to Mrs. X at the end of session by Allison and to Mr. X at home. Allison was asked to grade her parents on these skills every time they practiced them at home, and bring the "report card" back to session.
4. The "cognitive triad" was reviewed by acting out scenarios that happen within Allison's life such as finding a place to sit at lunchtime and listing different thoughts, feelings, and behaviors that could occur.
5. Throughout the first weeks, behavioral techniques were used to address the bedwetting, sleep problems, and clinginess.
6. The trauma narrative that Allison created started with a timeline drawing of "Before," "September 11," and "After—when the Ghosts and Goblins came." The therapist wrote down Allison's words, and then Allison drew accompanying pictures. Allison's

"hot spots" were seeing people jumping from the towers as she ran with her mom, and seeing adults around her with "scary and frantic" faces.

At the end of treatment, all presenting symptoms had dissipated. Allison was sleeping in her own bed and able to function without her mother by her side. Her school performance increased and her aggressive acts stopped.

FUTURE CLINICAL PRACTICE AND RESEARCH DIRECTIONS

It is clear from the foregoing review that more research is needed to determine optimal clinical interventions for children traumatized by disasters and mass violence. Studies that more accurately identify children at greatest risk for long-term problems might allow us to provide earlier focused treatments to those children. RCTs evaluating very early child and adolescent interventions such as debriefing are needed in order to determine whether these have any value, for whom, and which if any children should not receive these interventions. Conducting studies of TF-CBT after disaster situations may provide information about how this model might be modified specifically for community traumas. Determining the optimal timing of providing TF-CBT would also be helpful in planning treatment strategies. Studies are currently underway to determine the optimal dosage and critical ingredients of TF-CBT for children of different developmental levels and symptom severity, and these may also guide our efforts to better match treatments to individual children. Randomized controlled pharmacological trials are needed to determine whether offering medication in the hours or days after trauma exposure may protect some children from developing PTSD; if such treatments were found to be beneficial, they could be offered in a cost-efficient manner to large numbers of children. Treatments other than TF-CBT should also be evaluated in RCTs, for children who do not respond to TF-CBT and to offer therapists and families broader therapeutic alternatives. Finally, studies regarding best dissemination strategies will allow better adoption and implementation of EBTs by community therapists.

In summary, we have learned a great deal over the past decade about effective assessment strategies and treatments for traumatized children, which has advanced our ability to help children recover in the aftermath of disasters and mass violence. However, there is still much to be learned in order to ensure that all children receive the best possible care in these tragic situations.

REFERENCES

Brent, D. A., Moritz, G., Bridge, J., Perper, J., & Canobbio, R. (1996). Long-term impact of exposure to suicide: A three-year controlled follow-up. *Journal of the American Academy of Child and Adolescent Psychiatry, 35*, 646–653.

Brown, E. J., & Goodman, R. (2002). *Treating children with traumatic grief following 9/11.* Grant funded by the Silver Shield Foundation, New York, NY.

Butz, A., & Pulsifer, M. (2002). Research on the impact of the threat of war on children in military families: Where do we go from here? *Journal of Pediatric Health Care, 16*, 262–264.

Chemtob, C. M., Nakashima, J., & Carlson, J. G. (2002). Brief treatment for elementary school children with disaster-related PTSD: A field study. *Journal of Clinical Psychology, 58*, 99–112.

Chemtob, C. M., Nakashima, J. P., & Hamada, R. S. (2002). Psychosocial intervention for postdisaster trauma symptoms in elementary school children: A controlled community field study. *Archives of Pediatric and Adolescent Medicine, 156*, 211–216.

Cohen, J. A. (2003). Early mental health interventions for trauma and traumatic loss in children and adolescents. In B. T. Litz (Ed.), *Early interventions for trauma and traumatic loss* (pp. 131–146). New York: Guilford Press.

Cohen, J. A., Deblinger, E., Mannarino, A. P., & Steer, R. (2004). A multisite randomized controlled trial for children with multiple traumas and sexual abuse-related PTSD. *Journal of the American Academy of Child and Adolescent Psychiatry, 43*, 393–402.

Cohen, J. A., & Mannarino, A. P. (1996). A treatment outcome study for sexually abused preschool children: Initial findings. *Journal of the American Academy of Child and Adolescent Psychiatry, 35*, 42–50.

Cohen, J. A., & Mannarino, A. P. (1998). Interventions for sexually abused children: Initial treatment findings. *Child Maltreatment, 3*, 17–26.

Cohen, J. A., & Mannarino, A. P. (2004). Treating childhood traumatic grief. *Journal of Clinical Child and Adolescent Psychology, 33*, 820–832.

Cohen, J. A., Mannarino, A. P., & Deblinger, E. (2001). *Individual trauma-focused CBT for children and parents.* Unpublished treatment manual, Drexel University College of Medicine, Pittsburgh, PA.

Cohen, J. A., Mannarino, A. P., & Deblinger, E. (2003). *Trauma focused CBT for children and parents, revised version.* Unpublished treatment manual, Drexel University college of Medicine, Pittsburgh, PA.

Cohen, J. A., Mannarino, A. P., & Deblinger, E. (in press). *Treating trauma and traumatic grief in children: A clinician's guide.* New York: Guilford Press.

Cohen, J. A., Mannarino, A. P., Greenberg, T., Padlo, S., & Shipley, C. (2002). Childhood traumatic grief: Concepts and controversies. *Journal of Trauma, Violence and Abuse, 3*, 307–327.

Cohen, J. A., Mannarino, A. P., & Knudsen, K. (2003). *Treating childhood traumatic grief: A pilot study.* Manuscript submitted for publication.

Cohen, J. A., Mannarino, A. P., & Knudsen, K. (2005). Treating sexually abused children: One year follow-up of a randomized controlled trial. *Child Abuse and Neglect, 29*, 135–146.

Cohen, J. A., Perel, J. M., DeBellis, M. D., Friedman, M. J., & Putnam, F. W. (2002). Treating traumatized children: Clinical implications of the psychobiology of PTSD. *Trauma, Violence and Abuse, 3*, 91–108.

Davidson, A. C., & Mellor, D. J. (2001). The adjustment of children of Australian Vietnam veterans: Is there evidence for transgenerational transmission of the effects of war-related trauma? *Australia and New Zealand Journal of Psychiatry, 35*, 345–351.

DeBellis, M. D., Keshavan, M. S., Clark, D. B., Casey, B. J., Giedd, J. N., Boring, A. M., et al. (1999). Developmental traumatology, Part II: Brain development. *Biological Psychiatry, 45*, 1271–1284.

Deblinger, E., & Heflin, A. H. (1996). *Treating sexually abused children and their nonoffending parents: A cognitive-behavioral approach.* Thousand Oaks, CA: Sage.

Deblinger, E., Lippmann, J., & Steer, R. (1996). Sexually abused children suffering posttraumatic stress symptoms Initial treatment outcome findings. *Child Maltreatment, 1*, 310–321.

Dowdney, L. (2000). Childhood bereavement following parental death. *Journal of Child Psychology and Psychiatry, 41*, 819–830.

Field, T., Seligman, S., Scafidi, F., & Schanberg, S. (1996). Alleviating posttraumatic stress in children following Hurricane Andrew. *Journal of Applied Developmental Psychology, 17*, 37–50.

Goenjian, A. K., Karayan, I., Pynoos, R. S., Minassian, D., Najarian, L. M., Steinberg, A. M., et al. (1997). Outcome of psychotherapy among early adolescents after trauma. *American Journal of Psychiatry, 154*, 536–542.

Hardin, S. B., Weinrich, S., Weinrich, M., Garrison, C., Addy, C., & Hardin, T. L. (2002). Effects of a long-term psychosocial nursing intervention on adolescents exposed to catastrophic stress. *Issues in Mental Health Nursing, 23*, 537–551.

Jensen, P. S., Grogan, D., Xenakis, S. N., & Bain, M. W. (1989). Father absence: Effects on child and maternal psychopathology. *Journal of the American Academy of Child and Adolescent Psychiatry, 28*, 171–175.

Jensen, P. S., Martin, D., & Watanabe, H. (1996). Children's response to parental separation during operation desert storm. *Journal of the American Academy of Child and Adolescent Psychiatry, 35*, 433–441.

Jensen, P. S., Xenakis, S. N., Wolf, P., & Bain, M. W. (1991). The "military family" syndrome revisited: By the numbers. *Journal of Nervous and Mental Disease, 179*, 102–107.

Kataoka, S. H., Stein, B. D., Jaycox, L. H., Wong, M., Escudero, P., Tu, W., et al. (2003). A school-based mental health program for traumatized Latino immigrant children. *Journal of the American Academy of Child and Adolescent Psychiatry, 42*, 311–318.

Kelley, M. L. (1994). The effects of military-induced separation on family factors and child behavior. *American Journal of Orthopsychiatry, 64*, 103–111.

King, N. J., Tonge, B. J., Mullen, P., Myerson, N., Heyne, D., Rollings, S., et al. (2000). Treating sexually abused children with posttraumatic stress symptoms: A randomized clinical trial. *Journal of the American Academy of Child and Adolescent Psychiatry, 39*, 1347–1355.

LaGrone, D. A. (1978). The military family syndrome. *American Journal of Psychiatry, 135,* 1040–1043.

Laor, N., Wolmer, L., & Cohen, D. J. (2001). Mothers' functioning and children's symptoms five years after a SCUD missile attack. *American Journal of Psychiatry, 158,* 1020–1026.

Layne, C. M., Pynoos, R. S., Saltzman, W. R., Arslanagic, B. G., Black, M., Savjak, N., et al. (2001). Trauma/grief focused group psychotherapy: School based post-war interventions with traumatized Bosnian youth. *Group Dynamics: Theory, Research and Practice, 5,* 277–290.

Layne, C. M., Saltzman, W. R., Savjak, N., & Pynoos, R. S. (1999). *Trauma/grief focused group psychotherapy manual.* Sarajevo, Bosnia: UNICEF Bosnia and Hercegovina.

Lieberman, A. L., & van Horn, P. (1998, July). *Assessing the effectiveness of an intervention model: Can parent child psychotherapy ameliorate the effects of witnessing family violence?* Paper presented at the Family Violence Research Conference, Durham, NH.

Motta, R. W. (1990). Personal and interfamilial effects of the Vietnam War experience. *Behavior Therapist, 13,* 155–157.

Peebles-Kleiger, M. J., & Kleiger, J. H. (1994). Re-integration stress for Desert Storm families: Wartime deployments and family trauma. *Journal of Traumatic Stress, 7,* 173–194.

Pfeffer, C. R., Jiang, H., Kakuma, T., Huang, J., & Metsch, M. (2002). Group intervention for children bereaved by the suicide of a relative. *Journal of the American Academy of Child and Adolescent Psychiatry, 41,* 505–513.

Pfefferbaum, B., Nixon, S. J., Krug, R. S., Tivis, R. D., Moore, V. L., Brown, J. M., et al. (1999). Clinical needs assessment of middle and high school students following the 1995 Oklahoma City bombing. *American Journal of Psychiatry, 156,* 1069–1074.

Pfefferbaum, B., Sconzo, G. M., Flynn, B. W., Kearns, L. J., Doughty, D. E., Gurwitch, R. H., et al. (2003). Case finding and mental health services for children in the aftermath of the Oklahoma City bombing. *Journal of Behavioral Health Services and Research, 30*(2), 215–227.

Pine, D. S., & Cohen, J. A. (2002). Trauma in children and adolescents: Risk and treatment of psychiatric sequelae. *Biological Psychiatry, 51,* 519–531.

Pynoos, R. S., Rodriguez, N., Steinberg, A. M., Stuber, M., & Frederick, C. (1998). *UCLA PTSD Index for DSM-IV.* Unpublished instrument, University of California, Los Angeles.

Robert, R., Blakeney, P. E., Villarreal, C., Rosenberg, L., & Meyer, W. J. (1999) Imipramine treatment in pediatrics burn patients with symptoms of Acute Stress Disorder: A pilot study. *Journal of the American Academy of Child and Adolescent Psychiatry, 38,* 873–882.

Rosen, L. N., Teitelbaum, J. M., & Westhuis, D. J. (1993). Children's reactions to the Desert Storm deployment: initial findings from a survey of Army families. *Military Medicine, 158,* 465–469.

Rosenheck, R., & Nathan, P. (1985). Secondary traumatization in children of Vietnam veterans. *Hospital and Community Psychiatry, 36,* 538–539.

Rosenheck, R., & Thomson, J. (1986). "Detoxication" of Vietnam war trauma: A combined family-individual approach. *Family Process, 25*, 559–570.

Ryan-Wenger, N. A. (2001). Impact of the threat of war on children in military families. *American Journal of Orthopsychiatry, 71*, 236–244.

Salloum, A., Avery, L., & McClain, R. P. (2001). Group psychotherapy for adolescent survivors of homicide victims: A pilot study. *Journal of the American Academy of Child and Adolescent Psychiatry, 40*, 1261–1267.

Saltzman, W. R., Pynoos, R. S., Layne, C. M., Steinberg, A. M., & Aisenberg, E. (2001). Trauma- and grief-focused intervention for adolescents exposed to community violence: Results of a school-based screening and group treatment protocol. *Group Dynamics: Theory, Research and Practice, 5*, 291–303.

Scheeringa, M. S., Peebles, C. D., Cook, C. A., & Zeanah, C. H. (2001). Toward establishing procedural criterion and discriminatory validity for PTSD in early childhood. *Journal of the American Academy of Child and Adolescent Psychiatry, 40*, 52–60.

Solomon, Z. (1988). The effect of combat-related posttraumatic stress disorder on the family. *Psychiatry, 51*, 323–329.

Solomon, Z., Waysman, M., Levy, G., Fried, B., Mikulincer, M., Benbenishty, R., et al. (1992). From front line to home front: A study of secondary traumatization. *Family Process, 31*, 289–302.

Stallard, P., & Law, F. (1993). Screening and psychological debriefing of adolescent survivors of life-threatening events. *British Journal of Psychology, 163*, 660–665.

Stein, B. D., Jaycox, L. H., Kataoka, S. H., Wong, M., Tu, M., Elliott, M. N., et al. (2003). A mental health intervention for school children exposed to violence: A randomized controlled trial. *Journal of the American Medical Association, 290*, 603–611.

Trowell, J., Kolvin, I., Weeramanthri, T., Sadowski, H., Berelowitz, M., Glasser, D., et al. (2002). Psychotherapy for sexually abused girls: Psychopathological outcome findings and patterns of change. *British Journal of Psychology, 160*, 234–247.

Vila, G., Porche, L. M., & Mouren-Simeoni, M. C. (1999). An 18–month longitudinal study of posttraumatic disorders in children who were taken hostage in their school. *Psychosomatic Medicine, 61*, 746–754.

Yule, W. (1992). Post-traumatic stress disorder in child survivors of shipping disasters: The sinking of the "Jupiter." *Psychotherapy and Psychosomatics, 57*, 200–205.

Yule, W., & Udwin, O. (1991). Screening child survivors for post-traumatic stress disorders: Experiences from the "Jupiter" sinking. *British Journal of Clinical Psychology, 30*, 131–138.

Rapid Development of Family Assistance Centers

Lessons Learned Following the September 11 Terrorist Attacks

GREGORY A. LESKIN, WILLIAM J. HULEATT, JACK HERRMANN,
LISA R. LaDUE, and FRED D. GUSMAN

This chapter provides practical suggestions for the rapid development of a family assistance center (FAC) following a large-scale disaster. These recommendations are drawn from the experiences of senior-level clinicians and seasoned administrators who cared for thousands of families following the tragic events of September 11, 2001.

Following a large-scale disaster involving death or injury to multiple individuals, the FAC serves as a central location to administer multiple services, such as providing emotional care for families, informational briefings, coordination of staff, and services to give comfort to the families. In addition, the FACs may serve to collect information about missing persons and to provide a single location for other legal, forensic, and financial services. This chapter focuses on the provision of mental health within the overall framework of the FAC.

We begin by describing the context and the development of FACs in New York City and the Pentagon. Before September 11, plans did exist to implement FACs following disasters.[1] However, these plans did not antici-

---

[1]For more information about previous FAC operations, the interested reader is referred to Bartone and Ender (1994).

pate the extreme magnitude of events or quantity of who would require emotional support, resources, and services. Our objective here is to describe the development of FACs and to share the lessons learned. Despite some similarities between the events in New York City and at the Pentagon, both were unique disasters that required coordinated planning among local, state, and federal disaster service providers. The description of operations in both FACs are not presented here to evaluate one against the other. We are critically analyzing both experiences to provide the reader with practical, real-world experiences to prepare for and coordinate comprehensive care in any future disaster.

In addition to practical information, we include vignettes to illustrate the types of care and challenges faced during these disasters. To respect the privacy of families that suffered tremendous personal loss on September 11, 2001, we changed names and details. Even so, the composites reflect real-life events.

BACKGROUND: AVIATION DISASTER FAMILY ASSISTANCE ACT

The Aviation Disaster Family Assistance Act of 1996 (Public Law 104-264, Title VII) assigned responsibility to the Department of Transportation's National Transportation Safety Board (NTSB) to develop contingency plans and procedures to care for victims and families following an aviation accident or disaster. The NTSB coordinates family assistance with multiple local, state, and federal government agencies, including the Department of Defense and the American Red Cross. Two plans were developed by the NTSB to provide an organizing framework for a coordinated federal response to domestic aviation disasters: (1) the Federal Family Assistance Plan for Aviation Disasters, and (2) the Federal Plan for Aviation Accidents Involving Aircraft Operated by or Chartered by Federal Agencies.

FAMILY CARE AND MENTAL HEALTH

Though the President did not enact the Aviation Disaster Family Assistance Act after September 11, 2001, these NTSB plans provided the framework for developing a comprehensive response to airline accidents. According to the federal Family Assistance Plan for Aviation Disasters, the American Red Cross (ARC) is responsible for family and mental health care following civilian aircraft disasters. ARC is responsible for the overall coordination and management of personnel and other organizations offering psychological, religious and other volunteer support. Apart from the FAC, ARC may set up a separate center to screen, monitor, and manage ARC staff and volunteers. Local resources work through the ARC staff-processing center to provide crisis and grief counseling, food and shelter services, and other support services as needed. ARC also works closely with the airline carrier to care for family members not present at the crash scene.

ATTACKS ON THE WORLD TRADE CENTER AND PENTAGON

At 8:45 A.M. on September 11, 2001, terrorists hijacked American Airlines Flight 11, out of Boston, and crashed it into the north tower of the World Trade Center. At 9:03 A.M., a second hijacked airplane, United Airlines Flight 175 from Boston, crashed into the south tower. Over 2,700 (including New York City Fire, Police, and Port Authority personnel) were killed or injured. At 9:43 A.M. on September 11, 2001, American Airlines Flight 77, also commandeered by terrorists, crashed into the Pentagon, headquarters of the U.S. Department of Defense and nerve center for the military's command. One hundred eighty-four military personnel and civilians were killed in the Pentagon and on the airplane. After these attacks, ARC and Pentagon personnel set up both centralized and local FACs to assist survivors and families members in coping with the devastation.

EXCEPTIONAL TRAGEDY AND UNIQUE CHALLENGES

The magnitude and extensive human toll created challenges never before encountered by the disaster relief community. The attacks required an immediate response by local government, Pentagon, ARC, and other agencies, to those individuals both directly victimized and indirectly affected. There was also the concern for national security issues and the need for criminal and forensic investigations. Furthermore, victims and survivors at each disaster scene included airline passengers and crew members; private citizens employed or located in or nearby the crash site; personnel from local, state, or federal government agencies; and active-duty military and government contract staff. The diversity of victims required an extraordinarily wide range of disaster relief specialists.

Major search and rescue/recovery operations immediately followed. Located near the World Trade Center and the Pentagon, FACs were established as centers for providing information and support to the families of the killed and missing. FACs also served as centers for coordinating disaster mental health volunteers and the military's Casualty Assistance Officers (CAOs) assigned to assist the primary next of kin. Multiple local, state, and federal agencies, including the New York City Office of the Mayor, ARC, Department of Veterans Affairs, Social Security Administration, Federal Emergency Management Agency, FBI Crime Victims Assistance, and other relevant agencies were brought into the FAC to optimize access, interagency coordination, and responsiveness to family members. The consolidation of support service personnel at FACs allowed grieving families to receive information about their loved ones, counseling and spiritual guidance, assistance in the forensic and investigative aspect of the disaster, and an opportunity to join together with other families to begin the healing process. Table 14.1 provides an overview of available services at each site.

NEW YORK CITY

New York City Command Structure

During the initial rescue and recovery efforts, the number of dead and injured in the collapse were feared to be in the tens of thousands. The New York City Offices of the Mayor and Emergency Management took ultimate command of all operations following the attacks on the World Trade Center (WTC), with the assistance and guidance of the New York City Police Department (NYPD), New York City Fire Department, New York City Office of the Chief Medical Examiner, New York State Emergency Management Office, Federal Bureau of Investigation, Federal Emergency Management Agency, ARC, and other local, state, and federal agencies.

Facility Operations: An Overview

With the anticipated number presumed dead or injured in the WTC attacks, it became apparent that an information hotline and FAC were needed to respond to the outpouring of friends, families, and coworkers who attempted to gain access to the WTC sites and area hospitals, trying to locate missing loved ones. Within hours the Office of Emergency Management established a 24-hour patient information hotline at a local television station. Staffed by ARC mental health volunteers, workers provided emotional support to callers while collecting demographic information on those reported missing. By evening, the Office of Emergency Management (OEM) and the Mayor's Community Assistance Unit (CAU) were exploring potential sites for a family compassion center near the WTC site.

By 4:30 A.M. on September 12, representatives from OEM, the CAU,

TABLE 14.1. Basic Composition of the New York City and Pentagon Family Assistance Centers

New York City Family Assistance Center	Pentagon Family Assistance Center
1. *Command structure*: New York City Office of the Mayor, Community Affairs Unit with assistance from multiple local, state, and federal agencies.	1. *Command structure*: Department of Defense with assistance from multiple local, state, and federal agencies.
2. *Site*: Multiple locations for FACs in New York City initially used private, city, and state buildings.	2. *Site*: Large hotel nearby Pentagon chosen immediately after disaster.
3. *Mental health staff*: American Red Cross coordinated all-volunteer mental health personnel. New York City Department of Health and Mental Hygiene, Disaster Psychiatry Outreach, and other local community mental health agencies proved additional mental health resources.	3. *Mental health staff*: Military, civilian, ARC, and volunteer counselors supervised by Department of Defense senior clinician.
4. *Services offered*: FACs provided multiple services including mental health counseling; forensics; information on deceased, injured, or missing; child care; financial/housing assistance; interpreter services; and transportation for families.	4. *Services offered*: Pentagon FACs provided multiple services including information about dead or missing, CAOs, spiritual care, mental health counseling, forensics, child care, insurance/financial benefits, housing, and transportation for families.
5. *Accommodations*: A large dockside warehouse was finally identified and transformed into a comprehensive facility offering numerous supportive services and included a large registration area, multiple meeting and interviewing areas, dining facilities, and a quiet room for families. Security provided by New York Police Department and the National Guard.	5. *Accommodations*: Large hotel allowed for single, secured space, including meeting rooms, restaurant, snack/beverage services, and sleeping rooms for staff and families. Security provided by Department of Defense police units.

the Office of the Chief Medical Examiner (OCME), the NYPD, and ARC toured what would be the first compassion center, located at NYU Medical Center. Within an hour of opening the first compassion center at 8:00 A.M. it was clear that a larger space was needed. By 12:00 P.M., ARC volunteers escorted families down the street to the new building with more interview space but less waiting-room space. This resulted in many, who had been waiting inside at the NYU Medical Center, now having to wait in line, back outside. Security services were required to temper the frustration of family members relegated to their outdoor waiting room. More interviewing personnel were brought in, moving the process along somewhat more swiftly, but the need for larger space quickly became apparent. By the end of Day 2, the third location for the family compassion center, located at the 26th Armory, was identified. This newly-relocated center was far superior to the previous one, though the conditions were still not optimal to meet the ever-growing needs.

By the end of Day 1 here, representatives from the Mayor's Office, ARC, and others were already discussing moving the compassion center for what many hoped would be the final time. They were challenged to identify a place sufficiently large to accommodate the growing number still in search of loved ones, to provide support services to those who had received the devastating news that their family member was confirmed dead, and to provide a centralized place for those been displaced from their homes or jobs to seek assistance. They also needed to identify a location that provided a private and secure place for those seeking services, away from the eyes of the media and the public at large, and a structure that could accommodate the host of support agencies and organizations.

On Friday, September 14, 2001, representatives from a multitude of agencies toured Pier 94, a cavernous dockside warehouse located at 57th and West Side Highway. The informal inspecting committee decided this would provide adequate space over a period of time to meet the multifaceted needs of those affected by one of the nation's worst tragedies. The FAC at Pier 94 opened 6 days after the first strike on the WTC. All FAC operations were coordinated by a representative of the Mayor's Office, CAU. ARC coordinated all volunteer mental health personnel. Mental health resources were provided by the New York City Department of Health and Mental Hygiene, the Disaster Psychiatry Outreach team, psychiatrists who volunteered to provide mental health support to children and youth, and other professionals from local hospitals and community mental health centers. Staffing was covered over 12–14-hour shifts and included mental health supervisors and line personnel. These volunteers provided grief and crisis counseling to bereaved families; the injured seeking emotional support, rescue, recovery; and law enforcement personnel who came to the FAC for respite.

Mental Health Counseling

Public concern quickly spread. ARC was deluged with spontaneous volunteers. Many were mental health professionals, though others were well meaning citizens of New York City and other places who wanted to reach out and lend support to those directly affected by this tragedy. The challenges of verifying professional credentials, providing minimal training and education on the policies and procedures of the Red Cross Disaster Mental Health function, and deploying volunteers to multiple sites throughout the city took great orchestration.

Due to travel restrictions, the national ARC leadership was delayed in their response, leaving the primary coordination to state and local Red Cross leaders. The New York State Disaster Mental Health Leader responded within hours to New York City from his home in Upstate New York. Upon arrival, he took responsibility for coordinating the mental health resources, which would be utilized in the patient information hotline, the family compassion center, and the subsequent FAC. An ARC disaster mental health leader from nearby Connecticut took responsibility for coordinating mental health resources for the other ARC service sites.

Within hours, ARC responded to the needs of thousands of New York City residents and visitors directly affected by the disaster and the suspension of transportation services by opening numerous emergency aid stations and shelters throughout downtown Manhattan and the outlying boroughs. Mental health volunteers were stationed at JFK, LaGuardia, and Newark airports to assist passengers and airline personnel stranded when the federal government decided to suspend all U.S. air travel.

One mental health volunteer reported spending a considerable amount of time with an inconsolable airline attendant who feared a friend was on one of the ill-fated flights that struck the WTC towers.

Temporary shelters throughout lower Manhattan provided a safe place for those evacuated from the towers and the surrounding area and unable to get back into their residences. Mental health volunteers offered emotional support to those in the shelter who were trying to notify family members of their whereabouts but were faced with the communications system failure of telephones and cell phones affected by the disaster. These volunteers assisted those in the shelter in finding alternate housing with family or friends, or assured those without such resources that shelter would be available until other accommodations could be sought.

The shelters proved sparsely populated as many found alternative accommodations. Those homeless prior to the disaster appreciated their newfound homes. Major transportation hubs throughout New York City became makeshift shelters for those trying to find their way back to their homes outside the city. Mental health volunteers dispatched to Grand Central Station, Port Authority, and Pennsylvania Station calmed fears and suggested more comfortable shelters while awaiting alternative transportation home.

Emergency aid stations provided respite for rescue and recovery workers and offered water, snacks, brief rest, and first aid for the minor burns, scratches, and other injuries sustained from working on the smoldering pile of cement, metal girders, and remnants of the WTC towers. Mental health volunteers stood by to offer grief and counseling services to those looking for missing brethren.

One New York City firefighter had been working "on the pile" for over 24 hours searching for three coworkers who were in one of the towers when they collapsed. Energized by his adrenalin, he avoided a mental health volunteer's attempts to show him compassion and encouragement to get some rest. He avoided any expression of feeling, instead insisting that he must return "to the pile" to bring these fallen firefighters back home to their families. His search, he said, would not be stopped, until they were found. Later that day, the remains of one of his colleagues were found and removed ceremoniously to an awaiting caravan of ambulances to bring them to the temporary morgue. Despite his exhaustion, he continued to search for his two remaining friends. On the second day of his search his Captain ordered him home to rest. Though initially resistant, he obeyed, but he returned the next day to continue searching. He followed the same routine for the next 2 days, working tirelessly before going home to rest. Eventually the bodies of his two colleagues were identified.

By 6:00 A.M., the day after the attacks, thousands lined up along 1st Avenue, hoping to enter the FAC at NYU Medical Center scheduled to open at 8:00 A.M. ARC mental health volunteers helped sign in family members and seat them in the NYU auditorium to await interviews with personnel from the OCME and NYPD.

The new FAC had limited waiting space so many family members lined up again. NYPD services had to prevent families from forcibly making their way inside in an attempt to make their outrage known. By day's end, arrangements were made for yet another move to the 26th Street Armory, to open the next morning.

The Armory, though not optimal, provided additional interviewing and waiting room space. A canteen for snacks and drinks was established. A private area in the Armory basement was established for those who were there to peruse the lists of injured that started to come in from local area hospitals. Family members were seated with mental health professionals and volunteers from the Disaster Psychiatry Outreach group to review these. Others were moved on to look at lists of the deceased provided by the OCME.

Those unsuccessful in finding their loved ones on either list were directed to the first floor to complete a missing person's report, assisted by personnel from the OCME and NYPD. Those painstakingly aware that their loved ones might not come home presented with personal items of the missing, such as a toothbrush, comb, or hairbrush, in hopes that DNA tests would lead to final identification. Others needed to be more assertively directed to bring in such items and left in tears.

As the days wore on, many more families of the missing came to the compassion center. By September 17, 2003, the fourth and final location for what would be renamed the FAC was opened. What was once a cavernous pier warehouse, virtually overnight had turned into a comfortable FAC. Led by the New York City Mayor's Office, the FAC housed representatives of ARC, New York State Office of Mental Health, New York City Department of Mental Health, NYPD, New York City Office of the Chief Medical Examiner, Federal Emergency Management Agency, New York State Crime Victim's Board, Salvation Army, and over 50 other agencies. Families of those confirmed dead, the injured, those displaced from housing or work, recovery workers, law enforcement officers, and relevant others used the FAC for emotional support, assistance with housing and other basic needs, or for respite.

> Mental health volunteers worked with children, adults, families, couples, and coworkers. One mental health worker described his interaction with a worker from the WTC who had been blown from the building when the first plane struck. Bruised and injured, he described the need to come into the FAC to tell families of those missing their loved ones that they did not die alone. He recalled that before the building collapsed, people were evacuating calmly, some unaware of what lay ahead, others joking with their friends and colleagues as they proceeded downstairs toward the lobby. A mental health volunteer found a young man while the man was sharing his story with those who were waiting to be interviewed. Instead of relief, he shared how guilty he felt that he survived. His listeners told him not to feel guilty and how lucky his parents were that their son survived.

THE PENTAGON

Pentagon Family Assistance Center
Command Structure

The Pentagon response differed from the New York City response in numerous ways. The military and community response followed a chain of command. Immediately following the attack, staff from the Deputy Under Secretary of Defense, Military Community and Family Policy Office

(MC&FP) began planning for the Pentagon Family Assistance Center (PFAC). The director of the Office of Family Policy contacted staff familiar with family support services, casualty affairs policy, and functional programs and people familiar with Department of Defense (DoD) policies and procedures, who could also call on others within existing networks to obtain supportive resources and personnel quickly.

From the time of its inception, an Army Lieutenant General (three-star rank) served as PFAC director to lead the operation and many organizations at the facility: primary care and mental health providers from Walter Reed Army Medical Center, 89th Medical Group at Andrews Air Force Base, 81st Medical Group at Keesler Air Force Base, Army Community Service, Navy Fleet and Family Support Centers, ARC, National Center for PTSD, Department of Veterans Affairs, Tragedy Assistance Program for Survivors, Salvation Army, TRICARE, Federal Bureau of Investigation, and many others.

Facility Operations: Overview

Military Community and Family Policy Office staff worked with local officials to identify a site for the PFAC. The basic requirements were accessibility, convenience, and security. The facility needed to provide adequate meeting space, lodging, parking, and food service to feed the numerous families, staff, and volunteers. The Sheraton Crystal City Hotel, 1 mile from the Pentagon, met the requirements. Working with hotel staff, DoD and military staff prepared the facility overnight.

On September 12, during the Pentagon press briefing, the Under Secretary of Defense for Personnel and Readiness announced the initiation and location of the PFAC. A toll-free number for families to speak with a Pentagon representative was also operational. The primary task of the call center was to compile and provide current, accurate information about missing persons and about the services available.

A colonel trained in social work from the U.S. Army Medical Department's North Atlantic Regional Medical Command (William J. Huleatt, the second author) was primarily responsible for coordinating and supervising the mental health operation at the PFAC. He was ideally suited to lead mental health's efforts here due to his ability to tap into a large network of local resources, knowledge of the military command structure, and previous experience rapidly developing complex military operations and programs. Originally staffed by active-duty Army, Navy, and Air Force personnel; government and nongovernmental behavioral health personnel, and volunteers, the center was soon augmented by other disaster relief experts. Staff from the Department of Veterans Affairs, National Center for PTSD, provided on-site consultation and assistance to DoD personnel. Also, the

Disaster Mental Health Services (ARC DMHS) and mental health volunteers from the community provided additional staffing to meet emerging demands. PFAC staff provided 24-hour crisis intervention services to victims' families

Several days after the attack, the separate agencies involved in the attack, such as the Army, Navy, American Airlines, and Department of Justice Office for Victims of Crime, consolidated their individual assistance centers within the PFAC. Dulles Airport was theoretically to provide an FAC for the airline victims, but it quickly became clear that airline staff were too overwhelmed to do that effectively, so it was rolled into the PFAC (E. C. Ritchie, personal communication, June 2004). Thus the PFAC became a single, convenient source for reliable, accurate information and comprehensive services.

Organizational Structures

The PFAC was organized into three main support components: (1) management, (2) administration, and (3) operations. Part of the success of the PFAC operation was to allow these different components to evolve and mature consistent with the changing needs of the families. As search and rescue operations evolved into search and recover, the PFAC mission evolved too, primarily focusing on helping bereaved families to cope In the end, the PFAC served as (1) the central point for up-to-date information for families, (2) the main source for government and private agencies to provide crises intervention services, (3) a single location to coordinate mortuary affairs and collect DNA samples to identify remains, and (4) a secure, environment for families to come together to begin the grieving process.

Management Components

By the second week, a formal PFAC organization took shape. Rather than a multilevel, pyramid design, the organization took on a more decentralized structure, allowing a wide span of control by leadership. This wide span of control allowed leadership to remain flexible and directly responsive to family needs. Daily staff meetings and family debriefings allowed for PFAC top leadership to hear from families and augment services to respond to emerging concerns and issues.

PFAC leadership was vital in fulfilling the high demands and emotional rigors of the operation. It was designed as a military operation with its primary goal to provide relief and comfort to the families. The officer in charge (OIC) demonstrated compassion, openness, and comfort while maintaining significant positional authority to keep staff and volunteers focused on the mission.

No blueprint or previous guidance was available at the time the PFAC was formed to manage a joint DoD FAC. Leadership chose to develop an uncomplicated system of operational procedures that included (1) conducting daily PFAC staff meetings to ensure adequate coordination and communication; (2) conducting daily family briefings; (3) responding quickly and accurately to their questions, needs, and concerns; (4) creating a safe haven for families; (5) quickly screening agencies and volunteers wishing to work at the PFAC; (6) restricting media access to PFAC and families; and (7) establishing procedures to safeguard victim and family member information.

Family Briefings

Located in the main ballroom of the Sheraton Crystal City Hotel, daily briefings provided continuous, accurate information to family members. The first part included the officer in charge providing critical, up-to-date information. The second part included questions and answers from family members and CAOs. Question-and-answer sessions sometimes lasted 2 hours, which reflected the commitment to allow all members to ask as many questions and to request clarification as much as possible. The OIC also offered to meet with families individually to answer any remaining questions. Briefing notes were provided before each session to all attendees.

Families were provided with information corresponding to different stages of their needs. Generally, these progressed from seeking basic information about their missing loved one (Stage 1); seeking specific information about the disposition of remains, benefits, and entitlements and seeking to bond with other families (Stage 2); CAOs seeking information to support families (Stage 3); and families seeking to move on with their lives (Stage 4). At the family briefings, the officer in charge provided the current status of the rescue and recovery operation, the number of missing, the number of victims recovered and identified, and available services inside and outside the PFAC. In addition to the OIC, subject matter experts were available to family members, including experts who discussed mortuary and identification process, eligibility requirements for burial at Arlington Cemetery, the investigative process, and the role of the casualty assistance officers.

Mental Health Counseling at the PFAC

The mental health officer in charge had broad responsibility for the mental health counseling mission, including screening and scheduling all counselors and coordinating behavioral health support services to families and staff. He approved staff from National Center for PTSD, Education and

Clinical Laboratory to provide on-site counseling services and educational materials for the PFAC. Mental health counselors from military units from across the country augmented clinical coverage. Behavioral health staff delivered counseling across a full spectrum of normal grief reactions, including crisis intervention, family counseling, management of "at-risk" family members, child/adolescent counseling, consultation services, psycho-education, and referrals for longer-term follow-up counseling.

Besides these types of direct care services, behavioral health staff monitored family members during especially difficult emotional times, such as family briefings and ceremonial events. When families visited the Pentagon crash site, teams of behavioral health staff accompanied them and were available for crisis intervention or immediate social support. Mental health services at the PFAC worked closely with ARC mental health and chaplain services to maximize available resources and minimize possible overlaps in coverage.

Screening of Mental Health Staff

The mental health officer in charge established a minimum baseline of experience for counselors at the PFAC. One main objective for mental health staff was to provide nonintrusive, largely unstructured, emotional support for families. An important qualification for counselors was the ability to distinguish between persons experiencing normal grief and those having more difficultly adjusting postdisaster, and to intervene appropriately. Furthermore, offering assistance to disaster victims who may not necessarily be seeking help, hesitate to receive help, or are unaccustomed to mental health support requires disaster personnel who are respectful and informed. Often, family members would initially request information about general procedures or services offered at the PFAC. Such conversations would lead in to more specific queries by mental health personnel about the victim's general well-being and adjustment. One primary characteristic for disaster personnel is the ability and sensitivity to respond to the victim's immediate needs and, if appropriate, deliver mental health support at a level consistent with the victim's background and openness for support.

It was important to screen volunteers according to their ability to deliver compassionate and appropriate crisis intervention within this context. Often it is difficult, without a preestablished procedure, to accomplish adequate screening of volunteers, such as reviewing professional credentials and skills, in the midst of tragedy.

The American Red Cross does maintain such a system. All ARC disaster response volunteers are required to take disaster-training classes, as well as to hold professional licenses as mental health professionals. The PFAC mental health coordinator personally screened and interviewed all potential non-ARC volunteers from the community. Those with appropriate credentials and prior disaster work experience were assigned duties as counselors, escorts, or reception staff according to their qualifications

Composition and Role of the Mental Health Staff

Mental health staff at the PFAC provided emotional support to families and friends of the victims from the airline and Pentagon. Mental health counselors also provided ongoing support to staff providing services at the PFAC and the Pentagon. Consistent with crises intervention theory, on-site practice of psychotherapy was not permitted. Typically, mental health care delivery occurred within informal contexts, such as when family members requested information about the location of a particular service and would be escorted by mental health personnel. Mental health staff were encouraged to circulate actively among families and staff during breaks from meetings, or during memorial visits to the crash site, and at daily informational debriefings. By providing verbal messages of condolences, compassionate listening, and tissues, mental health staff played an important role in maintaining a safe environment conducive to appropriate emotional expressions of grief, anger, loss, and sadness. If family members requested individual time with a counselor or for individuals experiencing more severe emotional reactions (intensive crying, panic, depersonalization), private space was available to assist them.

On a typical day, 20 military and civilian counselors and 2 administrative assistants worked across three 8-hour shifts. Staff consisted of a mix between social workers, psychologists, and psychiatrists. Mental health staff also keep records of their informal contacts, in order to document PFAC activities and provide ongoing needs assessment. During Phase I of the PFAC operation, 18,000 staff contacts were made. Volunteer and military counselors provided both written and verbal reports to the PFAC mental health coordinator. At first the ARC counselors reported to their family assistance officer in charge. Keeping with PFAC goal of minimizing duplication of effort and recognizing that these two operations were performing similar functions, ARC mental health was eventually incorporated into the overall PFAC mental health operation.

Role of the Casualty Assistance Officers

Every military and DoD civilian next of kin was assigned a casualty assistance officer. CAOs are active-duty military servicemen and -women who volunteer to serve in this capacity as a separate, unique part of their military career. The CAOs were responsible for addressing logistical requirements of the family, (e.g., transportation and lodging), acting as an official liaison between the family and the DoD, working with the family to complete compensation and death benefits paperwork, and serving as an escort throughout the death notification process. Because of the demanding nature of this detail, including long work hours and working closely with grieving families, routine mental health support was not typically available for the CAOs. However, CAOs were offered a comprehensive and structured debriefing at the end of their tour of duty.

During the PFAC operation, mental health staff provided on-site evaluation of the critical role played by these CAOs. National Center for PTSD staff worked closely with the mental health officer in charge and other military staff to develop, conduct and analyze a survey and program evaluation of the CAOs operation. A "CAO survey" was created to (1) examine the perspectives of the CAOs in terms of assistance offered at the PFAC, (2) gather insights and after-action information critical for planning future responses to mass casualty incidents, (3) find out specific needs for additional services as the PFAC moved toward a reduction in force during Phase II, and (4) determine the stress level and perceived self-efficacy of each CAO. Results of the survey were quickly reported to PFAC operational leadership to assist ongoing planning.

Additional Role of ARC
Disaster Mental Health Services at the PFAC

ARC DMHS volunteers initially responded to the PFAC as members of integrated care teams. ARC developed these teams to address the financial, emotional, and physical health issues often encountered by individuals impacted by injuries and/or deaths from disasters. The ARC FAC officer directed all services provided by ARC volunteers and staff at the PFAC but was accountable to the PFAC OIC.

ARC integrated care teams were composed of Health Services, Family Services, and DMHS volunteers. These teams were established at the PFAC to assist family members locate hospitalized victims of the Pentagon attack, to provide financial assistance to these victims and their family members, to provide financial assistance to families of deceased victims to attend memorial services other than the Pentagon memorial service provided by the DoD, and to provide supportive physical and mental health services to these individuals.

Brief Education and Support Services
for Workers and Staff

PFAC workers and staff met with mental health staff in small group sessions. Instead of providing formal debriefing sessions in which participants describe the details of their exposure to the disaster or its aftermath, PFAC staff provided educational materials and information about normal stress reactions and building resiliency to cope with stress. Participants shared their concerns about their own stress reactions, as well as positive personal experiences in which they appropriately managed difficult situations. For example, difficulties sleeping and fatigue are normal during the aftermath of disasters and are considered one of the most frequently endorsed features of the posttrauma experience.

Participants to these group sessions discussed their concerns about sleep loss and fatigue and their effects on their mood, concentration and ability to cope overall. Mental health staff worked together with the participants to normalize such reactions by finding out if others in the room were also suffering loss of sleep and its effects. Sleep hygiene practices were discussed, strategies (e.g., brief daytime naps and moderate exercise) would be encouraged, and educational materials would be provided. Those with more intense sleep problems (insomnia leading to exhaustion and repeated nightmares) were referred for more intensive mental health services or psychiatric care.

All staff at the PFAC plus hotel staff were informed of the time and place of these small group sessions. PFAC leadership recognized the importance of this psychoeducational intervention for all those working with families or those with close ties to the disaster.

Defusing Leadership

During the PFAC operation, National Center for PTSD senior staff led informal, group defusing sessions with PFAC leadership officials. Their purpose was to provide the opportunity for disaster-scene leaders to speak honestly about their own thoughts, feelings, and experiences regarding the disaster and the resulting PFAC operation. Often, senior leadership officials began the sessions by reflecting on their own experiences, such as the emotionally challenging role of taking care of families that have lost loved ones. Leadership reflected that those lost in the building were also their own friends and colleagues. Reflections on personal loss, expectations of personal safety, anger toward the criminal perpetrators, and guilt about feeling powerless to lessen the pain and hurt were all themes senior leadership voiced during these sessions. In addition to the direct therapeutic value of such defusing sessions, it was important to discuss the idea that the disaster response was finite and would eventually end. Reminding leadership that the operation will have an endpoint normalizes the situation and can encourage leadership to think about the meaning of the event within a larger context.

LESSONS LEARNED FROM THE FACs

The experiences from September 11, 2001, and the rapid response to set up FACs in New York City and Washington, DC, provided invaluable opportunities for addressing future mass casualty incidents.

Community Planning and Preparedness

Disaster history, especially following mass casualty incidents such as September 11, underlines the immediate need to provide information to families and other loved ones. The rapid establishment of a central location as a single source of authoritative information directed specifically to families proves a necessary first step for disaster responders. This centralized location must be flexible and expandable to meet survivors' needs. In New York City, a change of venue was necessary to accommodate the larger numbers the services required to support their needs. Locations that provide privacy and security work well to shield individuals from the media or others during the acute phase of the grieving process.

Coordination of Mental Health Resources

Mental health volunteers prove key resources in the psychological aftermath of disasters. Following September 11, large-scale disasters and mass casualty incidents result in large numbers of well-meaning volunteers, including mental health professionals, offering assistance. Credentialing verification and identification of professional backgrounds proves a daunting task when disaster strikes. Therefore, community mental health leaders should establish criteria for the education and training of disaster mental health workers as part of their disaster preparedness. Processes for verifying professional credentials and scheduling and deploying of such mental health resources should be preestablished.

Adequate Training and Experience

It may have been erroneously assumed that all mental health professionals are equally qualified to work with disaster victims. Disasters present unique challenges for those in the "helping" profession. While past experience in working with victims of disaster is optimal, this is not always a reasonable prerequisite. Seasoned disaster mental health responders suggest that the most important attributes of the mental health disaster worker are the ability to be clinically flexible; to provide nonintrusive, supportive, brief interventions; to distinguish between normal grieving and complicated grief responses; and to work in nontraditional settings (e.g., at a disaster scene and in hotel rooms). These qualifications cannot be overemphasized. Working with grieving families at a disaster requires a delicate balance and sensitivity to allow individuals time and space to grieve while also presenting to them the availability of supportive counseling.

Disaster mental health staff must also possess high levels of self-awareness. In the immediate aftermath, disaster response results in long hours, stressful interactions with victims and their family members, and, often, repressing one's own needs to meet those of others. Mental health professionals must possess the insight to recognize the impact of disaster environments on their ability to fulfill their obligations and duties and to take precautionary measures to prepare and care for themselves. Having a predetermined self-care plan is critical. Experienced disaster mental health responders take periodic breaks for self-reflection, maintain a healthy regimen of diet and exercise, and have a sense of flexibility and humor. It is equally important that disaster mental health responders maintain a positive support system. This is often accomplished through daily defusings, either formally established within the operational structure or informally with peers.

Interagency Collaboration and Cooperation

Disasters can illuminate or create tensions within or between organizations. Which will be the lead agency at the FAC? What services will be provided at the FAC? Who will direct mental health operations? How will other organizations provide resources? These are critical questions, even in the midst of considerable pressure to respond to survivors, their loved ones, and the community. Remembering that there is often more work than can be accomplished by any one agency, the success of an FAC often relies on interagency collaboration. Disaster management leaders should preidentify and train mental health resources within a community in their roles following a mass casualty. Knowing which agencies will provide mental health support staff is an important component to any community disaster mental health plan.

The FAC is only one aspect of a mass casualty response. Leadership must be aware of the command structure of the overall operation and that the command structure of the FAC is readily established and understood by all agencies involved in delivering services at the center. Providing mental health or emotional support services is only one aspect of the operations within the FAC. Mental health staff must understand clearly the roles they are to fulfill and the command structure within which they are working at the FAC. Multiple command structures and reporting responsibilities are likely to create complications in communication and service delivery. Leadership personnel from all agencies involved at the FAC need to meet as soon as possible, establish a command structure with clear communication channels, and reach an understanding of the roles of each agency or organization. Daily management staff meetings are necessary for effective problem solving; effective communication; and provision of appropriate, responsive care to the family members and staff at the FAC.

Media Relations

The media may be viewed as adversaries. Mental health professionals must preserve the confidentiality of those who confide in them, while the media search for those who are willing to tell their stories. Although the personal experiences of those who seek the services of mental health workers in the FAC are confidential, the media often play an integral role in getting loved ones to the FAC where they can obtain information and receive assistance. Working together, mental health responders can educate the media on the types of services offered at the FAC and the value of families using these services. Disaster mental health workers, through these media outlets, can also educate a community on the psychological impact of a disaster and provide information about ways to cope and enhance recovery, as well as encourage individuals to seek mental health support when necessary.

Summary

With the advancing knowledge of our nation's vulnerabilities, communities face numerous challenges in responding to the mental health needs following disasters. The threat of weapons of mass destruction presents significant hurdles in establishing FACs in the aftermath of such disasters. Such challenges include:

- Identifying venues with sufficient space to accommodate large numbers of families.
- Identifying the resources that will inevitably be needed at the FAC.
- Screening of mental health professionals to ensure they provide the appropriate level of care to victims, their loved ones, disaster responders, and the community.
- Establishing an interagency command structure that fits within the overall operational disaster response plan.
- Opening an FAC following a biological, chemical, or nuclear terrorist attack presents the risk of contaminated individuals coming for assistance, potentially contaminating others.
- The potential loss of electricity, communication systems, computers, transportation, and other basic services.

Whatever a community's vulnerabilities, the role of disaster planning and preparedness cannot be overemphasized. Planning and preparedness for the rapid establishment of an FAC requires extensive collaboration among all agencies and organizations involved in providing services for victims, family members, staff, and the community following a mass casualty disaster. This includes those agencies involved in the logistics of the plan (e.g., the facility, equipment, supplies, and feeding), the medical examiner/coroner's office, agencies providing supportive and financial assistance, law enforcement and other security services, health care facilities, and those providing spiritual and mental health services. The resources of each agency must be identified and its role within the FAC defined. Interagency communication, collaboration, and coordination are of the utmost importance in the establishment and effective operation of an FAC. Mental health services must be clinically flexible, nonintrusive, and centered primarily on crisis/trauma intervention modalities. The special needs of a culturally diverse population, of populations such as the elderly, children of various developmental stages, physically and mentally impaired individuals, and those with chronic psychiatric disorders must all be considered.

CONCLUSION

Disaster and mass casualty response requires preparation, coordination, and collaboration. Disaster response leaders must remain flexible throughout the disaster response in order to solve the numerous challenges and attend to the decision-making processes that continuously arise. Successful and rapid development of the FAC can provide much needed structure, comfort, and information for the community in the aftermath of disasters

RESOURCES

American Red Cross. *September, 11, 2001: Unprecedented events, unprecedented response—A review of the American Red Cross' response in the past year.* Retrieved from www.redcross.org/press/disaster/ds_pr/pdfs/arcwhitepaper.pdf

National Transportation Safety Board. *Federal Family Assistance Plan for aviation disasters.* Retrieved August 2000 from www.ntsb.gov/publictn/2000/SPC0001.pdf

Department of Defense. *Response to the Terrorist Attack on the Pentagon: Pentagon Family Assistance Center (PFAC) after action report.* Retrieved March 2003 from www.mfrc-dodqol.org/enduring_freedom/pfacrpt.htm

Department of the Army. (1987). *Casualty assistance handbook* (Pamphlet No 608-33). Washington, DC: Author.

SUGGESTED FURTHER READING

Bartone, P. T. (1996). *Family notification and survivor assistance: Thinking the unthinkable.* In Ursano, R. J., Norwood, A. E. (Eds.). *Emotional aftermath of the Persian Gulf War: Veterans, families, communities, nations* (pp. 315–352). Washington, DC: American Psychiatric Association Press.

Bartone, P. T., & Ender, M. G. (1994). Organizational responses to death in the military. *Death Studies, 18,* 25–39.

Bartone, P. T., Ursano, R. J., Wright, K. M., & Ingraham, L. H. (1989). The impact of a military air disaster on the health of assistance workers: A prospective study. *Journal of Nervous and Mental Disorders, 177,* 317–328.

Bartone, P. T., & Wright, K. M. (1990). Grief and group recovery following a military air disaster. *Journal of Traumatic Stress, 3,* 523–539.

Dodgen, D., LaDue, L. R., & Kaul, R. E. (2002). Coordinating a local response to a national tragedy: Community mental health in Washington, DC after the Pentagon attack. *Military Medicine, 167*(9 Suppl.), 87–89.

Geiling, J. A. (2002). Overview of command and control issues: Setting the stage. *Military Medicine, 167*(9 Suppl.), 3–5.

Hoge, C. W., Orman, D. T., Robichaux, R. J., Crandell, E. O., Patterson, V. J., Engel, C. C., et al. (2002). Operation Solace: overview of the mental health intervention following the September 11, 2001 Pentagon attack. *Military Medicine, 167*(9 Suppl.), 44–47.

Huleatt, W. J., LaDue, L., Leskin, G. A., Ruzek, J., & Gusman, F. (2002). Pentagon Family Assistance Center inter-agency mental health collaboration and response. *Military Medicine, 167*(9 Suppl.), 68–70.

Ritchie, E. C., & Stokes, J. (2002). Perspectives on coordination from the Office of the Assistant Secretary of Defense/Health Affairs. *Military Medicine, 167*(9 Suppl.), 31–32.

Ruzek, J. I. (2002). Providing "brief education and support" for emergency response workers: an alternative to debriefing. *Military Medicine, 167*(9 Suppl.), 73–75.

Thomas-Lawson, M., Whitworth, J., & Doherty, J. (2002). The role of leadership in trauma response: Pentagon Family Assistance Center. *Military Medicine, 167*(9 Suppl.), 71–72.

Psychiatric Intervention for Medical and Surgical Patients Following Traumatic Injuries

HAROLD J. WAIN, GEOFFREY G. GRAMMER, JOHN STASINOS, and CATHERINE M. DEBOER

The impact of trauma or disaster on the medical surgical patient can be overwhelming for the patient, his or her family, and caregivers. Providing ideal care while attempting to prevent disabling psychiatric comorbidity have been goals of providers for many years. Previous attempts with similar goals are described following Gulf War I, the Pentagon attacks, the bombings of the U.S. embassy in Nairobi, and the current wars in Afghanistan and Iraq (Wain, Grammer, & DeBoer, 2004; Wain, Grammer, Stasinos, & Miller, 2002; Wain & Jacaard, 1996; Wain & Stasinos, 1999).

To provide effective interventions, mental health care providers must ally themselves to the patient, the patient's family, and the patient's treatment team; offer services and implement interventions that will assist the patient in processing their trauma and its aftermath; support the family members who provide critical emotional support to the patient; and facilitate, along with their treatment team, an optimal clinical outcome. All this happens as patients undergo medical and surgical care and seek to adapt to the new realities imposed by their trauma. Thus, a comprehensive program designed to help the entire medical institution respond to the trauma must consider the needs of the patient, the patient's family, and medical staff involved.

This chapter focuses on the psychological issues of medical and surgical patients suffering from traumatic injuries. This approach to care for these patients, their families, and medical care providers was innovated by the Psychiatry Consultation Liaison Service (PCLS) and is based on the experience of the authors and their colleagues in the caring for these patients, their families, and treatment teams at Walter Reed Army Medical Center (WRAMC) over the past 20 years.

INJURIES AND IATROGENIC STRESSORS OF TRAUMA VICTIMS

Patients who present to WRAMC for definitive treatment of injuries suffered in combat or terrorist attack usually are evacuated by air, following medical stabilization by local medical resources near the scene of the trauma. This may be a long pipeline. Soldiers wounded in combat usually have received immediate lifesaving intervention on the battlefield or in the battalion aid station by a combat medic, further treatment at a mobile surgical hospital, then evacuation by plane to Landstuhl Army Medical Center (LAMC), prior to transfer from Europe to the United States. Most of the Kenya Embassy bombing victims were also routed through LAMC before arriving at WRAMC. After the 9/11 attack on the Pentagon casualties who required extended inpatient management of their injuries were admitted to hospitals closer to the Pentagon than WRAMC. Thus we exported teams to these facilities to assist in their clinical management.

The nature and severity of injuries vary depending on the event. Terrorist attack victims may suffer extensive burns, blunt trauma, multiple wounds from shrapnel or broken glass, and smoke inhalation. Combat trauma from the wars in Afghanistan and Iraq include gunshot wounds, shrapnel wounds, brain and spinal cord injuries (sometimes resulting in cognitive and/or neurological impairment), and amputations. In many cases, the trauma and the injuries represented the end of life as the patient knew it and the beginning of a painful, arduous ordeal with an uncertain outcome.

The surviving patient is subject to a broad range of stresses throughout the process of recovery. Pain is exacerbated by debridement, dressing changes, skin grafts, plastic surgery, and the need to exercise burned limbs to avoid contractures. Gastric stress ulcers are another source of pain. The patient may have to be isolated until the danger of infection has passed, and extensive bandaging further reduces environmental contact. A tracheostomy may interfere with communication. In a state of relative sensory isolation, all the patient's fears are magnified (Weinstein, 1990).

While medical and surgical care are essential to the recovery of the trauma victim, this clinical care may be experienced by patients and their families as a significant ongoing stressor and, in severe cases, as an extension of the trauma itself. The mental health care provider must weigh the effects of the traumatic event, and of stressors arising from their medical and surgical management in the wake of trauma, to prevent or minimize psychological sequelae and optimize clinical outcome.

Definitive care of severe and complicated injury may require prolonged hospitalization with uncertain outcome. Neurological and physiological disturbances and behavioral changes may follow major amputations, spinal cord injury with paralysis, facial disfigurement from missile wounds and burns, blindness, and mutilating and castrating wounds of the external male genitalia (Weinstein, 1990). Inpatient stressors include pain, complications arising in the course of the patient's treatment and recovery, infection, the need for repeated incision and drainage or revision of surgical wounds, development of decubiti in the bedridden, side effects from medications, hospital-acquired infections, delays in recovery and prolonged hospital stays, and uncertainty in the outcome and time course.

An example of a typical therapeutic intervention for PCLS is described next.

A 32-year-old single male injured in Iraq sustained a gunshot wound to the left posterior heel resulting in calceneal and midfoot fractures. The patient underwent fashiotomies in the field, was evacuated to Germany, and then to WRAMC. While at WRAMC the patient experienced significant pain and anxiety before and after surgery. Pain was well controlled with a sciatic block, Dilaudid PCA, fentanyl patch, MS Contin, and Percocet.

With pain controlled, the patient could engage in physical therapy following surgery and was eventually discharged to home without dependence on any medication. The possibility of using an selective serotonin reuptake inhibitor was discussed with the patient to help with persistent thoughts about the injury, fears about the future, and increased arousal. The patient declined at the time but agreed to think about starting medication, which he eventually declined.

The patient was seen within 36 hours of arrival at WRAMC without a formal consult. He was hospitalized for 20 days. His trauma experiences were quickly normalized. An empathic exposure approach, both individually and in group, was used to help him integrate his traumatic experiences into a normal stream. Relaxation and hypnotic techniques were used to decrease his pain, to aid his sleep, and to help work through his conflict.

The patient was seen daily while hospitalized and he attended group sessions for injured soldiers. He was able to use this empathic exposure and the normalization of his events to facilitate his recovery.

Follow-up occurred via telephone interventions 30, 90, and 180 days after discharge. The patient made a good adjustment to his discharge and reported no psychiatric complication.

THE IMPACT OF TRAUMA

By definition, trauma is an overwhelming experience that disrupts one's homeostasis. Furst (1967) suggests that adaptive mechanisms are compromised and normal psychological defenses cannot be utilized. The experience of trauma results in a threat to self-integrity, self-confidence, and self-esteem. One's sense of vulnerability is heightened, trust of others is diminished, and critical judgment is suspended, and feelings of helplessness, dependency, and regression may occur. Feelings of rage, anger, and frustration may also result. Personality structures and defenses are pushed to their limits. Trauma may also recreate previous maladaptive patterns of behavior, which have remained dormant until activated by the traumatic experience.

A life-threatening, traumatic, emotional, or medical event may produce both short- and long-term emotional trauma. Most often mentioned are acute stress reactions and posttraumatic stress disorder (PTSD). Other diagnoses to include affective, anxiety, and somatoform spectrum disorders may also occur (Wain, Grammer, & DeBoer, 2004). Trauma victims also experience various responses independent of and or simultaneously with the foregoing disorders. These include separation anxiety, grief, anger, rage, fear, frustration, regret, shame, dissociation, regression, denial, and shattered ego integrity.

Psychological symptoms that may also occur include difficulty sleeping, irritability, poor concentration, hypervigilance, exaggerated startle response, and motor restlessness. Cognitive symptoms consist of recurrent dreams, thoughts, flashbacks, distractibility, and cognitive distortions in which the victim applies illogical rules causing errors in drawing conclusions about experiences. Emotional symptoms consist of fear, helplessness, horror, anxiety, detachment, absence of emotions, and numbing. Behavioral symptoms exhibited include avoiding people, places, activities, thoughts, emotions, conversations, or television programs reminiscent of the event. The clinicians' awareness of the impact of these responses can be significant and empathic responses to the patient thus facilitate in developing alliances with the patient that could facilitate treatment outcomes.

The severity of the injury and body part affected may also determine the patient's response to the traumatic injury. Injury to parts of the body with realistic or perceived significance may increase the patient's stress (Lenehan, 1986). Physical trauma is frequently associated with pain

(Mohta, Sethi, Tyagi, & Mohta, 2003). Trauma patients who experience severe pain are then less likely to be amenable to psychotherapeutic interventions. Schreiber and Galai-Gat (1993) identify uncontrolled pain as a stressor of catastrophic proportions that if not treated effectively may result in the development of PTSD. Pain may also be associated with the severity of injury (Lenehan, 1986). Uncontrolled pain may also lead to anxiety, depression, loneliness, hostility, and sleep disturbances (Mohta et al., 2003).

The impact of a trauma resulting in physical injuries may extend beyond the bodily disruptions sustained by the victims to encompass the psychological realm. While treatment teams designed to respond to physical traumas have primarily focused on the physical injuries, increasingly more emphasis is being placed on the mental health interventions needed to assist the victims of physically traumatic events. Physical loss of a limb brings with it the added anxiety of potential social and interpersonal impact. Trauma patients are described (Blum, 2003) as experiencing a loss of identity, self-confidence, self-esteem, self-reliance, and ideal self. Traumatic experiences may also bring to reality unconscious dangers such as castration, object loss, or narcissistic mortification (Blum, 2003).

Horowitz (1982) and Landsman and colleagues (1990) noted that reactions to traumatic injury can be similar to bereavement. In addition to concern regarding physical appearance, the trauma patient sustaining an amputation may be concerned with the reactions from peers, ability to earn a living (Lenehan, 1986), socialization, dating, and sexual behavior (Wain, Cozza, et al., 2004). Trauma victims are at risk of developing psychiatric illnesses based on a predetermined set of risk factors (Armfield, 1994). Integrating psychiatry into the trauma team and providing routine preventive psychiatric interventions with trauma patients may prevent psychiatric symptoms from becoming disabling. It may also alleviate the stigma associated with being a psychiatry patient and allow appropriate psychiatric intervention when necessary.

> A 26-year-old patient sustained a left tibial plateau fracture after a motor vehicle accident. He experienced pain and inability to ambulate afterward. He was transferred from Landstuhl to WRAMC for definitive care. When approached by psychiatry he became defensive and withdrew. The patient then realized that psychiatric interventions were routine and preventive, and that no formal consult was generated. He then relaxed and participated in the evaluation and intervention. Survivor guilt and abandonment were then able to be normalized with this patient.

It has been written that "early intervention is the best hope" of preventing psychiatric illness in trauma victims (Titchener, 1970). Respecting these observations as well as our own experiences (Wain & Jacaard, 1996), the PCLS at WRAMC intervenes early in the patient's hospitalization. Following Gulf War I, psychiatric interventions consisted of requesting a consult on each patient, developing individual treatments and dispositions, and having frequent interdisciplinary meetings with other providers and group interventions for patients and staff.

HOSPITALIZATION AND THE MEANING OF INJURY

The perception of an injury to ones body disrupts one's homeostasis. Initially upon being injured, a sense of shock, denial, and disbelief may evolve. The feeling of being dependent on others can become intimidating and overwhelming. Trepidation over loss of life or limb or loss of capacity, as well as feelings of loss of control, is a common occurrence among injured individuals. Apprehension of being abandoned prior to control occurring or help approaching can be very overpowering. Once help has arrived and the fear of being alone is relieved, a sense of initial comfort develops with potential dependency needs. Based on the severity of the injury, the individual may not be aware of all that has transpired until he or she awakes in the hospital. Some patients upon awakening are elated at being alive. After a time, the elation may fade and anxiety and depressive symptoms may appear.

Medical patients with or without trauma generally can experience a threat to their narcissistic integrity. Loss of body parts and threat of death or annihilation are also significant fears for patients. They become helpless, vulnerable, and dependent. Fear or discomfort with strangers may also become prominent because of the unknown quality of the new relationship. Fear of not having loved ones around and leaving a safe environment is also a major concern. Patients' perceptions can result in childlike adolescent patterns of behavior, which lead to conflicts with the nursing and medical staff. Regression and dependency needs are frequently observed.

Complicating these factors are the anxieties of the loved ones who either may be at the bedside or may be calling frequently. At times, the families' needs must be attended to so their anxieties do not affect the patient, exacerbating an already tenuous position. When in the hospital, family members may even choose to sleep in the patient's room.

Physical injury usually taxes an individuals adaptive functioning. Personality features effective as coping styles may become compromised. Patients may not respond in the best way as medical or traumatic injuries can be an overwhelming stressor. The patient and family are vulnerable and need support and guidance from caring individuals. Developing a relationship with them is imperative. Utilizing warmth, caring, empathy, and support can go along way in attempting to form an alliance with the family and the patient.

THE ROLE OF PSYCHIATRY
WITH THE GENERAL MEDICAL PATIENT

In his excellent review, Lipowski (1974) described consultation to the medical–surgical patient. Evaluation and treatment of the psychiatric and psychological sequelae of medical and surgical patients is typically the main mission of a psychiatric consultation service. However, consults are typically received only after patients manifest problems.

Medical patients may exhibit psychological distress while undergoing treatment for their symptoms. Studies indicate that interventions such as psychotherapy, cognitive-behavioral therapy, hypnosis, relaxation techniques, and pharmacotherapy help to reduce or prevent relapse of depression and anxiety in the medical patient (Cottraux, 1993; Covino & Frankel, 1993; Postone, 1998; Spiegel, 1996).

Psychiatric intervention in the medical–surgical patient also supports the primary treatment team by offering recommendations to prevent further emotional distress for the patient. Additional benefits of psychiatry's involvement include decreased length of hospital stay and improved discharge disposition following surgery (Levitan & Kornfeld, 1981; Schindler, Shook, & Schwartz, 1989).

THE ROLE OF PSYCHIATRY FOLLOWING TRAUMA

The literature generally presents many questions regarding the psychiatrist or mental health specialist's role in the treatment of the medically injured patient. Often treatment for the trauma injured patient focuses on the physical trauma itself.

Nearly all survivors exposed to traumatic events briefly exhibit one or more stress-related symptoms (Morgan, Krystal, & Southwick, 2003). These symptoms usually dissipate within a reasonable amount of time. However, symptoms persisting for a prolonged period following a trauma increase the probability of developing PTSD or other stress-related psychiatric disorders. Facilitating medical treatment still remains the primary goal of any psychiatric intervention. The trauma of a medical disorder or physical injury by itself can be overwhelming. War or disaster can exponentially expand it. The role of psychiatry with the trauma patient may need to change if prevention and a decrease in psychiatric comorbidity is a goal. To meet the effective goals in treating the medical–surgical patient following a traumatic injury new approaches were adapted (Wain et al., 2002; Wain, Grammer, & DeBoer, 2005).

Psychiatry is dedicated to understanding the biopsychosocial approach to behavior and providing appropriate treatment when behavior becomes maladaptive. At times the preventive and treatment mode of psychiatry is not heard or appreciated. To the lay public being seen by a psychiatrist at times is perceived as being a stigma. Trauma patients' feelings of helplessness and vulnerability regarding their physical symptoms may be exacerbated by their perception of a psychiatry consultation; thus psychiatry may make them feel more vulnerable. In our experience, the perception of psychiatry's role needed to be changed with trauma victims.

Trauma victims may need more immediate intervention than is typically recognized by psychiatric consult teams. Many patients tend to downplay their distress and underreport their psychiatric symptoms for fear of being labeled a "psychiatric" patient. As a way to decrease the stigma and establish the working alliance with the trauma patient the PCLS at WRAMC developed a subsection of its service called "Preventive Medical Psychiatry" (PMP) (Wain, Grammer, Stasinos, Cozza, & DeBoer, 2005). Patients are routinely screened following their medical evaluation and treatment. No formal consult is required (Wain, Grammer, & DeBoer, 2005). All notes are written under the label PMP.

UTILIZING PMP RATHER THAN CONSULTATION–LIAISON PSYCHIATRY WITH TRAUMA PATIENTS

The metaphor of "preventive medical psychiatry" (PMP) was chosen when working with trauma patients for various reasons. Traditionally, consultation–liaison psychiatry focuses on diagnosing and treating an already present illness and serving as liaison between the patient and the primary care team to enhance the quality of care. Consults are made when deemed necessary by the primary care team. In contrast, the PMP team's intent is to join the early trauma team effort to identify risk factors for developing a psychiatric response and attempt to prevent those responses. Each patient is given a preventive therapeutic intervention described by Wain and colleagues (2002; Wain, Grammer, & DeBoer, 2005). The PMP team also follows patients from the beginning of their hospitalization and works in conjunction with the medical–surgical teams. The patient is also followed after discharge.

In an effort to facilitate the patient's positive response to psychiatry, moving away from the traditional diagnostic approach appears necessary. Typically, PCLS is consulted when the primary physician recognizes a major disruption in a patient's behavior. Physically traumatized victims are rarely referred for routine psychiatric screening, as this carries the assumption that the patient possesses a psychiatric disorder. Changing the stigma patient's associate with psychiatry necessitates changing their perception of psychiatry. The traditional psychiatric interview may increase the patient's suspicions.

A comment often reported suggests that a medical patient perceives that his doctors may feel he or she is not coping well or is embellishing. To avoid the psychiatric label, it is beneficial to approach patients as part of the trauma team and make initial contact routine. Making it routine for all patients' demythesizes psychiatry's role and further prevents patients from asking, "Am I being flagged?" or "Do they think I'm crazy?"

It behooves any clinician working with trauma patients to form a bond with them. In particular, a mental health specialist needs to establish an alliance so that the patient perceives the intervention as coming from an ally. This is necessary as many patients develop psychiatric symptoms after their medical injury has healed or emotional trauma has become dormant. Then, if psychiatric symptoms develop, patients may feel more comfortable reaching out to mental health providers. Ways of building an alliance, reframing symptoms, and strengthening coping techniques are thus used with trauma patients (Wain et al., 2002; Wain, Grammer, & DeBoer, 2004).

Therapeutic Intervention for the Prevention of Psychiatric Stress Disorders (TIPPS; Wain, Grammer, & DeBoer, 2005) was implemented to address the psychological needs of trauma victims, provide support, assess psychiatric status, and provide early intervention when needed without stigmatization and to support the staff. The major components of the TIPPS approach follow.

One should allow the patient to process the trauma through empathic supportive exposure therapy. To facilitate processing, it is imperative that the mental health team develops a positive rapport with these patients both to make the initial intervention and to have input if problems arise. This may ensure that patients would feel comfortable approaching psychiatry. Complicating the issue may be the patient's reluctance to acknowledge the need for mental health intervention. It is further incumbent upon the mental health team to recognize that at times somatic complaints rather than anxiety or depressive symptoms may be described by the patient as a way of avoiding the psychiatric stigma.

INTEGRATION AND A PRAGMATIC REVIEW
OF INTERVENTION WITH PATIENTS

Based on our experience that traditional debriefing techniques of medical–surgical patients were not productive and a new approach was needed.

TIPPS (Wain, Grammer, & DeBoer, 2005) was developed for interventions with medical–surgical patients to decrease psychiatric comorbidity and emergent psychiatric problems while hospitalized and engender an alliance with their patients. This response entails seeing patients routinely without a consult, forming a therapeutic alliance, and allowing for empathic exposure to the traumas they faced. Other significant components of the intervention include recognizing personality styles and psychological defenses, countertransference and transference issues, normalizing events, cognitive reframing, educating patients, appropriate pharmacology, and utilizing hypnotic and relaxation techniques. Reinforcing patient's strengths regarding their survival was essential.

The development of the therapeutic alliance cannot be underestimated. It facilitates treatment while in the hospital and allows for easier follow-up treatment if problems arise for the patient or their family even on discharge. The frequency of this empathic exposure also appears to allow for the normalization of the event.

A review of some of the principles of TIPPS follows. The patients are initially approached by saying, "Hello, I'm Dr. _____ from Preventive Medical Psychiatry (PMP). Welcome back, we are sorry you had to experience your injury and we all thank you for what you did. It is our turn to take care of you." We also greet family members in a similar manner. The provider is introduced to the family as staff of the PMP service: "We see all patients returning from the Gulf. It is routine."

After the acute medical condition has stabilized, intervention occurs. The family is seen separately from the patient. As the interview begins, clinicians respond to the patients in an empathic, caring, and genuine manner. Nonthreatening techniques are employed and confrontational approaches are avoided. Comments that demonstrate patients' positive assets are quickly reinforced, such as "Your responses were quick" or "Where did you get that know-how"? Understanding their position and problems is necessary. Patients are asked to rate how they are feeling, their pain, and their sleep.

It is necessary to understand patients' situations. They are asked to reflect on their traumatic experience, suggesting that description at present is helpful in the future. Empathic exposure may help patients integrate the past trauma into their normal stream of consciousness. Adjunctive interventions and techniques that can be facilitative can be viewed in Tables 15.1 and 15.2.

- "Let them bear witness."
- Avoid pathologizing their trauma or responses.
- Offer rapid empathic responses to their recall of their trauma and injury.

- Make empathic reinforcing statements about their assets.
- Reinforce their positive behaviors during their descriptions.
- Look at what helped them survive.
- Understand their psychological defenses without breaking them.
- Use their personality style to reinforce their assets.
- Reinforce their assets as rapidly as you can.

The following excerpts illustrate some of the TIPPS principles in action.

- Have them describe what brought them to the hospital or how they got injured.

  PATIENT: I picked up my dead-weight foot and applied it to the brakes and stopped the car.

  DOCTOR: How did you have the ability and strength to stop the car and recognize, despite all you went through, that you could move that leg?

- Focus on the patients' styles. Reflect and reinforce what is important to them. Look for ways of reinforcing their behavior, thoughts, or actions.

  PATIENT: As I called for help, I applied a tourniquet to his wound.

  DOCTOR: Taking care of others when you are hurt is a monumental feat.

- Reinforce personality characteristics.

  PATIENT: How could it happen? I checked the details over and over.

  DOCTOR: That talks about one of your assets.

- Normalize responses to the abnormal event.

  PATIENT: I woke up thinking the dead bodies were near me.

  DOCTOR: These are normal experiences that can be expected.

- Allow for and accept patients' experiences of survivor guilt, fear, dissociation, etc.

  PATIENT: I feel terrible, I left my buddy behind and he died.

  DOCTOR: I'm sorry he died but your genuine feelings of caring about others is very evident and a wonderful trait.

- Emphasize safety.

  PATIENT: I get scared sometimes.

DOCTOR: That's normal. You are now here at Walter Reed and you are safe, but it is normal to have these feelings.

- Encourage healthy defenses and stress management. Denial early on is OK.

PATIENT: I don't want to see my stump.

DOCTOR: That's OK for now. Whenever you're ready.

- Advocate for patients' needs.

PATIENT: My prosthetic sucks and they don't hear me.

DOCTOR: I appreciate your frustration. Would it be alright if I talk to the prosthetist?

- Help reframe conflict when present.

PATIENT: I should have shot them.

DOCTOR: That's what makes us so unique. We care about other people and we don't want to hurt innocent individuals.

- Educate patients about psychiatric symptoms (some patients wait for symptoms to emerge).

PATIENT: I was waiting to pass out when my leg was shot off.

DOCTOR: Sometimes that occurs, but other times it does not. Many people expect symptoms based on TV shows and movies but it does not always occur.

Hypnotic techniques can be taught while the patients are in bed. Simply have patients practice breathing, and then utilize a rapid hypnotic

---

TABLE 15.1. Adjunct Interventions and Techniques

- Ask the patient about pain and him or her rate it from 0 to 10.
- Ask the patient about sleep and ask him or her to rate it from 0 to 10.
- Normalize sleep patterns as based on the patient's own vigilance during combat.
- Normalize the patient's experience as much as possible.
- Discuss the use of medications and sleep hygiene and the patient's medical regimen.
- Interventions and treatments need to be flexible.
- Expect the unexpected.
- Help anchor.
- Teach relaxation, hypnotic, and distancing techniques.
- Be empathic.

**TABLE 15.2. Clinical Adjuncts to Help the Clinician
Employ Interventions**

- Keep listening and observe.
- Be aware of transference and countertransference issues.
- Think about the patient's trauma.
- Consider distancing the patient from the event by using breathing exercises and reinforcing the "here and now," imagery, and humor, and encourage the use of social supports.
- Reinforce the patient's assets.

induction that they can repeat to themselves. This can at times manage and control symptoms. It may also allow a distance from the trauma, giving patients some control in finding a safe or happy place where they can begin processing information. Here the clinician can facilitate the patient's learning to process and reframe traumatic events. This technique can also be used to control pain, help with sleep, and most important, begin helping patients master symptoms.

Traditional psychotherapeutic interventions aid the provider support the trauma patient. Acceptance, respect, empathy, warmth, advice, praise, affirmation, and a sense of hope are qualities and characteristics the clinician should display with these patients. Providers need to be viewed as genuine in their concern and support while offering empathic validation and encouraging patients to elaborate on reactions to the trauma.

Groups can help many of the victims begin the working through process. At WRAMC, groups held twice weekly are open to the medical–surgical patients. Topics such as anger, expectations, recognition of limitations, sexual fears, separation anxieties, survivor guilt, losses, family concerns, and public responses are discussed after initiated by the patient. To help with the clinical process, objective psychometric instruments are given to patients while in the hospital. The questionnaires help to provide data and facilitate follow up.

PHARMACOLOGICAL INTERVENTIONS

Pharmacological interventions can facilitate psychotherapeutic and medical–surgical treatments. Physical trauma frequently results in significant somatic pain. Schreiber and Galai-Gat (1993) identify uncontrolled pain as a stressor of catastrophic proportions that may lead to PTSD. Some patients associate pain with the severity of their injury, which may also lead to anxiety, depression, loneliness, hostility, and sleep disturbances

(Lenehan, 1986; Mohta et al., 2003). Patients experiencing pain are less likely to respond to traditional psychotherapeutic interventions (Mohta et al., 2003). Prompt pain control is thus imperative in trauma patients and must be addressed early with judicious use of analgesics.

Insomnia can foster pathological derealization and dissociation and prevent victims from sustaining attention to recovery. Benzodiazepines, anticholinergics, and antidepressants can interfere with clarity of thought and prevent psychological integration, favoring other sedative agents such as low-dose trazodone (Desyrel), quetiapine (Seroquel), or zolpidem (Ambien). When insomnia is associated with nausea and or depression, mirtazapine (Remeron) can offer relief. Daytime ruminations, hypervigilance, avoidance, or declining may respond well to selective serotonin reuptake inhibitors such as sertraline (Zoloft). Nightmares, when overwhelming, have been reported to respond well to prazosin (Minipress), though caution should be exercised due to its hypotensive properties. Providers should consider their utility and may liaison with the medical–surgical teams to remove any connotation of significant psychiatric pathology from their administration.

A 27-year-old married male was injured in Iraq and admitted for facial burns and traumatic amputation of left arm from an improvised explosive device blast. The patient was seen by psychiatry for anxiety, flashbacks, nightmares and poor sleep, hypervigilance, and avoidant behavior. Patient gave history of prior obsessive–compulsive disorder, which was responsive to Lexapro. Started on Celexa 10 mg nightly, trazodone 25 mg nightly, and Ativan 1 mg, his sleep improved but not significantly. Nightmares and anxiety persisted. He was switched from Celexa to Lexapro 5 mg nightly and Trazodone was increased from 25 to 50 mg nightly. He learned hypnotic techniques. He described a history of dyspepsia secondary to stress. Family history of dyspepsia and anxiety secondary to stress was reported in the father.

As part of his treatment the patient continued with individual and group psychotherapy. As a result of the psychiatric intervention, which included not only the pharmacological intervention and an empathic exposure to the trauma, individual therapy, and the development of a therapeutic alliance, dyspepsia and anxiety symptoms diminished and his sleep much improved. Upon discharge the patient was on trazodone 100 mg and Celexa 40 mg. He continued to use self-hypnotic techniques. He was followed by phone contact and his medication was monitored in his local community.

A 36-year-old male sustained a blast injury to the right hand and face resulting in a traumatic amputation of the right thumb, pinky, and ring finger plus multiple facial lacerations and ruptured right globe. He underwent revisions of the amputations and laceration repairs of the face and right eye before being evacuated to Germany. There a CT scan showing a right nasal fracture, ruptured right globe, medial wall orbit fracture, and interior floor orbital fracture. The patient was then transferred to WRAMC. Here an enucleation of the right eye and flap revisions of the amputated fingers was performed, and shrapnel was removed from his face. The patient participated in occupational therapy and his pain was well controlled with nonnarcotic medications and hypnotic interventions. He gained support from his empathic exposure to his trauma and the therapeutic alliance he allowed to develop. Initially he had some difficulty with a startle response but that resolved following our intervention. After several months he complained of sleep difficulties and 50 mg of Seroquel was prescribed, which helped resolve the problem.

FOLLOW-UP

Each patient is given a contact number and encouraged to call our office if and when concerns develop for the patient or their families. They are also called 30, 90, and 180 days following discharge from the hospital. One of the early goals has been to make psychiatry an ally to the patient. When patients return home they find it easier to respond and receive intervention, and when crises occur they appear more willing to accept referral recommendations.

A 29-year-old with a right below-the-knee amputation returned home on convalescent leave and found that his wife was requesting a separation. Medically he was beginning to use a prosthetic device and was ambulating. Sertraline had been prescribed early to help with his anxiety and sleep. He was overwhelmed by the news of the pending separation but was able to hear and accept interventions suggested at home. He was also willing to see a mental health provider after we made an appointment for him in his local community.

Patients who need treatment upon leaving WRAMC are generally referred to resources within their military, veterans health system, or civilian community.

TREATING THE TRAUMA PATIENT'S FAMILY

Trauma patients are not the only ones affected by traumatic events. Family members may also experience psychological trauma from the events (Alexander, 2002; Brown, 1991; Flannery, 1999; Solursh, 1990). Families typically know little about the extent of the injuries or the prognosis of the patient and therefore experience more anxiety and a feeling of helplessness (Lenehan, 1986).

It is difficult to predict how family members will react to the trauma and the patient's injuries. However, the treatment team can help them in coping with the traumatic event and lessen the family members' chance of developing secondary PTSD (Flannery, 1999).

Intervention strategies used with the families include assessing the basic needs. When initially meeting with the trauma victim, one must ensure that their family members have access to food, clothing, and shelter. This will alleviate additional stress and allows the family to focus on the patient and deal with the events (Flannery, 1999). Each institution needs to provide personnel to help with this task. PMP can be there as an advocate for the patient and their families.

During periods of trauma the families' built in support system may need to be augmented with professional help (Harvey, Dixon, & Padberg, 1995). Crisis intervention may be needed. The purpose of the family crisis intervention is to build up the family's coping skills and resolve symptoms associated with psychological trauma. Other activities such as sharing meals with families of other trauma patients provide them with additional support (Flannery, 1999).

The experience of having a family member injured and the resulting adjustments may exacerbate family malfunctioning (Landsman et al., 1990). Support groups formed specifically to assist families of trauma victims provide an outlet for them to address their needs and feelings (Harvey et al., 1995). When developing family groups, Harvey and colleagues (1995) found that families were more willing to attend when the group focus was on families sharing their stories and on education. Families attending these support groups realized that they were not alone and could offer mutual support. Additional benefits from attending these groups were the ability to share feelings, reduce anxiety, instill hope, and gain a better understanding of their family member's injuries, medical treatments, and hospital procedures. Brief supportive counseling has also been proven effective at reducing their anxiety (Lenehan, 1986).

Trauma patients need as much support as possible. Family members are often better than staff at providing emotional support and reassurance to the trauma patients (Brown, 1991). Effective therapeutic family interventions may help both the family and the patient cope with the traumatic events. Family's anxieties tend to exacerbate patients' conflict and have a deleterious impact on the nursing staff. If the family remains stable and supportive the patient's anxiety is decreased.

Based on our experiences, families are also seen by a PMP provider. Groups are offered weekly for spouses and parents. Topics include fear, frustration, the need to protect the injured patient, depression, anger, education, coping with disabled spouses, and feelings of alienation and disappointment. We further ask family members how their children are doing and how they informed them about the patient's injury. When problems arise for the children, members of our adolescent psychiatry service may intervene. Individual attention for some family members at times is preferred.

A 26-year-old male with a left above-the-knee amputation injured in Iraq. The patient was flown to Germany and then air-evacuated to WRAMC where his wife met him. His wife began having difficulty adjusting to his injury. Problems with her in-laws also came to the surface. Concerns regarding her ambivalent feelings toward her husband, which existed prior to his deployment, became even more prominent. Therapeutic interventions were undertaken and as a result the marriage and in-law issues were resolved. The wife and husband were given our phone number for follow-up.

SUPPORTING THE STAFF WHO CARE FOR THE MEDICALLY INJURED TRAUMA VICTIM

Offering psychological support to victims following trauma has become an accepted practice (Robbins, 1999). This support is geared toward assisting the victim in working through the traumatic events and returning to normal daily activities as soon as possible. However, relatively little research has been conducted on the psychological impact on workers who work with trauma victims (Robbins, 1999; Salston & Figley, 2003) and the resources available to them.

Taylor (1983) suggests that on average there are three major disasters a week worldwide. Responding to the needs of these disaster victims, nurses and clinicians may also be placing themselves at risk of experiencing secondary trauma. Dyergrov (1989) suggests that among disaster workers, 80% are likely to experience emotional disturbances following the event, although only 3–7% are likely to experience significant psychological disruptions.

Bamber (1994) debunks the long held myth that those in the helping profession are somehow immune to the stresses experienced by those they help. Professionals are perceived by the public as strong, resourceful, and in control. Thus these professionals may be reluctant to seek help (Collins, 2001).

To decrease conflicts for the staff and encourage mutual support, PMP has routinely visited with the nurses. Groups have been established to empathically have them retell their conflicts. One of our team members is a nurse and visits the wards daily to work with the respective head nurses. Education about stress and responses are given when appropriate. Formal lectures are also provided.

Often overlooked is the stress the physician staff goes through, which may be exhibited on curb-sided conversations (Wain, McLaughlin, et al., 2004). An example of a comment made by orthopedic surgeons, "I just cut off this kid's leg." This experience can continue to be overwhelming. Offering support and time to talk to them is necessary.

Physicians are sometimes reluctant to talk about their fears and frustrations. Giving lectures to the medical staff and maintaining a professional collegial relationship allows others to see PMP as a resource. At times, groups for physicians have been held prior to their morning rounds. Email messages and notes about stress are also distributed.

A similar approach needs to be undertaken with the administration and command. Keeping them informed as well as being available for their concerns is helpful.

A patient with a spinal cord injury was being sent to another hospital for rehabilitation, a distance from his support system. Command was notified and a request was made to change the referral. After evaluating the situation, command intervened and was able to refer the patient to a hospital closer to his home.

Last but not least, the mental health providers need support. Reinforcement of their skills and keeping them educated about providing new approaches is facilitative. Maintaining a positive esprit de corps and sensitivity to each other's needs also helps. Time off, humor, lunches, dinner, and eating together may also help. Leaders must keep an open door and be sensitive to the staffs' frustrations and counter transference issues.

PREPARATION AND MINIMAL REQUIREMENTS FOR A MENTAL HEALTH PROVIDER WORKING WITH TRAUMA PATIENTS

Any psychiatrist may find him- or herself at a disaster or terrorism scene. Military psychiatrists are highly encouraged to have and maintain Advanced Trauma Life Saving (ATLS) and Advanced Cardiac Life Support (ACLS) certification, as they may be required in a disaster or terrorist attack. Psychiatrists with this training can be highly effective in the disaster or emergency room setting when the time comes to evaluate potential victims. This training and certification provide credibility with medical–surgical colleagues because they speak the language inherent in ATLS and ACLS algorithms and understand the concepts of those approaches. Credibility with disaster leaders is the key to influencing leadership behaviors (Rundell, 2000).

Any mental health worker in a trauma unit needs to be familiar with the setting and not place his or her needs or skills above that of the initial medical stabilization and treatment. Mental health workers need to consult about psychiatric and psychological issues related to patient care. Credibility with the medical team is essential. In the initial triage following a trauma the mental health provider must focuses on the most common psychiatric sequelae and the psychiatric concerns most likely to adversely affect the medical–surgical outcome.

SUMMARY

Exposure to traumatic situations is a life-changing event. Although most trauma victims adjust well, others need some intervention. Based on our past experiences, we at WRAMC developed an early-intervention treatment plan for responding to injured soldiers. Traditional debriefing interventions were not effective for this population. A new approach described intervening early without a formal consult, stressing the importance of the therapeutic alliance, reinforcing patient assets, using relaxation–hypnotic techniques, prescribing medication when necessary, and using empathic exposure as part of the therapeutic intervention for prevention of disabling psychiatric stress symptoms. A similar plan can be developed at any hospital that treats large numbers of trauma patients. The goals are to decrease the impact of disabling psychiatric symptoms, speed recovery, ease symptoms, teach mastery or control techniques, and recognize and treat psychiatric illnesses early. Being able to refer patients for treatment if required after they leave the hospital is also a major component. All patients at WRAMC were seen as early as possible. In this chapter, we highlighted TIPPS and emphasized empathic exposure to the trauma and the significance of the therapeutic alliance. The development of a program for trauma victims necessitates the inclusion of patients' families, hospital staff, and hospital leadership, as well as the mental health team serving this population.

Becoming a part of a trauma team further expedited intervention and allowed psychiatric entry to the patient without the typical stigmatization. The therapeutic alliance was effective in facilitating the working through of some conflicts while patients were hospitalized and it was beneficial upon discharge. Maintenance of the therapeutic alliance may facilitate positive treatment outcomes. Furthermore, it appeared that when patients need intervention upon discharge they are more likely to accept recommendations based on the therapeutic alliance that has been established.

REFERENCES

Alexander, D. A. (2002). The psychiatric consequences of trauma. *Hospital Medicine, 63*, 12–15.

Armfield, F. (1994). Preventing post-traumatic stress disorder resulting from military operations. *Military Medicine, 159*, 739–746.

Bamber, M. (1994). Providing support for emergency service staff. *Nursing Times, 90*, 22, 32–33.

Blum, H. P. (2003). Psychic trauma and traumatic object loss. *Journal of the American Psychoanalytic Association, 51*(2), 415–431.

Brown, V. (1991). The family as victim in trauma. *Hawaii Medical Journal, 50*(4), 153–154.

Collins, S. (2001). What about us? The psychological implications of dealing with trauma following the Omagh bombing. *Emergency Nurse, 8*, 9–13.

Cottraux, J. (1993). Behavioral psychotherapy applications in the medically ill. *Psychotherapy and Psychosomatics, 60*, 116–128.

Covino, N., & Frankel, F. (1993). Hypnosis and relaxation in the medically ill. *Psychotherapy and Psychosomatics, 60*, 75–90.

Dyergrov, A. (1989). Caring for helpers in disaster situations: Psychological debriefing. *Disaster Management, 2*, 25–30.

Flannery, R. B. (1999). Treating family survivors of mass casualties: A CISM family crisis intervention approach. *International Journal of Emergency Mental Health, 1*, 243–250.

Furst, S. (1967). *Psychic trauma*. New York: Basic Books.

Harvey, C., Dixon, M., & Padberg, N. (1995). Support group for families of trauma patients: A unique approach. *Critical Care Nurse*, pp. 59–63.

Horowitz, M. J. (1982). Psychological processes induced by illness, injury, and loss. In T. Milton, C. Green, & R. Meagher (Eds.), *Handbook of clinical health psychology* (pp. 53–67). New York: Plenum Press.

Landsman, I. S., Baum, C. G., Arnkoff, D. B., Craig, N. J., Lynch, I., Copes, W. S., et al. (1990). The psychosocial consequences of traumatic injury. *Journal of Behavioral Medicine, 13*(6), 561–581.

Lenehan, G. P. (1986). Emotional impact of trauma. *Nursing Clinics of North America, 21*(4), 729–740.

Levitan, S. J., & Kornfeld, D. S. (1981). Clinical and cost benefits of liaison psychiatry. *American Journal of Psychiatry, 138*(6), 790–793.

Lipowski, Z. J. (1974). Consultation liaison psychiatry. *American Journal of Psychiatry, 131*, 623–650.

Mohta, M., Sethi, A. K., Tyagi, A., & Mohta, A. (2003). Psychological care in trauma patients. *Injury: International Journal of the Care of the Injured, 34*, 17–25.

Morgan, C., Krystal, J., & Southwick, S. (2003). Toward early pharmacological post traumatic stress intervention. *Biological Psychiatry, 53*(9), 834–843.

Postone, N. (1998). Psychotherapy with cancer patients. *American Journal of Psychotherapy, 52*(4), 412–424.

Robbins, I. (1999). The psychological impact of working in emergencies and the role of debriefing. *Journal of Clinical Nursing, 8,* 263–268.

Rundell, J. R. (2000). Psychiatric issues in medical–surgical disaster casualties: A consultation–liaison approach. *Psychiatric Quarterly, 71*(3), 245–258.

Salston, M., & Figley, C. (2003). Secondary traumatic stress effects of working with survivors of criminal victimization. *Journal of Traumatic Stress, 16*(2), 167–174.

Schindler, B., Shook, J., & Schwartz, G. (1989) Beneficial effects of psychiatric intervention on recovery after coronary artery bypass graft surgery. *General Hospital Psychiatry, 11,* 358–364.

Schreiber, S., & Galai-Gat, T. (1993). Uncontrolled pain following physical injury as the core-trauma in post-traumatic stress disorder. *Pain, 54,* 107–110.

Solursh, D. S. (1990). The family of the trauma victim. *Nursing Clinics of North America, 25,* 155–161.

Spiegel, D. (1996). Cancer and depression. *British Journal of Psychiatry, 168*(30), 109–116.

Taylor, A. (1983). Adjustment to threatening events: A theory of cognitive adaptation. *American Psychologist, 38,* 1161–1173.

Titchener, J. L. (1970). Management and study of psychological responses to trauma. *Journal of Trauma, 10,* 974–980.

Wain, H. J., Cozza, S. J., Grammer, G. G., Oleshansky, M. A., Cotter, D. M., Owens, M. F., et al. (2004). Treating the traumatized amputee. In National Center for PTSD, *Caring for the clinicians who care for traumatically injured patients: Iraq War clinician guide* (2nd ed., pp. 50–57). Washington, DC: National Center for PTSD.

Wain, H. J., Grammer, G., & DeBoer, C. (2005). *Therapeutic intervention and prevention of psychiatric stress disorders with medical surgical patients following traumatic injuries.* Manuscript submitted for publication.

Wain, H. J., Grammer, G. G., Stasinos, J. J., & Miller, C. M. (2002). Meeting the patients where they are: Consultation–liaison response to trauma victims of the Pentagon attack. *Military Medicine, 167*(4), 19–21.

Wain, H. J., Grammer, G., Stasinos, J., Cozza, S., & DeBoer, C. (2005). *From consultation–liaison to preventive medical psychiatry.* Manuscript submitted for publication.

Wain, H. J., & Jacaard, J. T. (1996). Psychiatric intervention with medical and surgical patients of war. In R. J. Ursano & A. R. Norwood (Eds.), *Emotional aftermath of the Persian Gulf War.* Washington, DC: American Psychiatric Publishing.

Wain, H. J., McLaughlin, E. C., DeBoer, C. M., Grammer, G. G., Oleshansky, M. A., Cotter, D. M., et al. (2004). In National Center for PTSD, *Caring for the clinician who care for traumatically injured patients: Iraq War clinician guide* (2nd ed., pp. 62–65). Washington, DC: National Center for PTSD.

Wain, H. J., & Stasinos, J. (1999). *Response to bombing victims*. Paper presented at the State Department, Washington, DC.

Watson, P. J., Friedman, M. J., Ruzek, J. I., & Norris, F. (2002). Managing acute stress response to trauma. *Current Psychiatry Reports, 4,* 247–253.

Weinstein, E. A. (1990). Disabling and disfiguring injuries. In F. D. Jones, L. R. Sparachino, V. L. Wilcox, J. M. Rothberg, & J. W. Stokes (Eds.), *Textbook of military medicine*. Washington DC: TMM Publications.

CHAPTER 16

Mitigation of Psychological Effects of Weapons of Mass Destruction

ROSS H. PASTEL and ELSPETH CAMERON RITCHIE

The importance of the psychological effects of "weapons of mass destruction," or "WMD," is increasingly being recognized in the post-9/11 era. WMD include chemical, biological, radiological/nuclear, and high-explosive weapons. However, with the exception of nuclear weapons and high explosives, most WMD do not cause large-scale physical destruction. Therefore, a better term would be "weapons of mass *disruption*," as these weapons can cause mass casualties along with extreme psychosocial effects. This chapter concentrates on psychological effects of chemical, biological, radiological, and nuclear (CBRN) weapons.

CBRN weapons differ from conventional weapons (such as bombs or shootings). For example, biological weapons can be delivered via the air, water, or food supply, or by mail. Many CBRN agents are invisible and odorless, thus leading to uncertainties of exposure and amount of exposure. Many of the initial or prodromal symptoms are nonspecific, which leads to problems of differentiating those exposed from those who fear they were exposed. This issue is a very important theme for planners, emergency departments, the public health system, and, of course, the population at large. For example, the sarin attacks in the Tokyo subway system killed 12, but led 5,000 people to seek medical attention (Asukai & Maekawa, 2002). The anthrax in the mail attacks in 2001 caused 23 cases of anthrax with 5 fatalities, but over 32,000 people with potential exposure sought prophylactic antibiotics (often on the advice of their employer) (Centers for Disease Control and Prevention, 2001a).

In the event of smallpox or pneumonic plague, the threat of contagion is very real, which brings up issues of quarantine and isolation. The 2003 SARS (severe acute respiratory syndrome) epidemic demonstrated the challenges of quarantine (Pastel, 2004). In a smallpox outbreak, isolation of patients, tracing and quarantine of contacts, and vaccination—either ring (i.e., contacts and contacts of contacts) or mass vaccination—will be required to halt an epidemic. Many of the CBRN agents can cause disfiguring injuries, which increases the psychological impact on those affected and on those witnessing the event.

Special equipment may be needed to detect contamination for many CBRN agents. Issues of evacuation from contaminated areas or even permanent relocation due to long-lasting contamination (e.g., Chernobyl) require attention. The long-term health consequences of exposures to trace amounts of CBRN agents are controversial. Are long-term effects psychological, psychophysiological, or physiological? Reviewing the literature on "Gulf War Illnesses," the simplest answer is that there was a combination of all of the above (Riddle et al., 2003).

Health risk communication will be important for both acute and long-term risks. Poor knowledge and public communication will increase psychological ill effects. For example, information about how to protect oneself from immediate attack is currently scanty or contradictory. In the spring of 2003, the U.S. government advised the use of duct tape and plastic sheeting for home protection. Criticisms of efficacy and the dangers of suffocation, as well as many jokes, quickly followed. The loss of governmental credibility was, perhaps, the most serious consequence of this episode.

For many years, the military has studied the medical effects of CBRN agents. In July 2000, an international conference on the "Operational Impact of Psychological Casualties from Weapons of Mass Destruction" was held, organized by Pastel (Pastel, Landauer, & Knudson, 2001). There have also been a number of recent reviews on the topic (Benedek, Holloway, & Becker, 2002; DiGiovanni, 1999; Ursano, Norwood, Fullerton, Holloway, & Hall, 2003). Fortunately, although acute and long-term psychological effects after CBRN events may differ in degree from effects seen after natural disasters or high explosives, they seem to exist on a continuum with no apparent unique psychological disorders (Scharf et al., 2001) Psychophysiological effects may well dominate the long-term picture (Hyams, Murphy, & Wessely, 2002).

Although there are historical data about the range of psychological effects, fewer data are available about mitigation of expected psychological reactions. Unlike responses to other episodes of mass violence, we do not have enough information to divide our therapeutic responses into early, intermediate, and late phases. Therefore, response is not delineated in a time-sequenced fashion. In addition, CBRN attacks do not always have a clear end of the attack—long-term contamination may lead to a perceived ongoing presence and fear of exposure. There may also be a continuing fear of potential long-term health consequences (e.g., radiation exposure).

A historical review of psychological effects following CBRN attacks and accidents begins the chapter, followed by a summary of the acute and long-term psychological effects. The last section has suggestions for mitigation of these psychological effects. For reference, the appendix contains a brief description of CBRN agents and their medical effects.

HISTORICAL EXAMPLES

Nuclear and Radiological Weapons

Of the WMD, nuclear weapons have the greatest destructive impact: They are the quintessential weapons of mass destruction. The atomic weapons dropped on Hiroshima and Nagasaki caused incredible devastation; outbreaks of local fires; and large numbers of dead, dying, and injured people (Janis, 1945). In interviews after the war, approximately two-thirds described intense fear, emotional upset, or depression. Nevertheless, there was only a single incident of mass panic reported at Hiroshima: A large group of frightened people in a park pushed some victims into a river and several died (Hersey, 1946).

Survivors witnessed severely injured people suffering from burns and blast injuries. The exposure to the devastation and human suffering constantly reminded survivors of the original event (Janis, 1945). Survivors were severely stigmatized, especially those scarred from severe burns. A study of over 7,000 Nagasaki atomic bomb patients done 15 years later showed long-term psychological effects in approximately 7%, with the majority complaining of fatigue, lack of spirit, poor memory, and introversion (Nishikawa & Tsuiki, 1961). These symptoms were twice as common in survivors who had shown acute radiation sickness (ARS) symptoms and were related to severity of symptoms.

According to the President's Commission that studied the Three Mile Island (TMI) accident, the only medical effect documented was mental distress (Kemeny et al., 1979). There were *no* cases of ARS. The estimated doses for people living within 10 miles of TMI were approximately the dose of an average chest x-ray and much lower than the annual background radiation dose (Fabrikant, 1981). Populations exhibiting the most distress were TMI workers, families with pre-school-age children, and those living within 5 miles of TMI. TMI residents, compared to controls, displayed significant stress on measures of performance; on anxiety, depression, and somatic complaints; on physiological measures of urinary norepinephrine, epinephrine, and cortisol and disturbed sleep; and on changes in immune system parameters for up to 6 years after the accident (Baum, Gatchel, & Schaeffer, 1983; Davidson, Fleming, & Baum, 1987). Studies of TMI workers reported only short-term acute effects, including nausea, stomach troubles, headaches, diarrhea, sleep disturbances, and loss of appetite (Fabrikant, 1981; Parkinson & Bromet, 1983). The TMI symptoms were *not* the result of exposure to radiation but to perceived radiation threat. Therefore, the *fear* of exposure to WMD not only causes significant distress but also can cause symptoms that mimic symptoms of exposure.

Unlike the TMI accident, the Chernobyl accident in 1986 did release significant amounts of radiation. Approximately 135,000 people were evacuated from a 30 km zone in the 2 weeks after the accident. Most had to be permanently relocated. In addition, an estimated 600,000 workers (so-called *liquidators*) were involved in the emergency actions on site during the accident and the subsequent clean-up operations (Nuclear Energy Agency, 2002). An important health effect was widespread psychological distress. However, that distress could also have been caused by other factors including the economic collapse and breakup of the Soviet Union, evacuation or relocation of communities, distrust of the government, and other problems (Ginzburg, 1993; Nuclear Energy Agency, 2002).

Acute health effects did occur to liquidators involved in the initial emergency response, including 31 deaths and 140 cases of ARS and other radiation-related acute health effects. An epidemiological study of over 4,700 Estonian liquidators found an increase in suicide but no increases in cancer, leukemia, or overall mortality (Rahu et al., 1997). Suicide accounted for almost 20% of mortality in the liquidator cohort. Reasons for the increased suicide rate are not currently known.

A study of over 1,400 Latvian liquidators found that 44% had ICD-9 coded mental–psychosomatic disorders (depression, physiological malfunction arising from mental factors, or unspecified disorders of the autonomic nervous system) (Viel et al., 1997). Due to lack of ICD-9 codes, anxiety, posttraumatic stress disorder (PTSD), and sleep disturbances were not diagnosed. A variety of psychoneurological syndromes characterized by multiple unexplained physical symptoms (MUPS) including fatigue, sleep and mood disturbances, headaches, impaired memory and concentration, and muscle and/or joint pain have been reported as sequelae of Chernobyl (Torubarov, 1991, Yevelson, Abdelgani, Cwikel, & Yevelson, 1997). These syndromes were reported both in liquidators who had suffered ARS and in those who had not (Torubarov, 1991). No significant correlations were found among physical symptoms, radiation dose, and physical examination data. PTSD and PTSD symptoms have been found in two studies (Cwikel, Abdelgani, Goldsmith, Quastel, & Yevelson, 1997; Tarabrina, Lazebnaya, Zelenova, & Lasko, 1996).

Biological Agents

Smallpox and plague have historically been associated with epidemics and large numbers of fatalities. The most recent smallpox outbreak in a nonendemic country was in Yugoslavia in 1972 and caused 175 cases of smallpox with 35 deaths (Fenner, Henderson, Arita, Jezek, & Ladnyi, 1988). Containment measures included strict isolation of patients, ring vaccination, prohibition of public meetings, restriction of movement to affected areas, and establishment of checkpoints to check vaccination certificates. A 3-week mass vaccination program immunized 18 million out of a total population of nearly 21 million. How the American public would respond to such measures today is unknown.

In 1994, there were two outbreaks of plague in India, a bubonic plague outbreak followed 1 month later by a pneumonic plague outbreak in Surat (John, 1994). There were over 5,000 suspected cases of plague, including 55 deaths (Mavalankar, 1995). The initial government response was denial and officials downplayed the situation. The local press and media helped fuel the anxiety with anxiety with exaggerated reports (Mavalankar, 1995). An estimated 400,000–600,000 people fled Surat, including hospital staff, private medical practitioners, and municipal workers (Ramalingaswami, 2001). In the city of Delhi, 1,200 km from Surat, people improvised surgical masks. There was widespread buying and hoarding of tetracycline (used to treat plague, available without prescription in India).

In 2001, the United States was shocked by anthrax letters in the mail that led to 23 cases of anthrax (Centers for Disease Control and Prevention, 2001b). Following September 11, 2001, and prior to the first case of anthrax, there had already been increased purchases of gas masks and ciprofloxacin ("cipro," used to treat anthrax). After the anthrax mail attacks, there were hundreds of prescriptions for cipro given to people with no credible exposure (Steinhauer, 2001). Hospitals reported that their already busy emergency rooms were filled with people anxious about anthrax, many demanding treatment.

Anthrax survivors suffered symptoms of fatigue, shortness of breath, chest pains, memory problems, nightmares, and rage 6–12 months after their illnesses (Broad & Grady, 2002). Only one of the inhalational anthrax survivors was well enough to return to work. At this date, no studies have determined whether these symptoms are medical and/or psychological consequences.

Acute respiratory distress syndrome (ARDS) may be caused by numerous biological weapons. Other infectious disease outbreaks causing ARDS have been reported to cause both PTSD and a decreased health-related quality of life (HRQL). For example, the majority of survivors of a Legionnaires disease outbreak reported fatigue, neurological symptoms, and neuromuscular symptoms 17 months after diagnosis (Lettinga et al., 2002). HRQL was impaired in seven of eight dimensions, and 15% of patients experienced PTSD. Other survivors of ARDS have also reported decreased HRQL and PTSD (Schelling et al., 1998).

Chemical Agents

World War I chemical warfare agents (CWA) caused 31% of battle injuries but only 2% of deaths in U.S. forces (Gilchrist, 1925). In the initial use of chlorine gas on the Western Front by the Germans in 1915, "A full-blown, blind, contagious panic swept portions of the line" (Hammerman, 1987, p. 91). However, there was no panic farther out on the line where there was little or no gas. In the next six gas attacks over the next 2 months, there were no mass panics, although protective equipment was rudimentary and not widely available. There were only four other gas panics documented in World War I.

The impact of CWA casualties was powerful: "A field hospital full of freshly and badly gassed men is . . . the most horrible and ghastly sight of the war . . . to see a hundred or more men, hale and hearty a few hours before, slowly strangling to death from pulmonary edema, with gradually increasing dyspnea, cyanosis and pallor, making futile efforts to expectorate . . . " (Norris, 1919, p. 631). Mustard exposure required long convalescence—French mustard casualties at Ypres in 1917 typically required 45–70 days before return to duty (Wachtel, 1941). Even perceived CWA exposure could cause symptoms. In one incident following desultory gas shelling, 500 battle-tested troops drifted into medical aid stations over a 1-week period, suffering from chest pain, fatigue, dyspnea, coughing, husky voice, and indefinite eye symptoms (Salmon & Fenton, 1929). The divisional gas officer found no evidence of gas inhalation or burning.

Three years after World War I, approximately one-half of gassed veterans claimed subjective complaints in medical examinations (Wachtel, 1941). There were reports of large numbers of men who had recovered from acute gas poisoning and had good physical examinations but suffered from serious sequelae (e.g., easy fatigability and difficulty breathing on exertion) (Haldane, 1919). This condition was variously known as effort syndrome and neurocirculatory asthenia. In chronic gas cases, there were often acute attacks of breathlessness at night accompanied by nightmares, and patients usually reported insomnia and unrefreshing sleep (Haldane,

1919). PTSD has been reported in World War II American veterans exposed to mustard agent while participating in field trials and chamber tests of protective equipment (Schnurr et al., 2000).

Sarin, a nerve agent, was used twice by a terrorist cult in Japan. Over 5,500 people visited 280 medical facilities following the 1995 release of sarin in the Tokyo subway (Asukai & Maekawa, 2002). Of these, 1,046 were admitted to the hospital, 20 were treated in intensive care units, and 12 died (10 in the first 48 hours). No extensive mass panic was reported— victims waited in silence for help. The perplexing silence may have been a sign of psychic numbness (Asukai & Maekawa, 2002). Some patients reported sleep disturbances, nightmares, and anxiety. Whether these were due to acute stress disorder or to the cholinergic effects nerve agent exposure is not known. One study done 1 month after the event found that hospitalized patients reported fears when approaching the subway (20%), depressed feelings (18%), difficulty sleeping (16%), physical tension (13%), and emotional lability and irritability (7–9%) (Asukai & Maekawa, 2002). A long-term study of sarin patients hospitalized at St. Luke's Hospital found that somatic and psychological symptoms continued for 5 years after the incident (Kawana, Ishimatsu, & Kanda, 2001). PTSD was diagnosed in 2–3% and partial PTSD in 7–8%. MUPS (eye symptoms, fatigue, muscle stiffness, and headache) were reported by 10% of the study population.

ACUTE AND LONG-TERM PSYCHOLOGICAL EFFECTS

Although mass panic is common in disaster movies and headlines, evidence from CBRN events and natural disasters suggests that it is very rare (Glass & Schoch-Spana, 2002; Quarantelli, 1960). What is common in CBRN events are large numbers of patients reporting to the emergency room with mild or perceived exposure. These patients are not "worried well." They are worried—possibly with good reason—but they are not well for they have symptoms of pain and distress. *The use of the term "worried well" should be discontinued. The term is pejorative and suggests that nothing is wrong with the patient. Although these patients are worried, they are not yet known to be well.*

Unfortunately, prodromal symptoms of CBRN weapons are often nonspecific symptoms (e.g., headache, difficulty breathing, nausea, dizziness, fatigue, and malaise). These symptoms can also be caused by anxiety or hyperventilation. However, some CBRN agents may induce these same symptoms directly (DiGiovanni, 1999). After exposure to pulmonary agents, respiratory distress may precede measurable physical signs (Chemical Casualty Care Division, 2000). Symptomatic ambulatory cases with mild or perceived exposures will present difficulties for CBRN event triage.

Ubiquitous, nonspecific symptoms can also occur with the perception of exposure to a CBRN agent. Outbreaks of these symptoms are often referred to as mass hysteria, mass psychogenic illness, or mass sociogenic illness. However, these terms have a pejorative connotation and should not be used. A more neutral term has been suggested—outbreaks of multiple unexplained symptoms (OMUS) (Pastel, 2001). One review found that the most common symptoms included nausea, vomiting, headache, and dizziness or lightheadedness (Boss, 1997). Not all outbreaks occur in female school-age children! For example, over 1,000 male military recruits reported at least one symptom following a suspected exposure to a toxin in the dining hall (Struewing & Gray, 1990).

OMUS can co-occur with a CBRN event. A dramatic example occurred following a radiological contamination incident in Goiania, Brazil, in 1987 in which 4 people died, 20 required hospital care, and 50 required medical surveillance (Petterson, 1988). However, over 125,000 people demanded to be screened for radiological contamination. Only 249 had any radiological contamination. Interestingly, 5,000 of the first 60,000 people screened had symptoms of vomiting, diarrhea, and/or rashes around the face and neck. Although consistent with radiation sickness symptoms, none were contaminated.

The available data suggest that more patients will present with mild or psychological symptoms than will present with moderate or severe injury/illness. Unfortunately, when talking with various experts, most disaster exercises have few psychological casualties and what few casualties they have are typically "psychotic"—not the expected type of casualty. Furthermore, experience from various disasters demonstrates that the ambulatory patients show up at the hospital first—before the severely injured can be transported (Bleich, Dycian, Koslowsky, Solomon, & Wiener, 1992).

CBRN victims may present with ill-defined, chronic fatigue-like syndromes with MUPS, as was seen after the first Persian Gulf War in 1991. A review of Gulf War illness may be found elsewhere (Riddle et al., 2003). Similar syndromes have appeared in veterans following many wars. or following infectious diseases, CWA exposures, and nuclear/radiological exposures (Ayres et al., 1998; Bleich et al., 1992; Broad & Grady, 2002; Davidson et al., 1987; De Roo et al., 1998; Hyams, Wignall, & Roswell, 1996; Kawana et al., 2001; Nishikawa & Tsuiki, 1961; Petterson, 1988; Torubarov, 1991; Viel et al., 1997). These may be stress-related somatization disorders, but at this point, there are no definitive studies.

In natural disasters and terrorist attacks with conventional weapons, survivors are commonly seen with PTSD, depression, generalized anxiety disorder, and substance/alcohol abuse (Norris, 2002; North et al., 1999).

We can probably expect similar results from CBRN agents. For example, PTSD has recently been recognized in people recovering from sepsis and ARDS and following the Chernobyl accident and the sarin attacks in Tokyo (Kawana et al., 2001; Lettinga et al., 2002; Pastel, 2002).

MITIGATION OF EFFECTS

Preparation in Advance

Planning before a CBRN event occurs can help prevent and/or mitigate both medical and psychological effects. This should be done in many forms: education of the public, table-top exercises, disaster drills, practice performing tasks in protective equipment, and full-scale "mass casualty" exercises (DiGiovanni, 2001). The mass casualty exercises need to be realistic, and they need to role-play with large numbers of minimally injured and traumatic stress casualties (Campanale, 1963).

The difficulty will be to alert the public to the risks but not unduly alarm them. Planning and disaster drills can improve the resilience of the public. Accurate information should be released on the effects of the different CBRN agents. Currently, federal and state governments are implementing disaster planning on a wide scale.

In planning for a large-scale disaster, there are numerous scenarios to consider. Is this a chemical or biological or radiological incident? Is it an act of war, terrorism, or an industrial accident? Is there warning, or is it unexpected? Where does it take place? Who is in charge?

In all cases, there will be multiple agencies responding to the attack. Jurisdictional issues will be paramount. As much as possible, these should be thought through in advance on the local, state, and federal level. For example, in the national capitol area, deemed a high-threat target, there will be the local governments of northern Virginia, the District of Columbia, and Maryland, plus numerous federal agencies, including the military and the Department of Homeland Security.

Emergency departments should be prepared to handle large numbers of people who are very concerned about exposure. Rather than dismissing concerned citizens by using the pejorative term "worried well," cases must be taken seriously. A triage area outside the emergency room can be set up so that many casualties can be screened quickly but thoroughly.

Care should also be paid to the concerns of the health care workers. Risks of secondary contamination from chemical agents or infection by biological agents have to be planned for. During the SARS epidemic, many health care workers did not show up for work (Pastel, 2004). A number of studies have also demonstrated that victims of a CBRN event consist of more than those on-site during the event. Rescue workers, first responders, health care providers, and body handlers are also at risk, as are those who lost family or friends to the event (Fullerton, Ursano, Kao, & Bharitya, 1999; North et al., 2002). The SARS epidemic has demonstrated potential vulnerabilities in our assumption that the health care system is capable of a comprehensive response.

The federal government on February 10, 2003, began to issue guidelines for the general public to prepare for a chemical or biological attack. These contained commonsense recommendations, such as a supply of water, food, flashlights and radios with extra batteries, and mechanical can openers. They also recommended purchasing a roll of plastic, duct tape, and scissors for sealing off a room in the home from chemical attacks, but these are problematic. There is a risk of suffocation in complete sealed rooms, as was seen in the Scud missile attacks on Israel in 1991 (Bleich et al., 1992).

Training of medical and mental health care providers is critical, as stressed in other chapters. Further issues for mental health care providers include identification of medical and psychological effects of different CBRN agents, differentiation of medical from psychological effects, recognition that infected/injured patients may also suffer psychological consequences and require social support, desensitization of claustrophobia from protective gear, and other issues as described elsewhere (DiGiovanni, 1999; Ursano et al., 2003).

Protective Equipment Issues

The protective gear used for chemical and biological weapons varies; e.g., surgical masks, Mission Oriented Protective Posture (MOPP) gear used by the military, and self-contained suits used by HAZMAT personnel. Previously, issues of wearing the protective gear were limited to military personnel and first responders. However, civilians may also need to wear protective gear.

Issues can be problematic because the protective gear may obscure recognition of faces and garble communication. Labels on the outside of the suits should clearly identify the wearer and potential communication difficulties should be anticipated.

In the military setting, some users of MOPP gear develop symptoms of claustrophobia, which has been termed "gas mask phobia" (Ritchie, 1992, 2001). This is characterized by feelings of anxiety or panic, which may lead to hyperventilation. In turn, the hyperventilation and anxiety lead to the eyepieces clouding up and to difficulty breathing, which further contribute to anxiety. In training exercises, occasionally the mask is pulled off, which gives immediate relief. However, during a chemical attack, that may cause injury or death. Aside from the psychological effects, the equipment is hot and clumsy. The thermal burden may contribute to the psychological effects described previously. Most equipment allows one to drink through a water bottle, but eating and elimination of body wastes remain problematic.

"Gas mask phobia" may be treated like other phobias, with the mainstay of treatment being relaxation and desensitization. In practice, that means initially wearing the equipment in quiet situations for short periods of time and building up to longer periods with more intense activity. Emphasis should be placed on activities that replicate the actual duties a person would perform in the event of an attack, which may include strenuous activity or working on a computer. Activities of daily living, such as eating, drinking, and going to the bathroom, should also be practiced.

Firefighters and other first responders who routinely train in personal protective equipment are probably self-selected to tolerate the equipment. However, those applicants who are initially unable to tolerate the protective mask should be given a trial of the aforementioned techniques.

Risk Perception and Health Risk Communication

In a CBRN event, public health authorities must calculate the extent of the threat and release information via the media. However, the extent of the danger will not be known immediately and initial information will be incomplete, fragmented, and sometimes contradictory. Health risk communication will be essential and principles include having a consistent message delivered by a knowledgeable and credible official, listening and responding to the concerns of the public, and avoiding the appearance of defensiveness or concealment (Sandman, 1993). Experience from 9/11, the anthrax attacks, and the sniper in the Washington, DC, area, has demonstrated the value of daily or twice daily scheduled briefings with the media and the public, even if there is no new information to disseminate. Mayor Giuliani of New York City was extremely effective following the September 11.

After toxic accidents, there is anxiety about health effects of the release. Such anxieties will be multiplied after a CBRN event. Following 9/11 and the anthrax attacks, the news media was full of devastating descriptions of the results of a potential smallpox attack and suggested that in the event of anthrax, "Your next breath may kill you." The "scare-tactic' information was *not* helpful—instead the public should be provided with accurate hazard communication and workable solutions, especially with measures that protect self and family.

According to one approach, risk equals hazard plus outrage (Sandman, 1993). Hazard is the scientifically based risk assessment, but outrage is made up of nonquantifiable factors related to the public's concern and perception of the event. The Centers for Disease Control has developed a course on "Emergency Risk Communication Training," which contains more in-depth information on the topic. For more information, visit the website at www.cdc.gov/cdcynergy/emergency/. Outrage following a WMD attack will significantly influence both acute and long-term psychological effects.

Triage and Issues of Differential Diagnosis

During the Scud missiles on Israel during the first Gulf War in 1991, large numbers of people reported to the emergency room for treatment (Bleich et al., 1992; Rotenberg, Noy, & Gabbay, 1994). Approximately 70–80% of the patients in the early attacks were seen for stress-related symptoms. Unfortunately, emergency medicine physicians do not spend much time in residency learning how to evaluate psychological casualties (Williams & Shepherd, 2000). Only recently has there been inclusion of neuropsychiatric casualties in triage (Burkle, 1996). Mental health care providers must become better integrated with emergency rooms. An important lesson from the Israeli experience is the importance of a separate stress center at hospitals, so that psychological casualties can be removed from the emergency room and taken to a less stressful environment (Rosenbaum, 1993).

Initial treatment of psychological casualties may have profound consequences for long-term effects. Military experience from World War I demonstrated the need for early treatment of psychological symptoms, rather than waiting until the symptoms became ingrained (Hyams et al., 1996). Also important was the positive expectancy of the staff that the patient would get better, that he was suffering a normal response to an abnormal event. Military experience has continued to demonstrate the effectiveness of this treatment (PIES—proximity, immediacy, expectancy, and simplicity) in reducing PTSD and enhancing the return of soldiers to duty (Jones, 1995; Solomon & Benbenishty, 1986). Other chapters in this book cover this treatment in greater detail.

CONCLUSION

The use of CBRN weapons will result in mass disruption and lead to a complex of effects, including acute psychological casualties, long-term psychological casualties, and large-scale psychosocial consequences such as economic disruption, evacuation, and/or relocation. The psychological effects will not be unique but will resemble those seen after disasters and attacks with conventional weapons. Ill-defined, chronic fatigue-like syndromes with MUPS will appear. Many of these effects can be prevented or mitigated by proper planning and practice prior to a CBRN event. Mental health care providers will need to become better integrated with disaster response plans and emergency rooms. Early recognition of psychological casualties with prompt supportive treatment in an area separate from medical treatment may be very useful. Effective health risk communication will be critical.

APPENDIX: CHARACTERISTICS OF CBRN AGENTS

Chemical Weapons

Chemical warfare agents (CWA) had their first widespread use in World War I (Chemical Casualty Care Division, 2000). Chemical agents caused one-third of the estimated 5 million casualties of World War I (Newmark, 2001). Although not used in World War II, CWA were used on a large scale in the Iran–Iraq war in the 1980s, where they caused at least 45,000 casualties (Newmark, 2001).

Five types of CWAs are of most concern: lung-damaging or pulmonary agents, cyanides, vesicants, nerve agents, and incapacitating agents (Chemical Casualty Care Division, 2000). Pulmonary agents, such as phosgene and chlorine, are nonpersistent gases that produce local pulmonary effects—ARDS and pulmonary edema (Newmark, 2001). They are toxic industrial chemicals, which are possible terrorist weapons. Cyanides are also nonpersistent gases that can quickly poison cellular metabolism. High exposures cause seizures, and both respiratory and cardiac arrest. Vesicants (e.g., sulfur mustard, lewisite, and phosgene oxime) are persistent agents that produce delayed effects—blisters (vesicles)—with a latent period of hours following exposure. The most common effects are on the skin, eyes, and upper respiratory system (Chemical Casualty Care Division, 2000). Nerve agents (tabun, sarin, soman, and VX) are the most potent CWA. They were invented during World War II but not used until the Iran–Iraq war in the 1980s. They were also used by Iraq against the Kurdish minority and by a Japanese terrorist cult in the 1990s. Nerve agents can cause death in minutes by causing a cholinergic crisis. Signs and symptoms vary somewhat after small exposures of vapor versus small exposures of liquid on skin, but large exposures of vapor or liquids result in sudden loss of consciousness, convulsions, apnea, flaccid paralysis, and copious secretions (Chemical Casualty Care Division, 2000).

Biological Weapons

Biological warfare (BW) and bioterrorism (BT) use microorganisms (bacteria or viruses) or toxins (products of living organisms) to induce death or disease. Unlike CWA, BW agents require an incubation period before they can cause symptoms. Toxins do not require incubation, but they do have a latent period before symptoms occur (Kortepeter et al., 2001). BW agents cause a prodrome with nonspecific, flu-like symptoms that can make early diagnosis problematic. The Centers for Disease Control (CDC) has differentiated biological agents into different categories of concern. Category A agents are of most concern because of lethality, public fear, and public health requirements and include botulinum toxin and the organisms responsible for anthrax, smallpox, plague, tularemia, viral hemorrhagic fevers (e.g., Ebola and Marburg).

Bacterial agents can be treated with antibiotics. Few antidotes to the viral agents and toxins are available, so supportive care is often the only treatment. Smallpox and pneumonic plague are contagious, meaning that they can be transmitted from person to person. Viral hemorrhagic fevers can be transmitted by contact with blood or other body secretions. Licensed vaccines are available for smallpox and anthrax.

Radiological and Nuclear Weapons

Nuclear weapons can cause death and injury by three mechanisms: blast and thermal and radiation effects (Jarrett, 1999). Blast and thermal effects are the most prevalent causes of death and injury, but radiation is the most feared effect. Radiological weapons are often referred to as "dirty bombs" or radiological dispersal devices (RDD) and are typically a mix of a radiological source and an explosive. Another type of RDD would be an attack on a nuclear power reactor resulting in a release of radiological material into the environment. In the United States, the strong containment of nuclear power reactors makes this an unlikely scenario (Pastel, Kahles, & Chiang, 2001).

ARS occurs following exposure to high doses of ionizing radiation. ARS is actually a combination of different clinical syndromes: hematopoietic, gastrointestinal, and both cardiovascular and central nervous system effects. The higher the radiation dose, the shorter the asymptomatic period and the more intense the initial symptoms. The initial symptoms are nonspecific—nausea, vomiting, fatigue, headache, and weakness. A long-term sequela of large doses of radiation is an increased incidence of cancer, perhaps the most feared effect (Patterson, 1987).

REFERENCES

Asukai, N., & Maekawa, K. (2002). Psychological and physical health effects of the 1995 sarin attack in the Tokyo subway system. In J. M. Havenaar, J. G. Cwikel, & E. J. Bromet (Eds.), *Toxic turmoil: Psychological and societal consequences of ecological disasters* (pp. 149–162). New York City: Kluwer/Plenum Press.

Ayres, J. G., Flint, N., Smith, E. G., Tunnicliffe, W. S., Fletcher, T. J., Hammond, K., et al. (1998). Post-infection fatigue syndrome following Q fever. *Quarterly Journal of Medicine, 91*(2), 105–123.

Baum, A., Gatchel, R. J., & Schaeffer, M. A. (1983). Emotional, behavioral, and physiological effects of chronic stress at Three Mile Island. *Journal of Consulting and Clinical Psychology, 51*(4), 565–572.

Benedek, D. M., Holloway, H. C., & Becker, S. M. (2002). Emergency mental health management in bioterrorism events. *Emergency Medical Clinics of North America, 20*(2), 393–407.

Bleich, A., Dycian, A., Koslowsky, M., Solomon, Z., & Wiener, M. (1992). Psychiatric implications of missile attacks on a civilian population. Israeli lessons from the Persian Gulf War. *Journal of the American Medical Association, 268*(5), 613–615.

Boss, L. P. (1997). Epidemic hysteria: A review of the published literature. *Epidemiology Review, 19*, 233–243.

Broad, W. J., & Grady, D. (2002, September 16). Science slow to ponder ills that linger in anthrax victims. *The New York Times.*

Burkle, F. M. (1996). Acute-phase mental health consequences of disasters: Implications for triage and emergency medical services. *Annals of Emergency Medicine, 28*(2), 119–128.

Campanale, R. P. (1963). Realism in disaster exercises—A true challenge. *Military Medicine, 128*, 418–427.

Centers for Disease Control and Prevention. (2001a). Update: Investigation of bioterrorism-related anthrax and adverse events from antimicrobial prophylaxis. *Morbidity and Mortality Weekly Report, 50*(44), 973–976.

Centers for Disease Control and Prevention. (2001b). Update: Investigation of bioterrorism-related inhalational anthrax-Connecticut, 2001. *Morbidity and Mortality Weekly Report, 50*(47), 1049–1051.

Chemical Casualty Care Division. (2000). *Medical management of chemical casualties handbook* (3rd ed.). Aberdeen Proving Grounds, MD: USAMRICD.

Cwikel, J., Abdelgani, A., Goldsmith, J. R., Quastel, M., & Yevelson, I. I. (1997). Two-year follow up study of stress-related disorders among immigrants to Israel from the Chernobyl area. *Environmental Health Perspectives, 105*(Suppl. 6), 1545–1550.

Davidson, L. M., Fleming, R., & Baum, A. (1987). Chronic stress, catecholamines, and sleep disturbance at Three Mile Island. *Journal of Human Stress, 13*(2), 75–83.

De Roo, A., Ado, B., Rose, B., Guimard, Y., Fonck, K., & Colebunders, R. (1998). Survey among survivors of the 1995 Ebola epidemic in Kikwit, Democratic Republic of Congo: Their feelings and experiences. *Tropical Medicine and Internal Health, 3*(11), 883–885.

DiGiovanni, C. (1999). Domestic terrorism with chemical or biological agents: Psychiatric aspects. *American Journal of Psychiatry, 156*(10), 1500–1505.

DiGiovanni, C. (2001). Pertinent psychological issues in the immediate management of a weapons of mass destruction event. *Military Medicine, 166*(12, Suppl.), 59–60.

Fabrikant, J. I. (1981). Health effects of the nuclear accident at Three Mile Island. *Health Phys, 40*(2), 151–161.

Fenner, F., Henderson, D. A., Arita, I., Jezek, Z., & Ladnyi, I. D. (1988). *Smallpox and its eradication.* Geneva, Switzerland: World Health Organization.

Fullerton, C. S., Ursano, R. J., Kao, T. C., & Bharitya, V. R. (1999). Disaster-related bereavement: Acute symptoms and subsequent depression. *Aviation, Space and Environmental Medicine, 70*(9), 902–909.

Gilchrist, H. L. (1925). *A comparative study of warfare gases.* Carlisle Barracks, PA: Medical Field Service School.

Ginzburg, H. M. (1993). The psychological consequences of the Chernobyl accident—Findings from the International Atomic Energy Agency Study. *Public Health Report, 108*(2), 184–192.

Glass, T. A., & Schoch-Spana, M. (2002). Bioterrorism and the people: How to vaccinate a city against panic. *Clinical Infectious Diseases, 34*(2), 217–223.

Haldane, J. S. (1919). Lung-irritant gas poisoning and its sequelae. *Journal of the Royal Army Medical Corps, 33*, 494–507.

Hammerman, G. (1987). The psychological impact of chemical weapons on combat troops in World War I. In R. W. Young & B. H. Drum (Eds.), *Proceedings of the Defense Nuclear Agency symposium/Workshop on the psychological effects of tactical nuclear warfare* (pp. 84–108). Washington, DC: Defense Nuclear Agency, 1987.

Hersey, J. (1946). *Hiroshima.* New York: Knopf.

Hyams, K. C., Murphy, F. M., & Wessely, S. (2002). Responding to chemical, biological, or nuclear terrorism: The indirect and long-term health effects may present the greatest challenge. *Journal of Health and Political Policy Law, 27*(2), 273–291.

Hyams, K. C., Wignall, F. S., & Roswell, R. (1996). War syndromes and their evaluation: From the U.S. Civil War to the Persian Gulf War. *Annals of Internal Medicine, 125*(5), 398–405.

Janis, I. L. (1945, June 1). *Air war and emotional stress. Psychological studies of bombing and civilian defense* (R-212). Santa Monica, CA: Rand Corporation.

Jarrett, D. G. (1999). *Medical management of radiological casualties.* Bethesda, MD: AFRRI.

John, T. J. (1994). Learning from plague in India. *Lancet, 344*, 972.

Jones, F. D. (1995). Traditional warfare combat stress casualties. In F. D. Jones, L. R. Sparacino, V. L. Wilcox, J. M. Rothberg, & J. W. Stokes (Eds.), *War psychiatry* (pp. 35–62). Washington, DC: Borden Institute.

Kawana, N., Ishimatsu, S., & Kanda, K. (2001). Psycho-physiological effects of the terrorist sarin attack on the Tokyo subway system. *Military Medicine, 166*(12 Suppl.), 23–26.

Kemeny, J. G., Babbitt, B., Haggerty, P. E., Lewis, C., Marks, P., Marrett, C. B., et al. (1979). *Report of the President's Commission on the accident at Three Mile Island.* New York: Pergamon Press.

Kortepeter, M. G., Christopher, G., Cieslak, T. J., Culpepper, R., Darling, R., Pavlin, J., et al. (2001). *USAMRIID's medical management of biological casualties handbook* (4th ed.). Fort Detrick, MD: USAMRIID.

Lettinga, K. D., Verbon, A., Nieuwkerk, P. T., Jonkers, R. E., Gersons, B. P., Prins, J. M., et al. (2002). Health-related quality of life and posttraumatic stress disorder among survivors of an outbreak of Legionnaires disease. *Clinical Infectious Diseases, 35*(1), 11–17.

Mavalankar, D. V. (1995). Indian "plague" epidemic: Unanswered questions and key lessons. *Journal of the Royal Society of Medicine, 88*(10), 547–551.

Newmark, J. (2001). Chemical warfare agents: A primer. *Military Medicine, 166* (12, Suppl.), 9–10.

Nishikawa, T., & Tsuiki, S. (1961). Psychiatric investigations of atomic bomb survivors. *Nagasaki Medical Journal, 36,* 717–722.

Norris, F. H. (2002). 60,000 disaster victims speak. Part I: An empirical review of the empirical literature, 1981–2001. *Psychiatry, 65,* 207–239.

Norris, G. W. (1919). Some medical impressions of the war. *American Journal of Medical Science, 157,* 628–634.

North, C. S., Nixon, S. J., Shariat, S., Mallonee, S., McMillen, J. C., Spitznagel, E. L., et al. (1999). Psychiatric disorders among survivors of the Oklahoma City bombing. *Journal of the American Medical Association, 282*(8), 755–762.

North, C. S., Tivis, L., McMillen, J. C., Pfefferbaum, B., Spitznagel, E. L., Cox, J., et al. (2002). Psychiatric disorders in rescue workers after the Oklahoma City bombing. *American Journal of Psychiatry, 159*(5), 857–859.

Nuclear Energy Agency. (2002, March 15). *Chernobyl. Assessment of radiological and health impacts. 2002 Update of Chernobyl: Ten years on.* Paris, France: Organization for Economic Cooperation and Development.

Parkinson, D. K., & Bromet, E. J. (1983). Correlates of mental health in nuclear and coal-fired power plant workers. *Scandinavian Journal of Work and Environmental Health, 9*(4), 341–345.

Pastel, R. H. (2001). Collective behaviors: Mass panic and outbreaks of multiple unexplained symptoms. *Military Medicine, 166*(12, Suppl.), 44–46.

Pastel, R. H. (2002). Radiophobia: Long-term psychological consequences of Chernobyl. *Military Medicine, 166*(12, Suppl.), 134–136.

Pastel, R. H. (2004). Psychological effects of "weapons of mass disruption." *Psychiatry Annals, 34*(9), 679–686.

Pastel, R. H., Kahles, G. R., & Chiang, M. (2001, October 26). *Medical and psychological consequences of radiation dispersal devices* (SP 01-1). Bethesda, MD: AFRRI.

Pastel, R. H., Landauer, M. R., & Knudson, G. B. (Eds.). (2001). International Conference on the Operational Impact of Psychological Casualties from Weapons of Mass Destruction—Proceedings. *Military Medicine, 166*(Suppl. 2), 1–91.

Patterson, J. T. (1987). *The dread disease: Cancer and modern American culture.* Cambridge, MA: Harvard University Press.

Petterson, J. S. (1988). Perception vs. reality of radiological impact: The Goiania model. *Nuclear News, 31*(14), 84–90.

Quarantelli, E. L. (1960). Images of withdrawal behavior in disasters: Some basic misconceptions. *Social Problems, 8,* 68–79.

Rahu, M., Tekkel, M., Veidebaum, T., Pukkala, E., Hakulinen, T., Auvinen, A., et al. (1997). The Estonian study of Chernobyl cleanup workers: II. Incidence of cancer and mortality. *Radiation Research, 147*(5), 653–657.

Ramalingaswami, V. (2001). Psychosocial effects of the 1994 plague outbreak in Surat, India. *Military Medicine, 166*(12, Suppl.), 29–30.

Riddle, J. R., Brown, M., Smith, T., Ritchie, E. C., Brix, K. A., & Romano, J. (2003). Chemical warfare and the Gulf War: A review of the impact on Gulf veterans' health. *Military Medicine, 168*(8), 606–613.

Ritchie, E. C. (1992). Treatment of gas mask phobia. *Military Medicine, 157*(2), 104–106.

Ritchie, E. C. (2001). Psychological problems associated with mission-oriented protective gear. *Military Medicine, 166*(12, Suppl.), 83–84.

Rosenbaum, C. (1993). Chemical warfare: disaster preparation in an Israeli hospital. *Social Work Health Care, 18*(3–4), 137–145.

Rotenberg, Z., Noy, S., & Gabbay, U. (1994). Israeli ED experience during the Gulf War. *American Journal of Emergency Medicine, 12*(1), 118–119.

Salmon, T. W., & Fenton, N. (1929). Neuropsychiatry in the American Expeditionary Force. In T. W. Salmon & N. Fenton (Eds.), *Neuropsychiatry* (Vol. 10, pp. 217–474). Washington, DC: U.S. Government Printing Office.

Sandman, P. M. (1993). *Responding to community outrage: Strategies for effective risk communication.* Fairfax, VA: American Industrial Hygiene Association.

Scharf, T., Vaught, C., Kidd, P., Steiner, L., Kowalski, K., Wiehagen, B., et al. (2001). Toward a typology of dynamic and hazardous work environments. *Human Ecological Risk Assessment, 7*(7), 1827–1841.

Schelling, G., Stoll, C., Haller, M., Briegel, J., Manert, W., Hummel, T., et al. (1998). Health-related quality of life and posttraumatic stress disorder in survivors of the acute respiratory distress syndrome. *Critical Care Medicine, 26*(4), 651–659.

Schnurr, P. P., Ford, J. D., Friedman, M. J., Green, B. L., Dain, B. J., & Sengupta, A. (2000). Predictors and outcomes of posttraumatic stress disorder in World War II veterans exposed to mustard gas. *Journal of Consulting and Clinical Psychology, 68*(2), 258–268.

Solomon, Z., & Benbenishty, R. (1986). The role of proximity, immediacy, and expectancy in frontline treatment of combat stress reaction among Israelis in the Lebanon War. *American Journal of Psychiatry, 143*(5), 613–617.

Steinhauer, J. (2001, October, 21). Hysteria can be hazardous. *The New York Times.*

Struewing, J. P., & Gray, G. C. (1990). An epidemic of respiratory complaints exacerbated by mass psychogenic illness in a military recruit population. *American Journal of Epidemiology, 132*(6), 1120–1129.

Tarabrina, N., Lazebnaya, E., Zelenova, M., & Lasko, N. (1996). Chernobyl cleanup workers' perception of radiation threat. *Radiation and Protection Dosimetry, 68,* 251–255.

Torubarov, F. S. (1991). Psychological consequences of the Chernobyl accident from the radiation neurology point of view. In R. C. Ricks, M. E. Berger, & F. M. O'Hara Jr. (Eds.), *The medical basis for radiation-accident preparedness: Vol. III. The psychological perspective.* New York: Elsevier Science.

Ursano, R. J., Norwood, A. E., Fullerton, C. S., Holloway, H. C., & Hall, M. (2003). Terrorism with weapons of mass destruction. Chemical, biological, nuclear, radiological, and explosive agents. In R. J. Ursano & A. E. Norwood (Eds.), *Trauma and disaster responses and management* (pp. 125–154). Washington, DC: American Psychiatric Publishing.

Viel, J. F., Curbakova, E., Dzerve, B., Eglite, M., Zvagule, T., & Vincent, C. (1997). Risk factors for long-term mental and psychosomatic distress in Latvian

Chernobyl liquidators. *Environmental Health Perspectives, 105*(Suppl. 6), 1539–1544.

Wachtel, C. (1941). *Chemical warfare.* Brooklyn, NY: Chemical Publishing.

Williams, E. R., & Shepherd, S. M. (2000). Medical clearance of psychiatric patients. *Emergency Medicine Clinics of North America, 18*(2), 185–198.

Yevelson, I. I., Abdelgani, A., Cwikel, J., & Yevelson, I. S. (1997). Bridging the gap in mental health approaches between east and west: The psychosocial consequences of radiation exposure. *Environmental Health Perspectives, 105*(Suppl. 6), 1551–1556.

Promoting Disaster Recovery in Ethnic-Minority Individuals and Communities

FRAN H. NORRIS and MARGARITA ALEGRÍA

People who identify as African American, Native American, Asian American, or Hispanic/Latino accounted for 30% of the U.S. population in 2000 and are projected to account for almost 40% of the population in 2025 (U.S. Department of Health and Human Services [DHHS], 2001). The mental health system in general and the disaster mental health system in particular are challenged to meet the needs of this increasingly diverse population. The issues are complex because the effects of ethnicity and culture are pervasive. They may influence the need for help, the availability of help, comfort in seeking help, and the appropriateness of that help. In this chapter, we review the evidence regarding each of these points to draw conclusions regarding how to promote disaster recovery in ethnic-minority individuals and communities.

NEED FOR MENTAL HEALTH SERVICES

Ethnicity and the Epidemiology of Mental Disorders

Consistent with the Surgeon General's Report, *Mental Health: Culture, Race, and Ethnicity* (DHHS, 2001), need is defined here as the prevalence of psychiatric disorder or elevated distress in the population. Prevalence rates are clearly imperfect measures of need, but they may serve reasonably

319

as population-level markers of relative need for help. The inclusion of elevated levels of distress allows us to examine whether immigrants, particularly those who are less acculturated, are more likely to express their reactions to disaster by higher levels of distress, including cultural idioms, such as *ataque de nervios* or *neurasthenia*. Because research has pointed to posttraumatic stress disorder (PTSD) and depression as the two most likely adverse psychological consequences of disasters (Norris, Friedman, et al., 2002), we paid particular attention to the epidemiology of these two conditions. Findings from disaster research are best interpreted in light of the general epidemiology of mental disorders.

Holzer and Copeland (2000) presented a useful review of the role of ethnicity in the epidemiology of mental disorders in the United States and presented results from reanalyses of data from the Epidemiologic Catchment Area Survey (ECA) and the National Comorbidity Survey (NCS), two well-known national studies. In rank order, annual prevalence rates of major depressive disorder (MDD) were highest for Hispanics (4.0%, ECA; 14.1%, NCS), next highest for non-Hispanic whites (3.6%; 10.2%), somewhat lower but not very different for African Americans (3.2%; 8.4%), and lowest for Asian Americans (2.5%; 6.3%). More recent results of the National Comorbidity Survey Replication (NCS-R) indicate no ethnic differences in the rates of MDD between Hispanics and non-Hispanic whites (Kessler et al., 2003), but lower odds ratios for non-Hispanic blacks (odds ratio = 0.6, 95% confidence interval = 0.5–0.8). Perhaps because they composed the smallest subsample in the ECA and NCS, results were least consistent for Native Americans; their rate of MDD was lowest in the ECA (1.9%) but equivalent to that of African Americans in the NCS (8.5%).

These national surveys are supplemented by studies of particular or more localized populations. The Washington Needs Assessment Household Survey (WANAHS, also described by Holzer & Copeland, 2000) included over 1,000 Native Americans and, in this case, their MDD rate was the highest of all groups (11.7%, compared to 7.9% of white Americans). The Chinese American Psychiatric Epidemiology Study (CAPES; Takeuchi et al., 1998) replicated findings showing that Asian Americans had lower than average MDD prevalence rates. In the Mexican American Prevalence Study (MAPS; Vega et al., 1998), rates of MDD were comparable to those seen in the NCS but varied by place of birth, being higher for U.S.-born Mexican Americans than for Mexican-born participants. In general, researchers find that recent Latino and Asian immigrants tend to experience better physical and mental health outcomes than more established Latino and Asian residents (Takeuchi et al., 1998; Vega et al., 1998). Whether these outcomes can be attributed to selection processes or to acculturation into American lifestyles is open to conjecture. Overall, the available data on the need for mental health care suggest that prevalence rates of depression are similar or lower among ethnic minorities than among white Americans.

Estimating the relative vulnerability of culturally diverse groups to trauma is more challenging. The PTSD measure used in the ECA is generally considered to have been insensitive to the disorder regardless of ethnicity (e.g., Solomon & Canino, 1990). The NCS did not detect ethnic differences in the prevalence of PTSD (Kessler, Somnega, Bromet, Hughes, & Nelson, 1995), nor did Norris (1992) in a survey of black and white residents of four midsize southeastern cities. CAPES found extraordinarily low rates of PTSD (1.1% of men and 2.2% of women reported by Norris, Foster, and Weisshaar, 2002, with the assistance and permission of CAPES investigators). MAPS, unfortunately, did not assess PTSD, but an epidemiological study of PTSD in Mexico (Norris, Murphy, Baker, Perilla, et al., 2003) found the lifetime prevalence of PTSD (11% after and 13% before the criterion of functional impairment was applied) to be substantially higher there than in the United States (8%). Using data from the National Vietnam Veterans Readjustment Survey (NVVRS), Ortega and Rosenheck (2000) found Puerto Rican and Mexican American veterans, but not other Hispanic veterans, to have higher probabilities of PTSD and more severe symptoms than non-Hispanic white veterans.

The Detroit Area Survey of Trauma (Breslau et al., 1998) showed African Americans to be at increased risk for PTSD relative to whites, but this effect dropped out when central city residence was controlled. Inner-city Americans are disproportionately exposed to community violence (Osofsky, 1997; Parson, 1997). These findings suggest that more than minority status, living in urban inner cities with high exposure to community violence might pose increased risk for PTSD.

Limitations of the Epidemiological Research

Altogether, research on the epidemiology of depression and PTSD among American minorities is inadequate. The NCS Hispanic, Asian, and Native American samples were small in size, heterogeneous in terms of national origin, and limited to English-speaking persons. Supplementary surveys provided good data for specific subpopulations but can be generalized past them only with the utmost caution. The results quite obviously do not apply to the various smaller populations of Asian, African, Latino, and European refugees who live in the United States precisely because of violence and trauma in their home countries. Moreover, a number of investigators have argued that health data should be disaggregated by using subethnic groups (e.g., African Caribbean within the African Americans in the United States) because of considerable differences within groups (e.g.,

Srinivasan & Guillermo, 2000). For example, whereas Asian Americans as a group may appear similar to whites on a number of health-related and socioeconomic indicators, such statistics disguise higher rates of health problems and poverty among Asian American subgroups, such as the Vietnamese. These studies point to the complexity of understanding diverse subgroup process and the need to distinguish the impact of culture from minority status or poverty.

In addition to sampling, assessment raises a host of challenges. There is evidence to suggest that responses to screener items in diagnostic batteries may vary as a function of ethnicity/race, gender, education, and socioeconomic status of the respondent (Alegría & McGuire, 2003). A strict focus on traditional diagnoses may cause the clinician to miss "culturebound syndromes" and somaticized distress (Kirmayer; 1996; Norris, Weisshaar, et al., 2001). Zheng and colleagues (1997) provided an excellent example of this in their research on *neurasthenia*, a condition that is recognized among Chinese Americans and is characterized by fatigue or weakness accompanied by an array of physical and psychological complaints, such as diffuse pains, gastrointestinal problems, memory loss, irritability, and sleep problems. Over half of those meeting criteria for neurasthenia did not meet criteria for any DSM-III-R (American Psychiatric Association, 1987) diagnoses. Another example is *ataques de nervios*. In a Puerto Rican disaster study, 14% of the sample reported experiencing these acute episodes of emotional upset and loss of control, although the rate of disaster specific PTSD was quite low (Guarnaccia, Canino, Rubio-Stipec, & Bravo, 1993). With these caveats, the available data appear to suggest that Latinos most consistently show elevated mental health needs and that black and white Americans do not consistently differ. Data for Asian and Native Americans are too sparse, contradictory, or both to draw any comparative conclusions.

Ethnicity, Culture, and Disaster Recovery

Despite a few exceptions, most disaster studies that have examined the effects of ethnicity on outcomes have found that minority ethnic groups fare worse than persons who are of majority group status (Bolton & Klenow, 1988; Galea et al., 2002; Garrison et al., 1995; Green et al., 1990; March, Amaya-Jackson, Terry, & Costanzo, 1997; Palinkas, Downs, Petterson, & Russell, 1993; Perilla, Norris, & Lavizzo, 2002; Webster, McDonald, Lewin, & Carr, 1995). A few noncomparative studies have similarly shown that postdisaster stress was quite high in particular ethnic communities (Chen, Chung, Chen, Fang, & Chen, 2003; Hough et al., 1990; Thiel de Bocanegra & Brickman, 2004). Ethnic differences in posttraumatic stress may point to effects of various risk factors, such as low socioeconomic status, chronic adversities, and differential exposure to the event itself that have little to do with culture per se. Nonetheless, culture can also shape the experience and consequences of disaster exposure.

Palinkas and colleagues' (1993) study of the aftermath of the *Exxon Valdez* spill is a case in point. The investigation revealed significant differences between Native Alaskans and others in rates of postdisaster major depression, generalized anxiety, and PTSD that were not explained by exposure alone. The spill interrupted subsistence activities, and these disruptions had greater impact on natives because they feared losing long-held traditions that defined their culture and community.

Perilla and colleagues (2002) explicitly tested whether *differential exposure* or *differential vulnerability* best explained their results showing that Latinos and non-Hispanic blacks were more adversely affected by Hurricane Andrew than were non-Hispanic whites. Consistent with the differential exposure hypothesis, non-Hispanic whites were less often personally traumatized and far less exposed to neighborhood-level trauma than the other groups. The severity of their exposure accounted for much of minority group members' higher posttraumatic stress. However, the interaction of trauma and ethnicity indicated that differential vulnerability also would have to be considered, and, in fact, some of minorities' disproportionate distress was explained by their higher levels of fatalism and acculturative stress. Fatalism refers to beliefs that fate plays a disproportionate role in life circumstances and that events are not under a person's control. Perilla and colleagues' findings are consistent with a large literature showing that external control is a risk factor for poor psychological outcomes following stressful life events (leading to increase vulnerability). It is reasonable to speculate that the intergroup tensions manifested in acculturative stress could exacerbate the effects of other stressors like job disruption or homelessness caused by a disaster. Theoretically, it was important to demonstrate that differential exposure and vulnerability can work in tandem and are not necessarily rival explanations.

Thiel de Bocanegra and Brickman's (2004) study was important for documenting the potential of disasters to affect the mental health of Asian Americans. In this sample of Chinese Americans seeking financial assistance after the September 11 terrorist attacks, 22% showed a pattern of symptoms consistent with PTSD, a rate strikingly higher than the presumed base rate of PTSD in this population. An additional study of Chinese Americans living in Chinatown, New York City, found that more than half of community residents reported one or more symptoms of psychological distress immediately following the event, but less than 4% received counseling from a mental health professional during the 5-month period after the disaster (Chen et al., 2003).

Also pertinent to this discussion are findings showing that culture shapes the effects of other important variables, such as gender and age, on postdisaster mental health outcomes. Norris, Perilla, Ibañez, and Murphy (2001) found that being of Mexican culture exacerbated gender differences and African American culture attenuated them. Webster and colleagues (1995) also found that sex differences in the effects of the Newcastle earthquake in Australia were greatest within the non-English-speaking immigrant portion of their sample. Norris, Kaniasty, Inman, Conrad, and Murphy (2002) examined age effects in three disaster-stricken samples. Among Americans, age had a curvilinear relation with PTSD such that middle-age respondents were most distressed. This was consistent with the other findings from the United States (Norris, Friedman, et al., 2002). Among Mexicans, however, age had a linear and negative relation with PTSD such that younger people were most distressed. Forming yet a third pattern, age had a linear and positive relation with PTSD in Poland, such that older people were most distressed after the disaster. The authors interpreted the findings in light of anthropological research showing that the family life cycle is different in each of these societies. For our purposes here, the important lesson from this comparison is that there was no one consistent effect of disaster by age; rather, it depended on the cultural and historical context of the population and the country variance of social roles played at various ages (see also Chen et al., 2003).

USE OF MENTAL HEALTH SERVICES

Ethnic Disparities in Service Use

There are striking disparities for minorities in use of mental health services. To begin with, minorities in the United States are less likely than whites to seek mental health treatment until symptoms are more severe and less likely to seek treatment from mental health specialists, as they are more inclined to turn to primary care or to use informal sources of support (DHHS, 2001; Vega & Alegría, 2001). The disparities appear to hold specifically for PTSD as well as for mental disorders in general (Koenen, Goodwin, Struening, Hellman, & Guardino, 2003). There is substantial evidence that patients' views about health care differ by race, ethnicity, socioeconomic status, language, and literacy levels (Blendon et al., 1995; Carrasquillo, Ovar, Brennan, & Burstin, 1999).

Availability and Accessibility of Services

A number of explanations for these disparities have been offered, including insurance (Hargraves & Hadley, 2003) and inadequate detection of problems (Borowsky et al., 2000). The threshold for what is considered distressing or impairing may have strong cultural determinants, thereby producing an effect on reporting and ascertainment of symptoms that could have a bearing on diagnosis and detection. In many Hispanic and Asian cultures, communication in the absence of a relationship is not accepted or proper. Many immigrants have difficulties communicating in English or fear immigration or legal authorities, leading them to never receive care (Castaneda, 1994). Sue, Fujino, Hu, and Takeuchi (1991) concluded that an important cause of underutilization is the limited availability of culturally competent psychotherapists and culturally responsive services. Altogether, these facts point to a general problem in the availability and accessibility of mental health care for American minorities.

Help-Seeking Comfort, Stigma, and Mistrust

It is difficult to isolate *help seeking* from *help receiving* in most of the literature. It is often assumed that minorities possess more negative attitudes about seeking help because of the findings showing that they receive less help than white Americans. However, the issue for minorities is not help seeking per se. Kaniasty and Norris (2000) studied ethnic differences in help-seeking comfort after Hurricane Andrew. All ethnic groups reported feeling most comfortable requesting help from family, somewhat less comfortable seeking help from friends, and the least comfortable seeking help from outsiders (which would include formal sources). Overall, minorities held more rather than less positive views about seeking help from other people, and this effect was more rather than less pronounced for outsiders. If these findings at first seem surprising, they actually are in accord with cross-cultural descriptions noting the greater value that white Americans place on self-reliance. Still, most people prefer receiving help from natural, informal sources.

Of course, the preceding results did not specifically address willingness to acknowledge a mental illness and to seek professional help for that problem. The Surgeon General's Report (SGR) (DHHS, 2001) identified stigma as a critical barrier to the use of mental health services. Stigma refers to a cluster of negative attitudes and beliefs that motivate the general public to fear, reject, avoid, and discriminate against people with mental illness. People with mental problems internalize public attitudes and conceal symptoms to avoid embarrassment or shame. Stigma is pervasive in American society and prevalent among white Americans as well as among minority groups.

Mistrust is a somewhat different issue than stigma. As reviewed in the SGR, African Americans and Latinos are more likely to feel that a health provider has judged them unfairly and to be afraid of mental health treatment. Allen (1996) argued that shame and guilt were especially common in African American PTSD patients who may be hypersensitive to outsiders, including therapists, if they seem to stand in harsh judgment of them. Minorities also appear to have greater concerns around side effects and addiction potential of medication (Cooper-Patrick et al., 1997). For these and other issues of trust, even when offered, minorities may be less likely to opt for receiving evidence-based treatments such as antidepressant medication or specialty psychiatric care (Miranda & Cooper, 2002; Wang, Bergland, & Kessler, 2000; Young, Klap, Shelbourne, & Wells, 2001). More research is needed, but at present the data suggest that (1) stigma is a pervasive problem in America and (2) mistrust exacerbates its effects among minorities.

Promoting Service Use in the Aftermath of Disasters

The SGR noted that such negative attitudes could be addressed through public education efforts that are tailored to the languages, needs, and cultures of ethnic minorities. They proposed that one way to advance these efforts would be to involve representatives from the community in the design, planning, and implementation of services. On the basis of results from refugee programs, they concluded that successful programs do aggressive outreach and furnish a familiar and welcoming atmosphere (DHHS, 2001, p. 166). Disaster mental health services begin with critical assumptions (Flynn, 1994; Norris et al., Chapter 18, this volume) that match these recommendations quite well. First, crisis counseling programs assume that disaster victims are normal people responding normally to abnormal situations and therefore that services should be directed at normalizing individuals' experience and distress. By normalizing distress and help seeking, disaster services afford atypical opportunities to destigmatize mental health care. Second, crisis counseling programs assume that people prefer natural sources of assistance and therefore that services should be provided in schools, churches, and places of work. Third, these programs assume that people who need help the most may not necessarily seek it and therefore that services must assume a proactive posture to reach out to vulnerable groups.

There are few data that document whether these principles actually help to reduce disparities in service use. However, some data from Project Liberty in New York provide tentative support for the hypothesis that minorities are as likely as others to seek and receive care when other barriers are reduced (stigma, mistrust) or eliminated (cost). The ethnic breakdown of crisis counseling recipients matched the demographics of New York quite well (Felton, 2002). Moreover, in a diverse sample of 800 adults receiving crisis counseling services, and with the intensity of psychological reactions controlled, African American and white clients were equally willing to accept a referral to "enhanced services" (treatment). Hispanic ethnicity actually increased the likelihood that the referral was accepted (Norris, Donahue, Felton, Watson, & Hamblen, 2004).

Although Project Liberty was generally successful in reaching out to minority communities in the aftermath of 9/11, there was room for improvement (Norris et al., Chapter 18, this volume). Sometimes trust was difficult to establish. Most often mentioned was the difficulty in engaging the Muslim community. Sometimes hostilities were encountered in communities that had a multitude of predisaster problems and histories of neglect (Battery Park and Harlem were mentioned as two good examples in New York) but were overcome by involving community members in generating strategies and solutions.

APPROPRIATENESS OF MENTAL HEALTH SERVICES

Shortcomings of the Evidence Base for Minorities

The challenge for serving American minorities is to be both scientifically and culturally appropriate. The SGR concluded that the evidence base regarding effective treatments for minorities has remained quite poor (DHHS, 2001). Although effective treatments are available for many mental disorders, they are not being translated into community settings and are not being provided to everyone who comes in for care. The gap between research and practice is worse for minorities. The evidence base is meager but improving for trauma and PTSD. Zoellner, Feeny, Fitzgibbons, and Foa (1999) found no ethnic differences in completion rates and achieved equivalent results for 60 white and 35 black female assault victims who had been randomly assigned to active cognitive-behavioral treatment (CBT) or wait-list control. Kataoka and colleagues (2003) showed that an eight-session CBT intervention for Latino students exposed to community violence produced significant declines in depression and PTSD symptoms compared to a wait-list control. Many more studies like these are needed to establish the efficacy of various treatment approaches.

Ethnic Disparities in Quality of Care

A few studies have raised concerns about the overall quality of care being received by minority clients in community settings. Even after entering care, minorities face a higher risk of being misdiagnosed. This may be due to minorities being more likely to seek help in primary care as opposed to specialty care, where about one-third to one-half of patients with mental disorders remain undiagnosed (Williams et al., 1999). But even in psychiatric evaluation in emergency rooms, minorities are at greater risk of non-detection of mental disorders (e.g., Borowsky et al., 2000).

In many studies in the United States, members of minority groups are found to receive inferior health care compared to white patients. Using data from a large-scale survey, Wang and colleagues (2000) examined propor-tions receiving care that could be considered consistent with evidence-based treatment recommendations. This was defined operationally as attending at least four therapy sessions plus receiving medication or attending eight ses-sions in the absence of medication. African Americans were much less likely than white Americans to have received such care. Similarly, Young and colleagues (2001) showed that Latinos were less likely than non-Hispanic whites to receive treatment that was in accord with evidence-based guidelines.

Inappropriate prescription of medication is a source of significant con-cern. Clinicians in psychiatric emergency services prescribe both more and higher doses of oral and injectable antipsychotic medications to African Americans than to whites (Segel, Bola, & Watson, 1996), even when research recommends lower dosages to African Americans due to their slower metabolizing of some antidepressants and antipsychotic medications (Bradford & Kirlin, 1998). African Americans are less likely than whites to receive an antidepressant when their depression is first diagnosed and less likely to receive newer selective serotonin reuptake inhibitors (SSRIs), once medicated (Melfi, Croghan, Hanna, & Robinson, 2000).

Some studies suggest that retention and outcomes are superior when clients and clinicians are matched ethnically (Sue et al., 1991), but the crux of the matter may be *cognitive match*—that is, the congruence between therapist and client conceptions (Sue, 1998). One central dimension of care is the physician's or clinician's ability to communicate with the patient. The diagnostic formulation and treatment of mental disorders rely to a large degree on verbal communication between patient and physician about symptoms, the understanding of the possible causes of the problem, and the proper assessment of its impact on functioning. Miscommunication can lead to misdiagnosis, mismatch between the patient and the provider's expectation about treatment, and poor adherence to treatment. The assess-ment process is thus especially important when treating non-English-speaking populations.

Frameworks for Cultural Competence

The adoption of cultural competence as an overriding principle of services for minority populations is based in the premise that caregiver's or agen-cies' understanding of a person's cultural background and experience facili-tates a better match of services and thus more effective care and improved client outcomes. Siegel and colleagues (2000) provided a series of indicators that may serve to establish the performance of the agency or system in providing culturally competent services. Some of the indicators include consumer and family involvement in the design of services, training of staff in cultural competence, and number of services adapted for cultural or racial groups.

In recent years, various recommendations have appeared for creating culturally competent mental health services. Cultural competence refers to the behaviors, attitudes, skills, and policies that help mental health caregivers to work effectively and efficiently across cultures (New York State Office of Mental Health, 1997). Of these, the best known is the *Outline for Cultural Formulation* published in the appendix of DSM-IV (American Psychiatric Association, 1994). The process of applying DSM criteria across cultures involves several steps: (1) assessing the cultural identify of the client, including his or her degree of involvement with the culture of origin and host culture; (2) exploring cultural explanations for the individual's symptoms, including his or her perception of their cause; (3) exploring cultural factors related to the psychosocial environment and level of functioning, with particular attention to social stressors and social support and the role of religion and kin networks in the person's life; (4) identifying cultural elements in the relationship between the individual and clinician, such as differences between them in language and heritage; and (5) creating an overall formulation of diagnosis and care. The formulation has been criticized for not going far enough (e.g., Lopez & Guarnaccia, 2000), but it nonetheless represents a tremendous step forward for multicultural care.

Around the same time, the American Psychological Association (1993) established benchmarks for cultural competency. The competent provider is characterized by an awareness of his or her own assumptions and values, a respect for the worldviews of clients, and the ability to develop culturally appropriate interventions. Knowledge, beliefs, and attitudes must all be considered. Yet, there is evidence suggesting that clinician bias and stereotyping play a role in medical decision making. For example, broadly adopted stereotypes of Asian Americans as "problem free" may lead providers to miss an individual's mental health problems (Takeuchi & Uehara, 1996).

Fortunately, certain goals of psychotherapy can reasonably be assumed to be universal, such as the removal of distressing symptoms and communication of empathy (Draguns, 1996). Beyond these goals, standard practices are likely to need some adaptation across cultures. Vega (1992) summarized the challenges well by noting that "off-the-shelf" intervention materials are difficult to use in diverse settings because they are unknowingly embedded with cultural expectations and unsubstantiated assumptions about such issues as time orientation, social and occupational commitments, family structure, and gender roles. These issues are overlooked by interventionists with surprising regularity. Intervention materials, levels of respondent burden, and assessment protocols must be carefully reviewed by community judges before a program can be piloted and evaluated in the targeted community or population.

Sue (1998) advised that an important component is *scientific mindedness*, saying, "By scientific mindedness, I am referring to therapists who form hypotheses rather than make premature conclusions about the status of culturally different clients, who develop creative ways to test hypotheses, and who act on the basis of acquired data" (p. 445). Sue continued by noting:

> A good clinician who is uncertain of the cultural meaning of a symptom should engage in hypothesis testing. For example, if the symptom is a reflection of a psychotic episode rather than a culturally influenced characteristic, one would expect (a) the client to manifest other psychotic symptoms, (b) other individuals in the culture to be unfamiliar with the symptom, or (c) experts in the culture to indicate that the symptom is unusual in that culture. (p. 446)

However, this type of assessment might be particularly difficult to implement in the absence of cultural psychiatric liaisons, such as the ones proposed by Kirmayer and Young (1999).

On the basis of many years of experience working with traumatized refugees, Kinzie (2001) advised cross-cultural treatment programs to incorporate several key elements. These elements appear to apply to postdisaster clinical settings quite well. Such programs need to be able to treat major disorders in addition to PTSD because of high rates of comorbidity (e.g., depression and substance abuse) in some populations. Programs must address language needs, and they must be easy to access and perceived as credible. In addition, according to Kinzie, the program must have linkages with other services, integrate care for both physical and mental disorders, create mechanisms for feedback and advice, and be staffed by competent clinicians and bilingual mental health workers who can create bridges between the patient and professional staff.

Social Functioning as an Organizing Principle for Multicultural Interventions

Draguns (1996) speculated that cultural dimensions, especially individualism–collectivism, provided clues for the content of multicultural interventions. He reasoned that in individualist cultures that emphasize independence, it is appropriate for self-actualization to serve as the ultimate goal of psychological interventions, whereas in collectivistic cultures that emphasize interdependence, it would be more fitting to aim for the attainment of harmonious social relationships. Both objectives are inherently desirable; it is only their respective prominence that would differ given the cultural identify of the client. We agree with these points and would like to elaborate further on their implications for the content of multicultural postdisaster interventions. Individualist and collectivist cultures subsume strikingly different constructions of self (Markus & Kitayama, 1994). In collectivist cultures, such as found across most of Latin America and Asia, the self is unbounded and fundamentally interrelated with others. The goal is not to become autonomous but to fulfill and create obligation and, in general, to become part of various interpersonal relationships. In an important cross-cultural study, Kitayama, Markus, and Matsumoto (1995) distinguished between socially engaged emotions (e.g., feelings of closeness), socially disengaged emotions (e.g., pride), and generic emotions (e.g., happiness). They found that socially engaged emotions were more strongly related to emotional states than were socially disengaged emotions among the Japanese, whereas the reverse was true in the United States.

This finding is of particular interest for our purposes because perceptions of belonging and being cared for are critical to the well being of disaster victims (see Kaniasty & Norris, 2004, for a review of the literature on disasters and social support). Across a variety of settings both within and outside the United States, Kaniasty and Norris have shown that disasters exert their adverse impact on psychological distress both directly and indirectly, through disruptions of social relationships and expectations of support. This disruption of social supports occurs just when the need for them is at its highest. A disaster is an excellent example of a community event that alters the quantity and quality of social interactions. Because disasters affect entire indigenous networks, the need for support may simply exceed its availability, causing expectations of support to be violated. Relocation and job loss remove important others from victims' supportive environments. There are fewer opportunities for companionship and leisure. Physical fatigue, emotional irritability, and scarcity of resources augment the potential for interpersonal conflicts and social withdrawal. Interactions that are apparently supportive may be seen quite differently when one's obligations to help others in the network are taken into account; reciprocity is highly valued in many cultures. Furthermore, it needs to be recognized that disaster recovery can be a long process. The heightened level of helping and concern evident initially cannot be expected to last for the full length of the recovery process. Nor are supportive resources distributed equitably. Following several disasters, it has been found that disaster victims who had fewer economic resources or were members of ethnic minority groups received less emotional support than did their comparably affected counterparts who had greater economic resources or were members of ethnic majority groups (Kaniasty & Norris, 1995). Socially and economically disadvantaged groups are frequently too overburdened to provide ample help to other members in time of additional need.

From this research, a clear and deceptively simple recommendation for culturally responsive postdisaster interventions can be drawn. This is always to remember that *the individual is embedded in a broader familial, interpersonal, and social context.* (See Hobfoll, 1998, for an exceptional elaboration on this point.) The interventionist or practitioner must spend time assessing—and addressing—socially relevant cognitions and emotions as well as the person's social supports, network demands, and performed and expected social roles. On the positive side are constructs such as (1) perceptions of social support, social competence, belonging, and trust; (2) mutuality and marital satisfaction; and (3) social participation, sense of community, and communal mastery. On the negative side are constructs such as (4) withdrawal, loneliness, isolation, interpersonal estrangement, shame, and remorse; (5) familial obligations, caretaking burdens, and parenting stress; (6) domestic and other interpersonal conflicts; and (7) hostility, anger, societal alienation, perceptions of neglect, and acculturative stress. Broadly speaking, *the intervention goal is to enhance social functioning,* which indirectly addresses an important risk factor for chronic PTSD (Norris, Murphy, Baker, & Perilla, 2003).

Some previous recommendations in the multicultural treatment literature are consistent with our own. As Lindsey and Cuéllar (2000) noted, "African Americans will respond more favorably if therapy efforts are directed toward the environment or toward working with the extended family or toward spiritualistic and/or religious interventions or toward strengthening interdependency" (p. 199). They went on to say that cognitive therapy provides a good example. Similar recommendations to adjust cognitive-behavioral interventions to make them acceptable to Latino culture have been offered by Vera, Vila, and Alegría (2003). The therapist's techniques are essentially the same regardless of culture, but the client's explanatory models are culturally derived.

Community Action

To be culturally responsive in the aftermath of disasters, practitioners need to go beyond providing traditional services in nontraditional settings and embrace novel approaches to meeting community needs. Solomon (2003) summarized this well:

> The major concern is in fostering natural resiliency. For many survivors, removing obstacles to self-help, or providing for basic needs such as food, shelter, education, and health care may be the only intervention needed.

This type of secondary prevention may also involve reparations, provision of a safe and healthy recovery environment, and reunion of family and community members. The underlying goal is to empower victims to participate in their own recovery efforts so as to regain both a sense of control over their lives and an orientation toward the future. (p. 12)

Solomon went on to note, "Although professionals working in the mental health arena are seldom trained or prepared to work at a broader community level, the scale of these emergences may require abandoning dyadic interventions for those that can be implemented via community action using a public health approach" (p. 12). Somasundarum, Norris, Asukai, and Murthy (2003) and Hobfoll (1998) similarly advocated for community-level interventions that foster community competence and ownership of problems and solutions. Culturally based rituals and traditions sometimes can be used as the basis for innovative interventions (Manson, 1997; Nader, Dubrow, & Stamm, 1999). No one set of recommendations will apply to all communities cross-culturally, and activities must be developed from the "bottom up" to match the cultural context and needs of the group. Working collectively toward specific, achievable goals is helpful for many communities; community gatherings also help people to interpret and share their experiences and to establish social links (Somasundarum et al., 2003).

The evidence base supporting the effectiveness of community-oriented trauma programs is minimal, and building such a base is crucial for the advancement of culturally competent care. A few pilot studies are promising. For example, Weine and colleagues (2003) described the "Tea and Families Education and Support" intervention for Kosovar refugees. Three months after entering the program, participants demonstrated increases in knowledge about trauma and mental health, use of mental health services, perceived social support, and family hardiness.

RECOMMENDATIONS

Table 17.1 summarizes the following recommendations:

• *Assess community needs early and often.* Prior research indicates that minorities are at elevated risk for postdisaster mental health problems such as depression and PTSD. Small but important percentages will have mental health needs that predate the disaster. Assessment of needs in disaster-stricken communities is critical, and these assessments should oversample minority populations to determine the ways in which they were exposed and affected by the particular event. Because diagnoses may be less

TABLE 17.1. Guidelines for Culturally Sensitive Postdisaster Care

- *Assess community needs early and often.* Gaps in rates of recovery, awareness of services, and use of services can be noted and addressed.
- *Provide free and easily accessible services.* Minorities will be more likely to take advantage of services that are close to home, community-based, and offered in concert with other services and activities.
- *Work collaboratively and proactively to build trust and to engage minorities in care.* To reduce disparities in service use, practitioners must get out of the clinic into the community.
- *Validate and normalize distress.* Help seeking as well as symptoms can and should be normalized. Diagnosis of pathology should be deemphasized, relative to standard practice. An important task of the clinician is to help individuals identify and mobilize their natural resources.
- *Value interdependence as well as independence as an appropriate goal.* The intervention goal is to enhance social functioning, helping the person retain or resume his or her social roles.
- *Promote community action.* Novel and innovative strategies should be explored that involve minority communities in their own recovery by working toward specific, achievable goals.
- *Recognize that cultural competence is a process not an end-state.* Continuing education is key.
- *Advocate for, facilitate, or conduct treatment and evaluation research.* Researchers and practitioners should collaborate to test the efficacy and effectiveness of different intervention strategies for minority populations.
- *Leave a legacy.* Disasters create opportunities to educate the public, destigmatize mental health problems, and build trust between providers and minority communities.

valid for minority persons and because they represent only the tip of the iceberg in any case, needs assessments should include a focus on experienced emotional distress and impaired functioning, especially social functioning. Valid needs assessments for culturally diverse populations also require information on contextual and cultural variables such as trauma exposure in the country of origin, losing of social ties, level of comfort in host society, and level of English-language proficiency. Gaining support among policy researchers is the notion of surveillance. Needs evolve. Repeating the needs assessment periodically will provide invaluable information about the extent to which minorities are recovering from the disaster, have recovered, or still require help. Gaps in rates of recovery, awareness of services, and use of services can be noted and addressed.

- *Provide free and easily accessible services.* Minorities often lack insurance and other means of paying for mental health services. They will be more likely to take advantage of services that are close to home, community-based, and offered in concert with other services and activities.

This might translate in providing services in community-based organizations with sustainable relations with the minority community or offering services in schools or community facilities with easy access.

• *Work collaboratively and proactively to reduce stigma and mistrust and to engage minorities in care.* It should be anticipated at the outset that minority disaster victims, even those who have suffered intensely, will not necessarily seek professional mental health services, as they will tend to rely on families, friends, and other natural sources of help. Viewing this as an asset rather than a problem to be overcome reminds the interventionist to work collaboratively with natural helpers in the community, such as *promotoras* or paraprofessionals with experience and credibility in the community. To reduce disparities in service use, programs must build trust and be highly proactive; practitioners must get out of the clinic into the community. To the extent possible, programs should employ ethnic minority practitioners in the recruitment, retention in care, and recovery efforts. If such practitioners are scarce, they may serve the overall effort best in consultant, training, and supervisory roles. Local representatives of minority communities should be involved from the outset in preparing for and planning responses to disasters and terrorism.

• *Validate and normalize distress.* Over and over again, experienced disaster and trauma clinicians emphasize that some distress is a normal reaction to an abnormal event. But this does not mean that help cannot lessen that distress or hasten recovery. Help seeking as well as symptoms can and should be normalized. Diagnosis of pathology should be de-emphasized, relative to standard practice. Even when highly stressed, most people possess strengths they can draw on, and an important task of the clinician is to help individuals identify and mobilize their natural resources. At the same time, education regarding when dependence solely on self-reliance can be harmful to overcoming one's mental health problems or emotional distress should also be a task of disaster service providers. Self-reliance ("can handle the problem on my own") is a strong barrier to mental health care (Ortega & Alegría, 2002).

• *Value interdependence as well as independence as an appropriate goal.* As noted previously, the individual is embedded in a broader familial, interpersonal, and social context. The practitioner must spend time assessing and addressing socially relevant cognitions and emotions. The intervention goal is to enhance social functioning, helping the person retain or resume his or her social roles.

• *Promote community action.* Novel and innovative strategies should be explored that involve minority communities in their own recovery by working toward specific, achievable goals. Social marketing, advocacy, community organizing, train-the-trainer models, and mentoring programs are but a few examples that can be explored. By assuming a consultant or facilitator role, practitioners can help communities make informed choices while still recognizing that the choices are the community's own. At the same time, finding out about successful community interventions with similar communities and populations might help identify ingredients that can be used to enhance mainstream interventions.

• *Recognize that cultural competence is a process not an end-state.* Clinicians will only experience despair if they are expected to know everything that would be helpful about every culture that makes up the American whole. The importance of continuing education cannot be overstated.

• *Advocate for, facilitate, or conduct treatment and evaluation research.* There are still so few data on which to base recommendations for culturally responsive mental health care. Minorities will ultimately be better served if practitioners and researchers collaborate to test the efficacy and effectiveness of different intervention strategies.

• *Leave a legacy.* Notwithstanding the pain and stress they cause, disasters create opportunities to educate the public about trauma and mental health, to destigmatize mental health problems and mental health services, to build trust between service providers and minority communities, and to develop collaborative relationships that may serve the entire populace for years to come.

ACKNOWLEDGMENT

Preparation of this chapter was supported by Grant No. K02 MH63909 from the National Institute of Mental Health to Fran H. Norris.

REFERENCES

Alegría, M., & McGuire, T. (2003). Rethinking a universal framework in the psychiatric symptom–disorder relationship. *Journal of Health and Social Behavior, 44*(3), 257–274.

Allen, I. (1996). PTSD among African Americans. In A. Marsella, M. Friedman, E. Gerrity, & R. Scurfield (Eds.), *Ethnocultural aspects of posttraumatic stress disorder: Issues, research, and clinical applications* (pp. 209–238). Washington, DC: American Psychiatric Association Press.

American Psychiatric Association. (1987). *Diagnostic and statistical manual of mental disorders* (3rd ed., rev.). Washington, DC: Author.

American Psychiatric Association. (1994). *Diagnostic and statistical manual of mental disorders* (4th edition). Washington, DC: Author.

American Psychological Association. (1993). Guidelines for providers of psychological services to ethnic, linguistic, and culturally diverse populations. *American Psychologist, 48*, 45–48.

Blendon, R. J., Scheck, A. C., Donelan, K., Hill, C. A., Smith, M., Beatrice, D., et al.

(1995). How white and African Americans view their health and social problems: Different experiences, different expectations. *Journal of the American Medical Association, 273*(4), 341–346.

Bolton, R., & Klenow, D. (1988). Older people in disaster: A comparison of Black and White victims. *International Journal of Aging and Human Development, 26,* 29–43.

Borowsky, S., Rubenstein, L., Meredith, L., Camp, P., Jackson-Triche, M., & Wells, K. (2000). Who is at risk of nondetection of mental health problems in primary care? *Journal of General Internal Medicine, 15,* 381–388.

Bradford, L. D., & Kirlin, W. G. (1998). Polymorphism of CYP2D6 in Black populations: Implications for psychopharmacology. *International Journal of Neuropsychopharmacology, 1*(2), 173–185.

Breslau, N., Kessler, R., Chilcoat, H., Schulz, L., Davis, G., & Andreski, P. (1998). Trauma and posttraumatic stress disorder in the community: The 1996 Detroit Area Survey of Trauma. *Archives of General Psychiatry, 55,* 627–632.

Carrasquillo, O., Ovar, E. V., Brennan, T. A., & Burstin, H. R. (1999). Iimpact of language barriers on patient satisfaction in an emergency department. *Journal of General Internal Medicine, 14*(2), 82–87.

Castaneda, D. M. (1994). A research agenda for Mexican-American adolescent mental health. *Adolescence, 29*(113), 225–239.

Chen, H., Chung, H., Chen, T., Fang, L., & Chen, J.-P. (2003). The emotional distress in a community after the terrorist attack on the World Trade Center. *Community Mental Health Journal, 39,* 157–165.

Cooper-Patrick, L., Powe, N. R., Jenckes, M. W., Gonzales, J. J., Levine, D. M., & Ford, D. E. (1997). Identification of patient attitudes and preferences regarding treatment of depression. *Journal of General Internal Medicine, 12,* 431–438.

Draguns, J. (1996). Ethnocultural considerations in the treatment of PTSD: Therapy and service delivery. In A. Marsella, M. Friedman, E. Gerrity, & R. Scurfield (Eds.), *Ethnocultural aspects of PTSD: Issues, research, and clinical applications* (pp. 459–482). Washington, DC: American Psychiatric Association Press.

Felton, C. (2002). Project Liberty: A public health response to New Yorkers' mental health needs arising from the World Trade Center terrorist attacks. *Journal of Urban Health, 79,* 429–433.

Flynn, B. (1994). Mental health services in large scale disasters: An overview of the Crisis Counseling Program. *NCPTSD Clinical Quarterly, 4,* 1–4.

Galea, S., Ahern, J., Resnick, H., Kilpatrick, D., Bucuvalas, M., Gold, J., et al. (2002). Psychological sequelae of the September 11 terrorist attacks in New York City. *New England Journal of Medicine, 346,* 982–987.

Garrison, C., Bryant, E., Addy, C., Spurrier, P., Freedy, J., & Kilpatrick, D. (1995). Post-traumatic stress disorder in adolescents after Hurricane Andrew. *Journal of the American Academy of Child and Adolescent Psychiatry, 34,* 1193–1201.

Green, B., Lindy, J., Grace, M., Gleser, G., Leonard, A., Korol, M., et al. (1990). Buffalo Creek survivors in the second decade. *American Journal of Orthopsychiatry, 60,* 43–54.

Guarnaccia, P., Canino, G., Rubio-Stipec, M., & Bravo, M. (1993). The prevalence of *ataques de nervios* in the Puerto Rico disaster study. *Journal of Nervous and Mental Disease, 181,* 157–165.

Hargraves, J. L., & Hadley, J. (2003). The contribution of insurance coverage and community resources to reducing racial/ethnic disparities in access to care. *Health Services Research, 38*(3), 809–829.

Hobfoll, S. (1998). *Stress, culture, and community: The psychology and philosophy of stress.* New York: Plenum Press.

Holzer, C., & Copeland, C. (2000). Race, ethnicity, and the epidemiology of mental disorders in adults. In I. Cuéllar & F. Paniagua (Eds.), *Handbook of multicultural mental health* (pp. 341–357). San Diego, CA: Academic Press.

Hough, R., Vega, W., Valle, R., Kolody, B., Griswold del Castillo, R., & Tarke, H. (1990). The prevalence of symptoms of posttraumatic stress disorder in the aftermath of the San Ysidro massacre. *Journal of Traumatic Stress, 3,* 71–92.

Kaniasty, K., & Norris, F. (1995). In search of altruistic community: Patterns of social support mobilization following Hurricane Hugo. *American Journal of Community Psychology, 23,* 447–477.

Kaniasty, K., & Norris, F. (2000). Help-seeking comfort and the receipt of help: The roles of context and ethnicity. *American Journal of Community Psychology, 28,* 545–582.

Kaniasty, K., & Norris, F. (2004). Social support in the aftermath of disasters, catastrophes, and acts of terrorism: Altruistic, overwhelmed, uncertain, antagonistic, and patriotic communities. In R. Ursano, A. Norwood, & C. Fullerton (Eds.), *Bioterrorism: Psychological and public health interventions* (pp. 200–229). Cambridge, UK: Cambridge University Press.

Kataoka, S., Stein, B., Jaycox, L., Wong, M., Escudero, P., Tu, W., et al. (2003). A school based mental health program for traumatized Latino immigrant children. *Journal of the Academy of Child and Adolescent Psychiatry, 42,* 311–318.

Kessler, R., Berglund, P., Demler, O., Jin, R., Koretz, D., Merikangas, K. R., et al. (2003). The epidemiology of major depressive disorder: Results from the National Comorbidity Survey Replication (NCS-R). *Journal of the American Medical Association, 289*(23), 3095–3105.

Kessler, R., Somnega, A., Bromet, E., Hughes, M., & Nelson, C. (1995). Posttraumatic stress disorder in the National Comorbidity Survey. *Archives of General Psychiatry, 52,* 1048–1060.

Kinzie. J. D. (2001). Cross-cultural treatment of PTSD. In J. P. Wilson, M. J. Friedman, & J. D. Lindy (Eds.), *Treating psychological trauma and PTSD* (pp. 255–277). New York: Guilford Press.

Kirmayer, L. (1996). Confusion of the senses: Implications of ethnocultural variations in somatoform and dissociative disorders for PTSD. In A. Marsella, M. Friedman, E. Gerrity, & R. Scurfield (Eds.), *Ethnocultural aspects of posttraumatic stress disorder: Issues, research, and clinical applications* (pp. 165–182). Washington, DC: American Psychiatric Association Press.

Kirmayer, L. J., & Young, A. (1999). Culture and context in the evolutionary concept of mental disorder. *Journal of Abnormal Psychology, 108,* 446–452.

Kitayama, S., Markus, H. R., & Matsumoto, H. (1995). Culture, self, and emotion:

A cultural perspective on "self-conscious" emotions. In J. P. Tangney & K. W. Fischer (Eds.) *Self-conscious emotions: The psychology of shame, guilt, embarrassment, and pride* (pp. 439–464). New York: Guilford Press.

Koenen, K., Goodwin, R., Struening, E., Hellman, F., & Guardino, M. (2003). Posttraumatic stress disorder and treatment seeking in a national screening sample. *Journal of Traumatic Stress, 16,* 5–16.

Lindsey, M., & Cuéllar, I. (2000). Mental health assessment and treatment of African Americans: A multicultural perspective. In I. Cuéllar & F. Paniagua (Eds.), *Handbook of multicultural mental health* (pp. 195–209). San Diego, CA: Academic Press.

Lopez, S., & Guarnaccia, P. (2000). Cultural psychopathology: Uncovering the social world of mental illness. *Annual Review of Psychology, 51,* 571–598.

Manson, S. (1997). Cross-cultural and multiethnic assessment of trauma. In J. P. Wilson & T. M. Keane (Eds.), *Assessing psychological trauma and PTSD* (pp. 239–266). New York: Guilford Press.

March, J., Amaya-Jackson, L., Terry, R., & Costanzo, P. (1997). Posttraumatic symptomatology in children and adolescents after an industrial fire. *Journal of the American Academy of Child and Adolescent Psychiatry, 36,* 1080–1088.

Markus, H., & Kitayama, S. (1994). The cultural construction of self and emotion: Implications for social behavior. In S. Kitayama & H. Markus (Eds.), *Emotion and culture: Empirical studies of mutual influence* (pp. 89–130). Washington, DC: American Psychological Association.

Melfi, C. A., Croghan, T. W., Hanna, M. P., & Robinson, R. L. (2000). Racial variation in antidepressant treatment in a Medicaid population. *Journal of Clinical Psychiatry, 61*(1), 16–21.

Miranda, J., & Cooper, L. (2002). *Disparities in care for depression among primary care patients.* Unpublished manuscript.

Nader, K., Dubrow, N., & Stamm, B. (1999). *Honoring differences: Cultural issues in the treatment of trauma and loss.* Philadelphia: Brunner/Mazel.

New York State Office of Mental Health. (1997). *Crisis counseling guide to children and families in disasters.* Retrieved January 10, 2004, from www.omh.state.ny.us/omhweb/crisis/crisiscounseling.html

Norris, F. (1992). Epidemiology of trauma: Frequency and impact of different potentially traumatic events on different demographic groups. *Journal of Consulting and Clinical Psychology, 60,* 409–418.

Norris, F., Donahue, S., Felton, C., Watson, P., & Hamblen, J. (2004). *Making and monitoring referrals to clinical treatment: A psychometric analysis of Project Liberty's Adult Enhanced Services Referral Tool.* Manuscript under review.

Norris, F. H., Foster, J. D., & Weisshaar, D. L. (2002). The epidemiology of sex differences in PTSD across developmental, societal, and research contexts. In R. Kimerling, P. Ouimette, & J. Wolfe (Eds.), *Gender and PTSD* (pp. 3–42). New York: Guilford Press.

Norris, F., Friedman, M., Watson, P., Byrne, C., Diaz, E., & Kaniasty, K. (2002). 60,000 disaster victims speak, Part I: An empirical review of the empirical literature, 1981—2001. *Psychiatry, 65,* 207–239.

Norris, F., Kaniasty, K., Inman, G., Conrad, L, & Murphy, A. (2002). Placing age differences in cultural context: A comparison of the effects of age on PTSD after disasters in the U.S., Mexico, and Poland. *Journal of Clinical Gero-psychology* [Special issue], *8,* 153–173.

Norris, F., Murphy, A., Baker, C., & Perilla, J. (2003). Severity, timing, and duration of reactions to trauma in the population: An example from Mexico. *Biological Psychiatry, 53,* 769–778.

Norris, F., Murphy, A., Baker, C., Perilla, J., Gutierrez-Rodriguez, F., & Gutierrez-Rodriguez, J. (2003). Epidemiology of trauma and posttraumatic stress disorder in Mexico. *Journal of Abnormal Psychology, 112,* 646–656.

Norris, F., Perilla, J., Ibañez G., & Murphy, A. (2001). Sex differences in symptoms of post-traumatic stress: Does culture play a role? *Journal of Traumatic Stress, 14,* 7–28.

Norris, F., Weisshaar, D., Kirk, L., Diaz, E., Murphy, A., & Ibañez, G. (2001). A qualitative analysis of PTSD symptoms among Mexican victims of disaster. *Journal of Traumatic Stress, 14,* 741–756.

Ortega, A., & Alegría, M. (2002). Self-reliance, mental health, need and the use of mental health care among Island Puerto Ricans. *Mental Health Services Research, 4,* 131–140.

Ortega, A., & Rosenheck R. (2000). Posttraumatic stress disorder among Hispanic Vietnam veterans. *American Journal of Psychiatry, 157,* 615–619.

Osofsky, J. D. (1997). Community-based approaches to violence prevention. *Journal of Developmental and Behavioral Pediatrics, 18*(6), 405–407.

Palinkas, L., Downs, M., Petterson, J., & Russell, J. (1993). Social, cultural, and psychological impacts of the Exxon Valdez oil spill. *Human Organization, 52,* 1–13.

Parson, E. R. (1997). Postraumatic child therapy (P-TCT): Assessment of treatment factors in clinical work with inner-city children exposed to community violence. *Journal of Interpersonal Violence, 12,* 172–194.

Perilla, J., Norris, F., & Lavizzo, E. (2002). Ethnicity, culture, and disaster response: Identifying and explaining ethnic differences in PTSD six months after Hurricane Andrew. *Journal of Social and Clinical Psychology, 21,* 28–45.

Pynoos, R. S., Frederick, C., Nader, K., Arroyo, W., Steinberg, A., Eth, S., et al. (1987). Life threat and posttraumatic stress in school-age children. *Archives of General Psychiatry, 44*(12), 1057–1063.

Segel, S. P., Bola, J. R., & Watson, M. A. (1996). Race, quality of care, and antipsychotic prescribing practices in psychiatric emergency services. *Psychiatric Services, 47,* 282–286.

Siegel, C., Davis-Chambers, E., Haugland, G., Bank, R., Aponte, C., & McCombs, H. (2000). Performance measures of cultural competency in mental health organizations. *Administration, Policy, and Mental Health, 28*(2), 91–106.

Solomon, S. (2003). Introduction. In B. L. Green, M. J. Friedman, J. T. V. M. De Jong, S. D. Solomon, T. M. Keane, J. A. Fairbank, et al. (Eds.), *Trauma interventions in war and peace: Prevention, practice, and policy* (pp. 3–16). New York: Kluwer/Plenum Press.

Solomon, S., & Canino, G. (1990). The appropriateness of DSM-IIIR criteria for post-traumatic stress disorder. *Comprehensive Psychiatry, 31,* 227–237.

Somasundarum, D., Norris, F., Asukai, N., & Murthy, R. (2003). In B. L. Green,

M. J. Friedman, J. T. V. M. De Jong, S. D. Solomon, T. M. Keane, J. A. Fairbank, et al. (Eds.), *Trauma interventions in war and peace: Prevention, practice, and policy* (pp. 291–318). New York: Kluwer/Plenum Press.

Srinivasan, S., & Guillermo, T. (2000). Toward improved health: disaggregating Asian American and Native Hawaiian/Pacific Islander data. *American Journal of Public Health, 90*(11), 1731–1734.

Sue, S. (1998). In search of cultural competence in psychotherapy and counseling. *American Psychologist, 53*, 440–448.

Sue, S., Fujino, D., Hu, L., & Takeuchi, D. (1991). Community mental health services for ethnic minority groups: A test of the cultural responsiveness hypothesis. *Journal of Consulting and Clinical Psychology, 59*, 533–540.

Takeuchi, D., Chung, R., Lin, K., Shen, H., Kuraski, K., Chung, C., et al. (1998). Lifetime and twelve-month prevalence rates of major depressive episodes and dysthymis among Chinese Americans in Los Angeles. *American Journal of Psychiatry, 155*, 1407–1414.

Takeuchi, D., & Uehara, E. (1996). Ethnic minority mental health services: Current research and future conceptual directions. In B. L. Levin & J. Petrila (Eds.), *Mental health services: A public health perspective* (pp. 63–80). New York: Oxford University Press.

Thiel de Bocanegra, H., & Brickman, E. (2004). Mental health impact of the World Trade Center attacks on displaced Chinese workers. *Journal of Traumatic Stress, 17*, 55–62.

U.S. Department of Health and Human Services. (2001). *Mental health: Culture, race, and ethnicity—A supplement to Mental health: A report of the Surgeon General.* Rockville, MD: U.S. Department of Health and Human Services, Public Health Service, Office of the Surgeon General.

Vega, W. (1992). Theoretical and pragmatic implications of cultural diversity for community research. *American Journal of Community Psychology, 20*, 375–392.

Vega, W., & Alegría, M. (2001). Latino mental health and treatment in the United States. In M. Aguirre-Molina, C. Molina, & R. Zambrana (Eds.), *Health issues in the Latino community* (pp. 179–208). San Francisco: Jossey-Bass.

Vega, W., Kolody, B., Aguilar-Gaxiola, S., Alderette, E., Catalano, R., & Caraveo-Anduaga, J. (1998). Lifetime prevalence of DSM-III-R psychiatric disorders among urban and rural Mexican Americans in California. *Archives of General Psychiatry, 55*, 771–778.

Vera, M., Vila, D., & Alegría, M. (2003). Cognitive-behavioral therapy: Concepts, issues, and strategies for practice with racial/ethnic minorities. In G. Bernal, J. Trimble, A. Berlew, & F. Leong (Eds.), *Handbook of racial and ethnic minority psychology* (pp. 1–18). Thousand Oaks, CA: Sage.

Wang, P., Bergland, P., & Kessler, R. (2000). Recent care of common mental disorders in the United States. *Journal of General Internal Medicine, 15*, 284–292.

Webster, R., McDonald, R., Lewin, T., & Carr, V. (1995). Effects of a natural disaster on immigrants and host population. *Journal of Nervous and Mental Disease, 183*, 390–397.

Weine, S., Raina, D., Zhubi, M., Delesi, M., Huseni, D, Feetham, S., et al. (2003). The TAFES Multi-Family Group Intervention for Kosovar refugees: A feasibility study. *Journal of Nervous and Mental Disease, 191,* 100–107.

Williams, J. W. J., Rost, K., Dietrich, A. J., Ciotti, M. C., Zyzanski, S. J., & Cornell, J. (1999). Primary care physicians' approach to depressive disorders: Effects of physician specialty and practice structure. *Archives of Family Medicine, 8,* 58–67.

Young, A., Klap, R., Shebourne, C., & Wells, K. (2001). The quality of care for depression and anxiety disorders in the United States. *Archives of General Psychiatry, 58,* 55–61.

Zheng, Y., Lin, K., Takeuchi, D., Kurasaki, K., Wang, Y., & Cheung, F. (1997). An epidemiologic study of neurasthenia in Chinese-Americans in Los Angeles. *Comprehensive Psychiatry, 38,* 249–259.

Zoellner, L., Feeny, N., Fitzgibbons, L., & Foa, E. (1999). Response of American and Caucasian women to cognitive behavioral therapy for PTSD. *Behavior Therapy, 30,* 581–595.

CHAPTER 18

Toward Understanding and Creating Systems of Postdisaster Care

A Case Study of New York's Response to the World Trade Center Disaster

FRAN H. NORRIS, JESSICA L. HAMBLEN, PATRICIA J. WATSON,
JOSEF I. RUZEK, LAURA E. GIBSON, BETTY J. PFEFFERBAUM,
JENNIFER L. PRICE, SUSAN P. STEVENS, BRUCE H. YOUNG,
and MATTHEW J. FRIEDMAN

The terrorist attacks of September 11, 2001, generated acute and ongoing concerns regarding the capacity of federal, state, and local mental health systems to address the psychological consequences of terrorism. It has become increasingly recognized that disasters, especially those involving mass casualties, have various adverse effects on mental health that necessitate the provision of crisis intervention services to survivors of these events (Norris et al., 2002). Disaster mental health services thus have emerged as an integral component of federal and local emergency management (Flynn, 1994).

The response to the attacks of New York's mental health system was multifaceted, with Project Liberty, a federally funded crisis counseling program, at its heart. Federal disaster areas are eligible for a wide range of services, including the Crisis Counseling Assistance and Training Program. Funded by the Federal Emergency Management Agency (FEMA) and administered by the Center for Mental Health Services (CMHS), the crisis counseling program (CCP) is designed to address short-term mental health needs of communities affected by disasters through public education, outreach, and crisis counseling. Because the CCP was designed primarily for natural disasters, it was not clear how well its guidelines would match the needs of New York. Our case study was conducted to learn lessons from New York's experience that could be useful to other communities that must respond to major disasters and terrorism. The purpose was not to evaluate the impact or effectiveness of Project Liberty but rather to document the challenges it faced.

The impact of postdisaster services rests not only on their clinical efficacy but also on the capacity of the system to deliver those services in an appropriate way. Hodgkinson and Stewart (1998, pp. 95–96) outlined a set of service characteristics that serve as useful criteria for process evaluation of disaster mental health services. These criteria relate to maximizing the reach of a program to those in need of it, regardless of the program's content or underlying rationale. These characteristics include *credibility* (the service must be seen by survivors as offering something that will be of use), *acceptability* (help must be offered in a way that does not demean the survivor), *accessibility* (help must be offered in the heart of the affected community), *proactivity* (the service must reach out to those most affected), *continuance* (the service must be present for a sufficient period to meet the need), and *confidentiality* (survivors must believe that their privacy is assured). In a previous case study of the Oklahoma City bombing (Norris, Watson, Hamblen, & Pfefferbaum, 2005), participating providers agreed that the proposed characteristics were valuable goals for service delivery in disaster stricken settings.

Figure 18.1 illustrates the conceptual framework for the project. Disaster mental health systems are inherently complex because they *are mesosystems,* (i.e., networks of other systems). Disaster mental health systems, such as Project Liberty, are imposed upon *host systems* that have preexisting missions and vary in their preparedness, their trauma expertise, and the extent to which they are disrupted by the focal event. Both New York State's Office of Mental Health (NYS OMH) and New York City's Department of Mental Health (NYC DMH) were host systems, yielding a remarkable level of complexity. Host systems are both assisted and constrained by the federal system of emergency management and CCP guidelines. In addition to the host system(s), the new system is composed of a variety of *microsystems* (i.e., participating agencies, clinics, and hospitals that provide direct services). There were over 100 of these in New York. These organizations vary in their centrality to the overall mission, linkages and competition with one another, and fit between their orientations and disaster mental health principles. Turf boundaries, poor interagency linkages, communication gaps, confusion, and ambivalence regarding outsiders

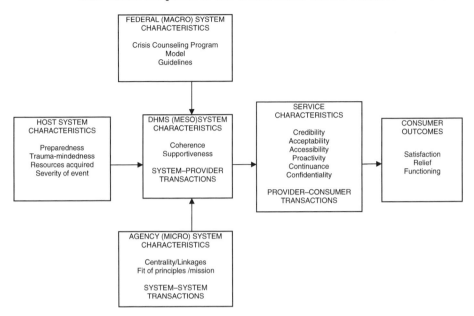

FIGURE 18.1. Conceptual framework.

have been identified previously as issues that interfere with service delivery and add to the stressfulness of disaster work (Allen, 1993; American Psychological Association, 1997; Bowenkamp, 2000; Call & Pfefferbaum, 1999; Canterbury & Yule, 1999; Gillespie & Murty, 1994; Lanou, 1993; Myers, 1994; Norris et al., 2005; Sitterle & Gurwich, 1998; Young, Ruzek, & Gusman, 1999). We began our work with the assumption that providers who function within coherent and supportive systems will deliver services that are perceived to be credible, acceptable, accessible, and proactive, thereby maximizing the reach of the program to those in need.

METHODS

Ninety-seven individuals were interviewed in person between January and March 2003. In December 2003, 11 participants were reinterviewed and 5 new participants were interviewed about the enhanced services initiative, which had not been implemented at the time the original interviews were conducted, and the phasedown of Project Liberty. Participants are classified as *leaders* (*n* = 21; primarily NYC DMH or NYS OMH), *directors* (*n* = 51; persons who often provided direct services but had broader administrative responsibilities), and *providers* (*n* = 31; individuals who provided direct services). In all, 103 participants from 50 agencies were interviewed. Interviews were audiotaped and transcribed, producing 3,010 pages of transcribed text.

Data analysis proceeded through several phases. *Data* refer to the verbatim transcriptions, *findings* to consensually agreed-on paraphrases or summaries of the data, and *conclusions* to investigator interpretations of the findings. Within each participant type, research assistants "chunked" the transcripts into broad topics (e.g., Leadership Roles/Actions). Within each topic, two to four investigators worked together to paraphrase comments, identify themes, and capture quotes that represented the themes well. The findings were organized into six broad categories: *Preparing for Disaster, Responding to the Crisis, Managing a Coordinated Long-Term Response, Training the Workers, Caring for the Providers, and Serving the Consumers*. Findings were shared and discussed with CMHS staff and Project Liberty leadership; their additional comments are attributed to *reviewers*. Findings were then analyzed collaboratively to yield conclusions and recommendations.

PREPARING FOR DISASTER

Summary of Findings

Various features helped New York City and New York State to be as prepared as any city and state could have been for a disaster of the magnitude of 9/11. The state had organized an incident command system and prepared its facilities to manage the transition to the year 2000 and more generally to respond to disasters. In New York City, mental health was "at the table" from the beginning of the response because the head of the NYC DMH was a psychiatrist who worked closely with the mayor to provide messages about mental health. New York City also had a crisis intervention unit in place, and the city had learned from several previous, smaller-scale disasters. LifeNet, a hotline and referral source that had relationships with government and service providers, was perhaps the "single most important asset in the response."

Despite these assets, New York was not adequately prepared for September 11. Statewide, the mental health system was underfunded, understaffed, geared toward the seriously mentally ill, and inexperienced in terms of prevention and outreach work. The educational system and mental health system were isolated from one another. Most important, the sheer magnitude of the event overwhelmed all systems. "The problem was scale. There was infrastructure; there just wasn't enough infrastructure."

Many provider organizations felt reasonably well prepared because they had a disaster response team, large infrastructure, or collaborative relationships with schools, their community, or the Red Cross. Agencies that responded quickly were more likely to view themselves as having been prepared (an interpretation that we would not make). However, providers often were unprepared for the community work and levels of stress and vicarious trauma they would experience.

Recommendations were plentiful. Participants viewed advanced planning and preexisting infrastructure as essential and commented on the necessity of having mental health professionals involved in the planning of the overall response. Planning itself requires education and coordination. As one director remarked, "We've been inundated with disaster planning with little education about how to do it." Another stated, "There are now too many planning groups. . . . We need one table rather than 10 splinter tables making different plans."

Specific comments about components of preparedness plans could be organized into four themes. *Program design* includes issues regarding the development and maintenance of infrastructure and technical assistance for creating staffing and service delivery plans. One leader remarked, "I don't even need the answers, just tell me the questions. I'll figure out the answers 'cause the answers are going to look different wherever you are." Planning is a complex process as plans must vary across locations, levels of government, and types of events. *Communication* includes the need for systems, such as LifeNet, and materials that make it easier to deliver messages to the public. *Information* resources include written and online materials, trained personnel, and knowledge of effective interventions. *Coordination, collaboration, networks, and partnerships* were mentioned by participants over and over again as essential aspects of preparedness.

Conclusions and Recommendations

- *At the federal level, policies, sufficient funding, and information resources must be generated and disseminated without delay to support state preparedness and eliminate deficiencies exposed by the September 11 attack.* Most states would find it difficult to prepare without federal guidance and support. After 9/11, federal support was provided to states to improve their preparedness, and it is essential that this support continue at adequate levels. In addition to providing preparedness funding, the federal government should ensure that states have easy access to current information on disaster effects, risk communication strategies, evidence-based interventions and best practices, and lessons learned from previous disaster responses.
- *At the state level, preparedness plans should address multiple levels of the response across relevant jurisdictions. It is essential for this plan to include mechanisms for communicating with the general public and providers.* At minimum, each state should have a full-time disaster coordinator.

Additional research should be conducted to identify the specific features of LifeNet that were helpful for New York.

• *Collaborative relationships and understandings must be formed in advance.* Most critical are relationships between mental health, public health, primary care, first responders, emergency management, schools, and various community-based agencies. Plans should identify the leadership hierarchy, specific roles, and linkages. School involvement is critical. Organizations should work together to avoid the creation of separate, uncoordinated preparedness plans. Collaboration in the planning process will foster collaboration during and after an incident. It would be helpful to develop contracts between state authorities and provider agencies that could be activated quickly in the event of a disaster.

RESPONDING TO THE CRISIS

Summary of Findings

Although the initial response to the crisis was highly stressful, the chaos turned fairly quickly into a coordinated response. The acute mental health response involved a variety of organizations, including but not limited to the Red Cross, Fire/Police Departments, and the New York City Crisis Intervention Unit. Rapid recognition and use of LifeNet and establishment of the Family Assistance Center had a very positive impact in the immediate aftermath of the attacks. Thousands of state and local clinicians were made available to the effort by governmental and nongovernmental organizations. Establishing control of the response was complicated by the rush of individuals wanting to assist. Comments were made about "wacko," "inappropriate," or "bizarre" groups showing up to work at Ground Zero without regulation in the early days. Legitimate volunteers often lacked clear guidance about what to do. Participants generally recognized the need for credentialing and supervision of volunteers.

It is a natural, understandable, and appropriately empowering phenomenon that local people feel ownership of and responsibility for disasters that occur in their communities. "Insider–outsider dynamics" emerged in New York at multiple levels of the crisis response. Tensions between the values of knowing disaster work and knowing the city were evident. Resentment of outsiders was manifest in comments regarding perceived differences between the New York experience of terrorism and the experience of communities that have experienced natural disasters.

Several directors and leaders noted that they were approached by many self-proclaimed experts who wanted to provide consultation in the aftermath of 9/11. Agency directors observed that a lot of money and time was spent with "experts" who did not ultimately prove to be useful or knowledgeable. Directors and leaders noted that it would have been helpful to have a system for identifying legitimate experts.

Early responses to the crisis embedded psychological first aid into concrete services and support. Mental health services ranged from "just being present" to more formalized interventions. There were ongoing uncertainties and controversies about whether or not debriefing was an appropriate intervention. Individual agencies experienced difficulty in locating easily digestible information.

Almost immediately, leaders began working on the federal grant application that would fund the longer-term CCP, Project Liberty. In daily meetings of senior management, a framework was developed that, in the words of one leader, "included the notion of tiers but also embraced that this model is for everybody." They had to modify the CMHS needs assessment formula substantially. In the end, they estimated that 3.1 million people in New York were affected by 9/11, 2 million of whom were children. It was a challenge to develop the Immediate Services Program grant application in the midst of the crisis, but the application was nonetheless submitted on time. Lack of familiarity with the program, a compelling need to respond to the ongoing crisis, and a reduction in staff accessibility due to the crisis itself made the work all the more difficult.

Conclusions and Recommendations

• *The operational plan for an acute response should identify local leadership, specify the command structure, define roles for local and national leadership, and develop linkages between the crisis team and familiar community-based agencies and organizations.* To decrease the initial chaos, plans need to be made in advance specifying who would be responsible for specific tasks. Local leaders should be in charge because they are the recognized leaders of their community, and the responsibilities and demands of leadership require continuity. Conflicts between "insiders" and "outsiders" could be reduced by having more clearly defined roles and responsibilities. Another key operational component is coordinating and regulating volunteers. Professionals who would work on site should be organized, trained, and credentialed before an incident. Better systems for identifying and selecting volunteer mental health workers are required. Supervision is needed on site.

• *Policies and guidelines must be derived that address programmatic components of an acute response so as to provide appropriate, effective, and evidence-based care for disaster victims.* Such policies could be described as incorporating "musts" and "mays," as the goal is to provide guidance while also encouraging local innovations. Experienced disaster workers generally believe that emphasis should be placed on the provision of basic support and assistance in providing essential resources, rather than on providing structured mental health interventions. While professionals should be available for victims who have severe reactions, the majority of individuals appear to need basic human comfort, kindness, and practical support in the immediate aftermath of disaster. Thus, overall, there is need for an appropriate blend of informal support (just being there, warmth, acceptance of emotions) and more structured acute interventions (medical screening, provision of medication, individual/group counseling) that address the needs of both children and adults.

• *Launching of programs for meeting victims' longer-term needs must be planned for as integral to the local acute response, and ample personnel and resources must be allocated to this component of the plan.* Project Liberty leadership recommended that states develop preapproved grant applications for federal crisis counseling funds that could be modified according to the size and scope of the disaster. This would prevent state agencies from having to start from scratch during a time of crisis. Best-practices guidelines should be distributed to state leaders in advance and again immediately postcrisis.

• *National efforts should focus on generating policies, disseminating practice guidelines, providing high-quality information resources to state and local governments and organizations, and coordinating national-level expertise.* Certainly, national experts should be called on to develop the aforementioned consensual guidelines and policies for meeting acute needs in the aftermath of terrorism, building on previous efforts (e.g., National Institute of Mental Health, 2002). National efforts can take several additional forms that share the common goal of making credible, accurate information resources readily available and accessible. It is important to develop a national clearinghouse that includes model grant applications, needs assessment materials, information about what services can and cannot be covered, training materials, and materials for the delivery of formal community educational presentations. Access to credible experts could be similarly organized by a trusted national source.

MANAGING A LONG-TERM COORDINATED MENTAL HEALTH RESPONSE

Summary of Findings

The magnitude of the September 11 attacks created the need for a large and effective administrative infrastructure, one of unprecedented size for a CCP. Leadership advised future programs to "take enough time in the beginning getting an administrative structure together so that it could run for the duration without having to be constantly tinkered with and expanded."

Leadership expressed a strong need for more technical assistance from the federal government with regard to fiscal and administrative issues. A leader recommended that CMHS develop a "flexible formula for estimating the administrative and staffing needs of the programs, with advice about how to scale up and scale down." On the other hand, one reviewer expressed skepticism that *a priori* anticipation of circumstances could match actual circumstances to provide a meaningful set of guidelines.

Staff shortages, especially in the beginning, created significant challenges for leaders and directors. In fact, this was often mentioned by participants as among the biggest challenges they faced. Many participants mentioned needing staff to assist with administrative aspects of the program. Like leadership, directors recommended the creation of mechanisms that would make staffing and hiring easier, such as websites for resumes and job descriptions.

The complexity and scope of the program generated difficult choices between alternative payment systems. For the Immediate Services Program in New York City, Project Liberty initially employed a fee-for-service model, in which eligible organizations were reimbursed for direct services performed, because there was not time to negotiate the 100+ contracts involved in service delivery. Later, with the transition to the Regular Services Program, Project Liberty switched to a "cost-based" model, in which agencies were paid agreed-on amounts for an agreed-on number of services that were to be provided. The service goals were set at a level believed by leadership to allow for planning, supervision, and training time. It was possible to include direct administrative costs in the contracts, but it appeared that some agencies did not understand this. The different systems posed different challenges for agency directors and providers: delays in reimbursements in the fee-for-service system, service levels in the cost-based system. Although the system was set up to provide financial support for a range of activities beyond direct service, many agency directors reported that the demand to "meet quotas" was so high that it was difficult to allow for trainings and additional supervision. Providers believed that service-level requirements harmed quality of care, fueled competition, and adversely affected morale.

Directors also had much to say about unallowable costs. Lack of funding for food or space caused problems for many. Lack of indirect funding for administrative costs created stress for many participating organizations (e.g., "You can't just finance direct costs *and* ask agencies to do all this. Either finance indirect costs or do these things centrally"). Issues such as these were mentioned very often by directors as the primary challenges of the work—far more often than were clinical issues.

Relative to previous CCPs, Project Liberty took tremendous steps forward in evaluation and quality management. The evaluation had several components, including encounter log data, a telephone survey, and several smaller initiatives. Local government units had to develop explicit quality management plans, as guided by a template created by leadership. Leadership also developed a site-visit protocol that covered operations, training, supervision, outreach, needs assessment, and the use of encounter logs. The sheer volume of data made it difficult to provide timely feedback to the agencies. Directors and providers complained often and loudly about the paperwork—a point that went hand in hand with the aforementioned complaints about lack of funding for administrative costs.

Decision making and control were ongoing challenges. According to many respondents, the primary issue was centralization of decision making and accompanying slowness. Directors wanted more control over their own programs and often complained about having to get approvals and the amount of time it took to get them. For the system as a whole, such concerns have to be balanced with retaining coherence and consistency across various settings. The New York City schools fought vigorously (but unsuccessfully) to have FEMA money allocated directly to them so that they could design their own response. Predictably, power struggles between the city and state emerged, although their relationship was also characterized as a "superb partnership."

Communication—the accurate transmission of information—was viewed as critical for the system as a whole. Leadership disseminated ideas from one agency to another. "It's like being Johnny Appleseed," one leader explained. Many directors described their communications with leadership as generally good. Some providers pointed to the regular meetings as examples of good communication. However, many others described program information and guidelines as confusing and constantly changing. A reviewer argued that it was absolutely not the case that rules were in flux. The comments may represent misunderstandings of the rules or evolving understandings of rules. These disagreements illustrate the natural challenges for communication in complex systems involving multiple levels.

One important system of communication was LifeNet, which served as one entry point into services and, for providers, was a resource for information on other services available in the community. LifeNet attempted to create a "seamless presentation of services and benefits," maximizing use of both charitable and federal dollars. Before 9/11 LifeNet handled about 3,000 calls per month. At approximately 16 months postdisaster, it was handling 6,000 to 7,000 calls per month. Calls peaked around the first anniversary at 12,000 calls in September 2002. The challenges for LifeNet were the types of calls (meaning the intensity and irritability of some callers) and the ever-changing resource map. Although there were a few complaints, many participants described it as one of the most essential and effective features of New York's mental health response.

Participants provided more examples of collaboration than of competition. Several participants commented on the general lack of "turf" issues among Project Liberty subcontractors. The problems that did arise were attributed to communication failures, lack of knowledge about one another, or competition to serve the same population or area. A few participants believed that cooperation decreased over time. Despite the inherent challenges, there were several extraordinary examples of collaboration throughout New York. The United Services Group and its September 11 fund and the New York Consortium for Effective Trauma Treatment stand out among the other various collaborative efforts in New York.

Conclusions and Recommendations

• *CMHS needs to increase its capacity to provide technical assistance with regard to administrative issues, including staffing, fiscal management, and decision-making structures.* The administrative structure of CCPs should be put in place immediately to avoid continuing changes in staff and organizational structures. A flexible formula for estimating the administrative needs of programs would be helpful. Decision making should either be less centralized, with program directors given more power to make decisions, or there should be more people in positions of power to reduce "bottlenecks."

In complex systems, control, communication, collaboration, quality management, and responsiveness almost inevitably emerge as challenges, and indeed these were prominent themes for the functioning of Project Liberty. The challenges can often be conceptualized as competing goods and trade-offs (e.g., program consistency vs. flexibility and sound evaluation efforts vs. increased administrative burden). Our recommendations recognize the complexities of achieving such balances in large-scale initiatives.

• *Building on Project Liberty's innovations, the federal government should designate evaluation and quality management activities as essential to the operation of CCPs, meaning that more effort is needed to (1) provide useful tools and strategies to leadership from the outset, (2) increase provider "buy-in," and (3) give participating agencies the administrative and financial support they need to do the work.* Evaluation is necessary for accountability, but approaches should avoid excessive paperwork, allow timely feedback to administrators, and inform ongoing program design and development.

• *Leadership needs to give providers consistent, specific guidance on allowable crisis counseling activities including clear explanations of where program flexibility is allowed. Timely answers and adequate lead time are important qualities of communication.* Providers wanted both more clarity and more flexibility, and both are necessary in balance. Especially after highly traumatic events, there may be confusion concerning where to draw the line between crisis counseling and more traditional mental health services.

• *State and local governments should promote collaborations among key stakeholders, including but not limited to those between mental health authorities and school systems.* Collaboration and linkages are essential elements of an effective mental health response to disaster. A search for model programs illustrating collaborations between schools and mental health systems should be undertaken to identify exemplary practices.

TRAINING THE WORKERS

Summary of Findings

Following the events of September 11, trainings were offered by several established organizations, such as the American Red Cross, FEMA/CMHS, the Mental Health Association, and Disaster Psychiatry Outreach, as well as by newly established organizations, such as Project Liberty, the New York Consortium for Effective Trauma Treatment, and the 9/11 Fund. Many directors and providers were not satisfied with the training they received. In interpreting this point, the diversity of training sources should be kept in mind. It was not usually possible for the authors to discern the particular training being referenced by the participant. Concerns included logistical issues, such as when and where the trainings were offered, as well as the quality of the trainings. Many providers viewed the majority of trainings as too basic, but Project Liberty reviewers noted that advanced trainings were not as well attended as basic, mandated trainings. Generally, paraprofessionals were more positive about the trainings than were professionals. Leadership believed that the trainings were true to what crisis counseling is and that what clinicians really objected to was not the training but the scope of practice. The FEMA/CMHS training was criticized by many as inadequately tailored to New York's context. (We revisit this point in a subsequent section.)

A variety of recommendations for training emerged. A leader remarked, "Training does more than teach needed skills; it provides clinicians with the confidence they need to handle potentially new and difficult clinical situations. Training is two parts reassurance, one part information." There was a general desire for the trainings to be run by people who had actual experience in responding to disasters and to incorporate hands-on examples, drills, and scripts. Sequencing trainings so that they begin with foundations and then become more specialized was recommended as well. Trainers should recognize that the people being trained may have themselves been affected by the disaster; acute emotions can interfere with trainees' understanding or acceptance of materials.

Conclusions and Recommendations

• *CMHS should develop a complete curriculum for disaster mental health that (1) covers both foundations and advanced topics, (2) incorporates scripts and simulations, and (3) can be adapted to the local context depending on the type and magnitude of the event.* Curricula must anticipate various types of disasters, consequences, settings, and providers. Different programs or sequences may be needed for paraprofessionals and licensed clinicians because of their different skills. Incorporation of scripts, scenarios, and various simulation exercises is advised. The potential topics are wide ranging, including foundations of crisis counseling and outreach, specific clinical issues, evidence-based interventions, special populations, and compassion fatigue.

• *State and local authorities need to attend carefully to the logistics of training programs offered after disasters.* Trainings should be held in convenient locations and provided in a timely manner. It should be clear to providers whether attendance is mandatory or optional. Trainings should be coordinated for consistency of message across trainers and sessions. They should be small enough to allow for interaction between trainer and trainees. Trainings should be offered by experts who have responded to disasters.

• *To assist local communities in coordinating trainings and selecting qualified trainers, a national system for credentialing trainers should be created.* Disaster-stricken settings are often besieged by self-proclaimed, and sometime self-serving, experts seeking entrée to offer training in specific clinical approaches. A resource that can help local people to identify good trainers and evaluate training proposals could be helpful.

CARING FOR THE PROVIDER

Summary of Findings

The work was stressful. Several participants experienced minor physical ailments. A provider observed, "Sleep was the universal problem." The stress arose from various sources, including providers' personal experiences and reactions to the event and ongoing stress in the environment, as well as work-related factors. Vicarious trauma from listening to horrible stories was commonly reported. One provider recalled, "It doesn't get easier. It really doesn't get easier. Stories are sadder, the stories are more intense, people aren't bouncing back, people are amazing that they have endured and survived so long. But usually when we're done it takes a toll absolutely. It's very stressful."

Organizational and program factors, such as hours, workload, staff tensions, and uncertain funding, added further to the stress. Many providers mentioned working long hours, including nights and weekends, which caused difficulties at home. Directors noted that quotas and uncertain funding were stressful for staff: "This whole drive for numbers, our energy is being exhausted running after the numbers, you don't get a lot of time to sit down and process what's going on." Another said, "I think some of the stress is the uncertainty about the funding and whether the project would continue." Tension emerged between people in the organization who did 9/11 work and the people who did other trauma work, because 9/11 workers had more resources. Working in the community raised unusual challenges. One provider reported, "When I go to the firehouse it's extremely stressful. It's different from clinic work, where there's a parameter around the session, and you plan ahead for a certain amount of time. It is stressful and I'm always cognizant of trying to make them comfortable and not being intrusive. This is their house."

Participants also described positive effects of their work. It was intense but rewarding and satisfying. Providers enjoyed making a difference and helping others, and one individual claimed that it was "by far the best work I've ever done." Another provider said that the focus on educating others about stress management and coping really provided a wealth of personal skills.

There was general consensus that formal, imposed stress management strategies are critical to the well-being of providers because mental health professionals tend to impose high standards on themselves. Self-care was often neglected because of the perceived needs of other people. Numerous examples of formal strategies emerged in New York, including group discussions, training, and support for complementary interventions such as writing, yoga, and massage. The importance of regular, ongoing, one-on-one supervision was highlighted by many providers. Overall, providers reported excellent support from their coworkers, supervisors, and program managers. Staff also implemented informal ways of supporting each other.

Conclusions and Recommendations

• *Mechanisms for provider supervision, support, and care should be incorporated into the disaster response structure, plan, and budget.* It should not be left to individual workers themselves to organize their own self-care. Plans should include arrangements for providers to support and learn from each other and to receive ongoing supervision and independent support. Emotional support should be recognized as an activity separate from case supervision and may best be provided by someone external to the organization. Organizations should strive to create compassionate work environments. Plans for caring for providers should be a required part of the application for federal crisis counseling funds.

- *Training programs should incorporate modules on self-care, compassion fatigue, and related concerns.* For direct service providers, such training would convey institutional support for setting boundaries, maintaining healthy habits and lifestyles, and cultivating relationships. For directors, it would provide guidance on options for scheduling, supervision, and best practices.

SERVING THE CONSUMER

Summary of Findings

Comments on services addressed a variety of issues ranging from the overall appropriateness of the crisis counseling model to service characteristics to the overall effectiveness of services provided. Participants identified numerous strengths of the CCP model. Most important, the model makes sense from a public health perspective because, in the words of participants, "it gets the word out" and "provides a low-level intervention for many people." The outreach component is critical because people who need help often do not seek it. Some providers initially resisted outreach but were subsequently convinced of its value. One director remarked, "One of the best things about Project Liberty is the message that it is okay to feel upset." Another said Project Liberty provided a "real opportunity to acknowledge the public education role of mental health authorities, e.g., concern for wellness, for entire range of the mental health continuum."

These strengths notwithstanding, participants expressed numerous concerns about the fit of the model for terrorism and an event of this magnitude. Participants often (correctly) concluded that the model was formulated for natural disasters, disasters that have clear beginnings and ends and seldom involve mass casualties in the United States. A related point, but one not necessarily confined to terrorist-caused disasters, was the appropriateness of the model for persons who were most severely affected or impaired. One director reported, "We have learned that a substantial minority of people would continue to experience stress even after receiving our services." Various miscellaneous limitations of the model were also raised. That the model allows for neither case management nor case finding was criticized by some. The model fits neither individuals nor communities that have many predisaster problems. Project Liberty's innovative response to many of these concerns was to advocate for the inclusion of "enhanced services" within the broader crisis counseling model. This was a new conceptual model that, in the words of one participant, is "attempting to fill the gap between those who need 1–2 crisis counseling contacts and the seriously mentally ill."

"Selling the model" was one of the most significant challenges faced by leadership, and, initially, it was a large part of the work. It was new to providers, "a different way of thinking about mental health work," as one leader said. Some in leadership positions observed that the model was less difficult to grasp for social workers and grassroots organizations. Altogether, leaders believed they had experienced some success at forging a new culture.

Whereas participants often criticized the "model," they resonated with the desired characteristics of disaster mental health work. *Credibility* was achieved by drawing on preexisting reputations, using the Project Liberty name, relying on professional credentials, fostering collaborative styles, and having a persistent presence in the community. Very few participants raised concerns about credibility, a notable difference between these findings and those from Oklahoma City (Norris et al., 2005).

Acceptability was achieved by offering services that were nontraditional and nonpathologizing. Destigmatizing mental health care appeared to be a notable strength of Project Liberty. Providers validated and normalized feelings and experiences, conveyed a genuine respect for diversity, and incorporated personal strengths into the work. A few providers expressed concern that normalizing responses might delay some people whose responses are not normal from seeking help, saying, "It's very important to normalize help-seeking behavior in tandem with normalizing reactions." Another provider observed, "What differentiates a normal reaction from a more serious one is whether it is interfering with functioning—to work or care for family."

Accessibility was achieved by the overall geographic dispersion of services across the system as well as by individual providers' efforts to make services available in a variety of settings, including schools, workplaces, malls, and homes. Providers "offered to go wherever people wanted us." Organizations worked evening and weekend hours or even "24/7."

Many participants commented on why *proactivity* is essential for disaster services. As one leader explained in a training session, "We know from previous disasters that people who are really suffering aren't going to come to your clinic. People may not recognize that their feelings are due to the disaster. You must get out of the clinic into the community." Nonetheless, sometimes directors and providers had to learn this lesson for themselves. One provider told us, "Everyone thought we were gonna have waiting lines of people to come in for counseling and we had almost nobody." A director noted, "We had a walk-in crisis counseling office for awhile, but it wasn't used as much as you would think. FEMA was very accurate to take the focus away from traditional mental health work, because most folks would not respond. We maybe saw 10–12 people in clinics." Still another noted, "We decided to establish a drop-in center for anybody who was scared and wanted to talk. Some people responded but not in the large numbers that we thought. 'So,' we said, 'we need to go to them.' " Another provider said that outreach was "very important because the worst of the worst are absolutely the ones who won't show up in the system." System-wide, proactivity was achieved by contracting with niche agencies to reach out to specific populations, employing indigenous workers, and effective use of media, as well as by individual providers' efforts to go everywhere to deliver the message.

Confidentiality was achieved by not keeping records and by adhering to professional standards of behavior. However, not keeping records was a problem for some providers. Psychiatrists, for example, were concerned about liability.

Of the various characteristics included in our framework as essential for disaster mental health, *continuance* was alone in eliciting concern, as the general view was that Project Liberty was not going to run as long as was needed to meet New York's mental health needs. Moreover, it was a challenge to adapt the program to changing community needs. Many providers emphasized the need to focus on the most seriously distressed in the latter phases of the project: "The 15-minute session at the supermarket—I don't see a huge need for that anymore." When they go out into the community they hear, "No we're fine, that happened a long time ago." More people are saying, "We're saturated, we've had enough; it's over." As a provider expressed, "Where do you go after that?... We need to find new ways to market our services."

Enhanced services refers specifically to an extension of the federal CCP that allowed New York to provide more intensive services than are usually permissible. Enhanced services were authorized by CMHS in August 2002 but not implemented until May 2003. Two cognitive-behavioral interventions were developed for adults, one generally targeted at postdisaster distress and one specifically targeted at traumatic grief. Four modules were developed for children on depression, anxiety, trauma, and behavior problems. A culturally sensitive psychoeducational intervention was also developed.

Participants reported dissatisfaction with the process and timing of the implementation of the new services. The good collaboration between state and city leaders was challenged, as city leaders reportedly felt left out of the planning process. Comments such as enhanced services "got started way too late," "should have been running within the first year," and "were needed 18 months ago" were frequent. That enhanced services started at the same time regular services were phasing down generated problems and misunderstandings. One leader said, "The program was not well coordinated. The State identified agencies to be enhanced service providers that the City was eliminating as part of their phase down process." The timing led some to believe (incorrectly) that regular services were phased down because of enhanced services, although the two processes were actually independent.

Despite implementation problems and delays, everyone seemed to agree that the enhanced services initiative was a good idea and that the interventions themselves were generally of high quality. Although many providers were initially apprehensive about using a manualized intervention, most reported that they liked the structure it provided. For the adult program, a referral tool was developed that was found to have good reliability and predictive validity. However, many fewer adults participated in the enhanced services program than qualified for it. Some participants commented that crisis counselors may not be making referrals either because clients are "too attached" to their counselors or because counselors do not want to "give up" their clients.

With few exceptions, participants were adamant that they had made a difference in people's lives. Leadership pointed to the successful branding of Project Liberty, the overall reach and responsiveness of the program, and the legacy of public mental health, especially its focus on outreach. Directors and providers shared numerous anecdotes and stories about lives that were changed. Limitations to effectiveness were also voiced. Most comments concerning limitations expressed concerns for certain populations believed to have been served less well than others, especially youth, immigrants, and Arab Americans. Many participants also believed that CCPs need to do more to build community resiliency by fostering natural supports in communities.

Conclusions and Recommendations

- *The service characteristics of credibility, acceptability, accessibility, proactivity, continuance, and confidentiality should be adopted as valuable goals for service delivery in disaster-stricken settings.* The extent to which these characteristics were perceived by providers to have been achieved was among the most impressive findings in this case study. If we were correct in proposing that such characteristics provide a window into the functioning of the entire system, then Project Liberty functioned exceedingly well. Applications for federal funding should address how they will be achieved by drawing on these documented practices as appropriate for their populations and context.

- *Progress toward more rigorous evaluation of crisis counseling programs must be continued by developing tools and strategies, mandating such activities, and funding them.* Despite New York's important efforts, participants still relied largely on anecdotal evidence to support their claims of program effectiveness. This state of affairs is highly inconsistent with the current zeitgeist that emphasizes evidence-based practices.

- *Mechanisms for ongoing community-based needs assessments should be incorporated into disaster programs, and funding for these provided by the federal government.* Leadership, program directors, and service providers work with little knowledge about the evolution of needs in their community. It is interesting to contrast the increasingly frequent reports from residents that "we're over it" to providers' beliefs that the program was not going to last long enough. Data are needed to plan and deliver services that match the distribution, severity, and duration of impairment in disaster-stricken settings.

- *The capacity of disaster programs to meet the needs of children and culturally different populations must be enhanced by (1) involving the schools, persons with appropriate expertise, and representatives of various communities in all phases of the response, including preparedness planning efforts, and (2) creating strong linkages between specialized and general service providers.* Children composed 2 of the 3 million persons targeted for services according to New York's needs assessment, yet working with schools and the school system posed an ongoing challenge. Participation of ethnic minorities and other populations with special needs should be increased.

- *The federal CCP model must be revised to match the contemporary context of terrorism by providing a continuum of care, ranging from recovery initiatives for the community at large to enhanced services for the minority of victims who are most adversely affected.* Issues of balance and timing are critical ones in redefining a continuum of care to encompass both broad community efforts and targeted clinical efforts.

- *At least on a trial basis, enhanced services should become a well-integrated and well-timed part of the overall package of services.* Despite many implementation problems, the enhanced services initiative was a significant advancement and an innovative effort to meet community-defined needs. The psychometrically sound referral tools, evidenced-informed interventions, and piloted evaluation strategies developed by and for Project Liberty make it possible for future programs to implement enhanced services in a manner that is integrated into the system and coherent to providers. These services should supplement, not supplant, regular services.

CONCLUDING REMARKS

Guided by a systems perspective on disaster mental health, we sought to learn lessons from New York's experience that could be useful to other communities that must respond to major disasters and terrorism. In discussing those lessons, we need to acknowledge the limitations of our study. We elicited only the perspectives of providers, and it will be critical for the voice of consumers to be heard before definitive recommendations can be made. There are no data that unquestionably establish whether or not the services offered matched consumers' needs or helped them. Perspectives were embedded in one state's experience and may not generalize. Our case study was both enhanced and limited by its qualitative methodology and its focus on process as opposed to outcome. Whereas standards for practice in this field ideally would rest on scientifically sound evidence of effectiveness, at present such data are not easily attainable because of various political, ethical, and practical constraints. In the absence of higher levels of evidence, conclusions regarding best practices legitimately rest on opinions of respected authorities, clinical experience, and descriptive accounts (Foa, Keane, & Friedman, 2000).

Viewed holistically, New York's response to the September 11 terrorist attacks was nothing short of remarkable. Despite the inherent challenges in responding to an event of this magnitude, despite whatever complaints and misunderstandings arose, despite the need for many to adapt to a different way of doing mental health work, most of these providers viewed themselves as having been well supported and described the services they delivered in the most positive of terms. Project Liberty delivered the services it intended to deliver and achieved its broad goals for public health.

Many elements of New York's response to the attacks were impressive and other communities would do well to emulate them—the early involvement of mental health; the strong communication infrastructure; the rapid evolution from frenzy to structure; the vision of what it means to do public mental health work; the serious attempt to evaluate services; the incredible collaborations; the number and diversity of training opportunities; the universal recognition of the need to support providers; the efforts to destigmatize mental health care; the creativity of outreach efforts; and the innovative enhanced services initiative, which may serve to redefine crisis counseling as we know it.

These accomplishments notwithstanding, there are strong needs nationally for improved preparedness, volunteer and expert credentialing, management strategies, program evaluation and needs assessment, training curricula, information resources, knowledge dissemination, community involvement, and models of care. It will take a sustained national commitment of unprecedented proportions to make a substantial difference in the state of the art. It will require collaboration between institutions that do not usually collaborate. It will require the courage to make mistakes and an ongoing commitment to evaluation and research.

The September 11 terrorist attacks challenged—and changed—the field of disaster mental health in untold ways. Those of us who had the privilege of observing New York's response from the outside must pause to recognize the dedication of the mental health professionals and paraprofessionals who were called on to serve on behalf of us all. We trust that the issues raised in this chapter will be attributed to the magnitude and complexities of the challenges they faced rather than to shortcomings of any of the actors involved. Indeed, this case study would not have been possible without the collaboration and candor of Project Liberty leadership, CMHS staff, and the various organizations that opened their doors to us despite numerous competing demands on their time. The attacks exposed numerous deficiencies in the system, but they also showed how willing we, as a people, are to commit human and financial resources to helping those who suffer the most, to do the best job we can under extremely trying circumstances, and to learn from our mistakes. There is reason in this for optimism.

ACKNOWLEDGMENTS

This work was funded through an interagency agreement between the Substance Abuse and Mental Health Services Administration/Center for Mental Health Services and the National Center for PTSD and by Grant No. K02 MH63909 to Fran H. Norris from the National Institute of Mental Health. Appreciation is extended to Melissa Hiller, Nancy Bernardy, Shira Maguen, and Madelyn Miller for their assistance in conducting the interviews; to Dan Almeida and Sherry Wilcox for coordinating the fieldwork and travel; and to Sheila Donahue, Chip Felton, April Naturale, and Trish Marsik of Project Liberty for their help in planning and sample selection.

REFERENCES

Allen, R. (1993). Organizing mental health services following a disaster: A community systems perspective. Handbook of post-disaster interventions [Special issue]. *Journal of Social Behavior and Personality, 8*, 179–188.

American Psychological Association. (1997). *Task force on the mental health response to the Oklahoma City bombing*. Washington, DC: Author.

Bowenkamp, C. (2000). Coordination of mental health and community agencies in disaster. *International Journal of Emergency Mental Health, 2*, 159–165.

Call, J., & Pfefferbaum, B. (1999). Lessons from the first two years of Project Heartland, Oklahoma's mental health response to the 1995 bombing. *Psychiatric Services, 50*, 953–955.

Canterbury, R., & Yule, W. (1999). Planning a psychosocial response to a disaster. In W. Yule (Ed.), *Post-traumatic stress disorders: Concepts and therapy* (pp. 285–296). New York: Wiley.

Flynn, B. (1994). Mental health services in large scale disasters: An overview of the Crisis Counseling Program. *NCP Clinical Quarterly, 4*, 1–4.

Foa, E. B., Keane, T. M., & Friedman, M. J. (2000). Introduction. In E. B. Foa, T.

M. Keane, & M. J. Friedman (Eds.), *Effective treatments for PTSD: Practice guidelines from the International Society for Traumatic Stress Studies* (pp. 1–17). New York: Guilford Press.

Gillespie, D., & Murty, S. (1994). Cracks in a postdisaster service delivery network. *American Journal of Community Psychology, 22,* 639–660.

Hodgkinson, P., & Stewart, M. (1998). *Coping with catastrophe: A handbook of post-disaster psychosocial aftercare* (2nd ed.). London: Routledge.

Lanou, F. (1993). Coordinating private and public mental health resources in a disaster. Handbook of post-disaster interventions [Special issue]. *Journal of Social Behavior and Personality, 8,* 255–260.

Myers, D. (1994). Psychological recovery from disaster: Key concepts for delivery of mental health services. *NCPTSD Clinical Quarterly, 4,* 1–7.

National Institute of Mental Health. (2002). *Mental health and mass violence: Evidence based early psychological intervention for victims/survivors of mass violence: A workshop to reach consensus on best practices* (NIH Publication No. 02-5138). Washington, DC: U.S. Government Printing Office.

Norris, F., Friedman, M., Watson, P., Byrne, C., Diaz, E., & Kaniasty, K. (2002). 60,000 disaster victims speak, Part I: An empirical review of the empirical literature, 1981–2001. *Psychiatry, 65,* 207–239.

Norris, F., Watson, P., Hamblen, J., & Pfefferbaum, B. (2005). Provider perspectives on disaster mental health services in Oklahoma City. In Y. Danieli & D. Brom (Eds.), *The trauma of terror: Sharing knowledge and shared care* (pp. 649–662). New York: Haworth Press.

Sitterle, K., & Gurwich, R. (1998). The terrorist bombing in Oklahoma City. In E. Zinner & M. Williams (Eds.), *When a community weeps: Case studies in group survivorship* (pp. 161–189). Philadelphia: Brunner/Mazel.

Young, B., Ruzek, J., & Gusman, F. (1999). Disaster mental health: Current status and future directions. *New Directions for Mental Health Services, 82,* 53–56.

Outreach Strategies

An Experiential Description of the Outreach Methodologies Used in the September 11, 2001, Disaster Response in New York

APRIL J. NATURALE

HISTORICAL BACKGROUND

The concept of outreach has its roots in early social services work conducted by such pioneers as Jane Addams, who founded Hull House in Chicago in 1889. Addams and her colleagues brought social services to various immigrant groups by establishing settlement houses within their neighborhoods. The reach of the staff was then expanded into the local places of worship and recreational areas throughout the city (University of Illinois at Chicago, n.d.).

In the 1930s during the New Deal era, President Franklin Roosevelt introduced the social welfare policies that allowed assistance to vulnerable populations, such as the poor, the disabled, and the elderly, which are still in force today. Outreach became the modality through which to deliver these social services and was actually conducted by the First Lady of that time, Eleanor Roosevelt, who visited the homes of poor families when their pride prohibited them from asking for assistance (Lash, 1971).

This governmental financial support developed as an outgrowth of the functionalist social systems theory, with the goal of ensuring stability within communities by protecting individuals (Gilbert, Specht, & Terrell, 1993). While the receipt of federal aid by the poor, the disabled, and the elderly has became more socially acceptable, pride is often still a deterrent to accepting services, particularly for those in some ethnic and cultural groups who view public assistance as a disgrace or failure.

Emergency and disaster mental health services, though, have a continuous history of being delivered in the community. While this is primarily due to the nature of the disasters, pervasive stigma and a lack of understanding of mental health counseling contribute significantly. Organizations such as the American Red Cross (ARC), which was founded in 1881, first focused on delivering first aid, water, and public health nursing to the armed forces and their families and then expanded its mission to include emotional care and support to disaster victims and their survivors after World War II (American Red Cross, n.d.). ARC assisted in the development of the arm of the federal government that serves to respond to federally declared disaster areas, the Federal Emergency Management Agency (FEMA).

FEMA's Crisis Counseling Assistance and Training Program, which is available to state mental health authorities once an area has been declared a disaster by the President, as authorized under the Robert T. Stafford Disaster Relief and Emergency Assistance Act (Public Law 93-288, as amended by (Public Law 100-707), is founded on the concept of outreach (Center for Mental Health Services, 2001). In keeping with the goal of ensuring the eventual restabilization of the community, crisis counseling delivered in an outreach modality after a disaster attempts to mitigate the development of serious emotional disorders such as posttraumatic stress, anxiety, and depression.

There is no empirical literature that guides the use of outreach strategies in a disaster situation. While a small body of studies exists that looks at outreach outcomes in health care settings around utilization of services, smoking cessation programs, screening programs, and treatment compliance (McFall, Malte, Fontana, & Rosenheck, 2000), these studies examine unique circumstances, none of which may be generalizable to a disaster. Many disaster research studies focus on the development of mental disorders such as posttraumatic stress, but none addresses the mode of service delivery. The nature of disasters does not easily afford an opportunity to conduct random controlled trials and there is some concern about conducting research with direct victims, family members, and others traumatized by disruptive events. Evidence-based and evidence-informed research is necessary to further support the current understanding of best practices in both the clinical outcomes and the success of outreach strategies in this area.

DEFINING AND DEVELOPING
OUTREACH STRATEGIES

The Urban Experience

A challenge in the disaster mental health response in New York after 9/11 was to define outreach and crisis counseling, operationalizing both the modality and the intervention. In a psychoanalytic and psychodynamic mental health delivery system such as the one that exists in Manhattan and several other large cities throughout the nation, outreach was relatively unknown as a mode of service delivery. The mental health community of New York seemed to have a picture of outreach (going door to door on "cold" calls) as applicable only to small, rural communities in Middle America. Some agencies working with people who are homeless or physically ill understood outreach, but they were in the minority.

In the immediate response, support services happened everywhere in the community and family assistance centers were rapidly set up at various sites, offering a continuum of disaster-related assistance. Once the grant funds were received and the contracting process was implemented, service provision at agency sites became the norm, primarily due to the requirement by the city that contracted agencies had to be licensed mental health clinics. As the agencies received FEMA training and technical assistance later in the program, they moved to embracing the practice of outreach.

If crisis counseling continues to be the model for the nation's disaster mental health response, it may be helpful as part of planning efforts to include discussions of how to frame the concept of outreach to the administrative public mental health and academic communities. Community building and partnering may be structured differently in larger cities to include more formal meetings and subcontracting rather than the informality usually seen in small communities, but they can still be accomplished using the basic outreach efforts conducted in prior disasters. These include one-to-one, face-to-face, personal contacts where disaster response managers and outreach staff make an attempt to engage key members of the community in planning how to address the needs of those affected (Young, Ford, Ruzek, Friedman, & Guzman, 1998).

Suburban and Rural Areas

The more rural and suburban areas of the counties in upstate New York had less difficulty with the idea of outreach and more easily accepted the recommendation that disaster response staff include a mix of professionals, paraprofessionals, and non–mental health workers indigenous to their communities. This was partly due to the lack of available professional mental health counselors in some areas but also due to the general acceptance in rural areas that everyone has something to offer and all who are able to assist are respected for what they bring to the effort.

The upstate county administrators provided solid support for the disaster relief project, encouraging the use of messaging on billboards located on major roadways and advertisements in movie theaters, in community newspapers, and on local radio spots. In Long Island and Staten Island, where there were extensive losses of rescue and recovery personnel and where several providers were well versed in disaster response due to their previous experiences with airplane disasters, outreach was operationalized rapidly. In many of the suburban counties, creative outreach staff who quickly identified the rescue, recovery, and construction workers' favorite hangouts started advertising the disaster response program on bar coasters and posting the program information in restrooms at local pubs. Diner placemat ads were also a successful route to getting people's attention as they sat waiting for their meals.

The counties that housed large numbers of military personnel and their families reported high levels of disaster anxiety responses that were being compounded by the possibility of family members going off to war. Military personnel indicated that they received debriefings as necessary from their respective units and refused any assistance from civilian outreach workers. Interventions with their families through family support groups and schools became the most successful routes to working with these populations.

Low-Socioeconomic versus High-Income Areas

The state mental health authority used the FEMA needs assessment formula to determine the grant allocation for each county. But the size and scope of the 9/11 disaster made it quite difficult to determine if each socioeconomic area received more or fewer services because of need or due to any of the following variables: the number of contracted providers that chose to participate in the program; how aggressively each agency implemented outreach; a higher allocation of dollars due to an area's high-risk designation; and how much the local community's altruism circumvented their need for federal funds.

Initial data reports from New York City indicated that the highest-income areas were the least penetrated by the outreach staff. The assumptions derived from these reports include the following: people in higher-income brackets may feel more stigmatized by the need to access mental health support and avoid doing so; people who could afford to would access private rather than public mental health support (which was found to be true of many children in the Ground Zero schools); and people who lived in high-income areas of the city were accessing services outside their residential area. The final analysis of the program's data collection may help to determine what variables may have most significantly influenced the penetration into various economic areas.

The General Population

Awareness of the various groups that reside within the boundaries of a particular community is a first step in planning outreach strategies. Outreach staff may easily overlook closed communities, populations that attract little attention to themselves and groups that may be invisible due to hidden bias (Lum, 2000). At key points in New York State's disaster response, the coordinator for outreach and special populations compared the percentages of different ethnic groups identified by the current census to the number of contacts documented in data collection reports. The subsequent penetration rates were shared with the local program directors to assist them in targeting areas that emerged as uncovered. This information also suggested the ethnicity of the outreach staff that would likely be successful in engaging those in the identified areas via mutual cultural and ethnic backgrounds.

Broad-Scale Public Media Campaign

As with any new program, marketing is an important outreach methodology that can accomplish the goal of letting the community know that services have been established. It is important to brand the disaster response program and normalize disaster distress responses. Marketing can provide the community with a sense of security knowing there is help available and it can legitimize outreach staff who are on the streets and might otherwise be perceived as suspicious characters.

Television, radio, and print media are primary sources of communication utilized throughout the country and are effective outreach tools. In the World Trade Center attacks in New York, a 30-second television commercial was developed within weeks of the disaster that identified the mental health response program. Within 2 months of the event a telephone survey reported that 25% of New Yorkers knew of the disaster mental health response program, and of those 25%, 70% knew of the program through the television commercial (Galea et al., 2002).

The commercials created to address the first-year anniversary prompted responses indicating that the culturally diverse and age specific images were highly effective. The utilization of well-known actors attracted the public's attention as they reported responding directly to the instruction to call the program (e.g., "Alan Alda told me to call"). It is recommended to avoid using controversial public figures whose presence may counteract the intent of delivering a benign message of assistance.

Brochures providing basic information about common disaster distress responses and simple coping techniques are a valuable outreach tool for individuals who more easily absorb information in print, especially if they have seen the program title in places they perceive as reliable sources of information. Brochures can eliminate human contact, which may be important for those who are not ready to engage directly, or whose defenses are weaved tightly.

General marketing techniques should be employed in the development of educational materials. In the federally funded crisis counseling program in New York, highlighting that services were "free" and "confidential" was especially important. The program's publicized affiliation with FEMA legitimized the service for many as FEMA is nationally recognized as the disaster response agency available to help. Over 20 million brochures in 10 different languages addressing resources, coping skills, and talking to children were distributed in total. The primary brochure was even added to *The New York Times* as an insert during the week of the first anniversary.

The advertising of a central hotline number in additional to geographic specific contact information is a good backup for smaller community service agencies that may not have the staffing to cover a 24/7 service. Telephones answered live are most effective in engaging callers, but recorded messages that address the disaster response program by name and give time frames within which phone calls will be returned have been reported to successfully invite callers to leave callback information.

As in all culturally competent outreach efforts, language diversity is as important in the written material as it is in the human contacts. Assuming that individuals of various ethnic and cultural backgrounds can speak, comprehend, and read the primary language of the area is an error that can undermine any disaster response outreach efforts. Brochures need to be translated into common usage languages in the affected communities. This is where disaster preparedness is key as translation is usually very time-consuming. Utilizing the available general disaster-related materials that have already been translated and adding brief, customized messages and symbols appropriate to a particular culture can save valuable material development time.

Web-based outreach was a new modality with which to deliver disaster mental services, and concerns had to be addressed in the New York experience by dealing with problems as they arose. The goal of the website was to provide information and referral, but significant numbers of affected individuals emailed the disaster response program communicating a need for an immediate crisis counseling response.

Web-based services are similar to telephone services, but there is even less of an opportunity to establish a human connection to the individual out in cyberspace. Telephone counseling can allow for a certain level of auditory observation of emotional intensity, but email relies solely on what the individual chooses to write. Outreach workers utilizing this type of engagement should be trained in how to convey a human quality to their writing and how to accurately reflect their responses through the written language, leaving minimal space for assumed understanding or misinterpretations. Many individuals who accessed the 9/11 disaster mental health response website for support were those who were extremely concerned about confidentiality. This was especially true of the rescue and recovery workers, who feared they would lose their jobs if they expressed any type of disaster distress symptoms. Thus, offering Web crisis counseling may be a successful way to engage those who otherwise would not accept such support.

Cultural Competence

The definition of cultural competence has evolved to encompass the concepts of knowledge, values, behaviors, attitudes, respect and the ability to provide services addressing all of these (Substance Abuse and Mental Health Services Administration [SAMHSA], 2003). Stamm and Friedman (2000) indicate that culture does not have a universally accepted definition. What becomes evident in a disaster is that culture takes on the broad description that is inclusive of ethnicities, professions, businesses, organizations, individual schools and neighborhoods, community groups, religious groups, age groups, and so on.

There is no one formula that dictates exactly how to work with various ethnic groups, cultures, or organizational structures. One key to successful outreach is to partner with knowledgeable members of the particular culture, group, or organization so they may act as cultural brokers in opening communication doors. It is vital to the effort that they are bilingual where needed and, ideally, bicultural as well (SAMHSA, 2003). They should be willing to share the unspoken rituals, routines, and rules of the membership. Many such individuals are often leaders of some kind, formally, socially, or politically. They may be in managerial positions in some business but are still perceived as peers. They may be coworkers who have leadership skills that are informally acknowledged by the group and they may be the best people to suggest how to engage the population in crisis counseling.

Cultural competency also requires that staff become aware of the economic, social, and historical problems as they work with community leaders to elicit information on the culture and values of a particular group (Lum, 2000). Although this topic was addressed more fully in a previous chapter, we discuss brief examples in the following sections, addressing high-risk groups, ethnic cultures, and closed communities.

High-Risk and Special Populations

The identification of high-risk populations in a disaster should be based on the type of disaster, the scope, each population's relationship to the disaster, and the demographic composition of the community. Known high-risk populations in a catastrophic disaster include the families of victims, physically injured, evacuees, rescue and recovery workers, children, individuals with a prior history of trauma, those in a low socioeconomic status, immigrant groups, and some adults in the middle and older age ranges (Norris, Byrne, & Diaz, 2001; Norris, Phifer, & Kaniasty, 1994; Young, 2002). In addition, people who suffer with major mental illnesses and other disabilities that may increase their vulnerability have the potential to develop posttraumatic stress disorder (Jankowski & Hamblen, 2001). Persons who fall within one or more of the identified high-risk categories may develop more severe disaster distress responses based on their comorbidity. Outreach staff needs to be open to the possibility that individuals may have more than one context affecting their ability to recover from the current loss or disaster experience. Staff must explore each separately as well as in combination.

Directly Impacted Groups and Family Members

The most clearly identified groups in need of emotional support after a disaster (e.g., the injured and their loved ones and families of the deceased) may be somewhat more receptive to supportive counseling, but outreach approaches to each of these groups must still be sensitive to the vulnerable position in which these individuals find themselves. People coping with trauma and loss have emotional responses of differing types at time frames that are their own rather than at predetermined periods and this must be respected. Those suffering with significant physical losses or the death of a loved one as a result of a terrorist attack may experience significant distress for several years or longer (Solomon & Green, 1992). It is not unusual that people who experience a common, significant physical trauma or loss often form a tight bond very quickly and intensely. Many of the families of victims of disasters naturally come together to console one another and share emotions as well as information. This type of bonding, peer support, and self-help can be encouraged and reinforced by staff. Mental health professionals who are well versed in crisis intervention and supporting the grieving process are most appropriate in working with this population.

The Adult and Elderly Populations

Some in the elderly population may be at high risk after a disaster and others may be a resource. Studies indicate that the middle-age group responsible for child care, aging parents, and nuclear-family economic support may be more stressed in a disaster situation than some elderly, but certainly older adults who are physically restricted from accessing support services are at higher risk of developing problems that, if left unaddressed, may become more severe (Green & Solomon, 1995; Norris et al., 1994).

Primary care physicians, who currently provide over 70% of treatment for mental disorders in this age group are most likely to have contact with the elderly population, making outreach to geriatricians, internists, and general practice physicians a good first point of contact. Questions asked in the course of a routine physical assessment that explore for common disaster distress reactions such as sleeplessness; anxiety symptoms such as hypervigilance, or depressive symptoms such as changes in appetite and listlessness, as well as symptom exacerbation of current illnesses, may assist in identifying those suffering with disaster-related distress (Center for Mental Health Services, 1995).

Outreach in the medical arena may include having mental health staff in waiting areas, in consultation rooms, and in emergency rooms available for discussion and leaving disaster-related brochures. Crisis workers may accompany Meals-on-Wheels and visiting nurse services as outreach to the elderly. In one of New York's upstate counties, this was the only point of contact with some reclusive or physically frail community members. Skilled nursing facilities and senior centers were another successful point of contact as residents and their family members were quite accustomed to visitors bringing useful information.

Seriously and Persistently Mentally Ill Persons

Crisis counseling services are not meant to take the place of formal mental health treatment already being provided to persons with serious and persistent mental illnesses, people with a history of substance abuse, and people who have suffered from some type of prior trauma. Due to their history, such populations may be at risk for developing an exacerbation of symptoms or destabilization impeding their ability to function well. Mental health recipients also have a high possibility of having experienced the trauma of some type of abuse, the distress of institutionalization, and/or social stigmatization (McFarlane & Piveral, 1996), further increasing their risk status. If included in outreach efforts, these individuals may be able to maintain the emotional stability and functional abilities achieved prior to the disaster event.

The clinical guidelines set up during the 9/11 disaster indicated that these individuals would need to have their preexisting conditions stabilized sufficiently to allow them to benefit from crisis counseling, including continuing with the level of treatment that would assist in keeping their prior condition(s) stable and continued participation in any ancillary services that supported the stabilization of their preexisting condition(s) such as Alcoholics Anonymous or Narcotics Anonymous meetings. Recipients of mental health services were educated to the concerns that the disaster may add to the stress of their current struggles to stay well, and the importance of maintaining existing physician relationships and compliance with routine treatment was stressed.

A peer training was designed to address the specific needs of this population. The peer outreach workers addressed the concerns of recipients, arranging for them to spend time talking on the phone without tying up the disaster hotline by setting up "warm lines." This helped reduce the fear of being stigmatized or hospitalized due to their discussion of symptoms. An important concern for the recipient community is that peers must know when it is necessary to refer a recipient of mental health services to his or her psychiatrist or psychotherapist as serious setbacks or psychosis can require a long recovery period. For many who rely on pharmacological interventions to keep their mental illness under control, it is suggested that they consider temporary medication adjustments during times of known or anticipated stress (McFarlane & Piveral, 1996). Staff must be trained to identify counterproductive or overlapping service delivery and assurance of referring to the appropriate levels of care in a timely manner.

Ethnic Cultures

The Immigrant Population

Many individuals who have migrated to areas outside their country of origin have done so to escape poor economic conditions, war, torture, and other life-threatening events. Entering a country without speaking the primary language and leaving family and other supports behind undoubtedly creates a sense of loss and vulnerability (Lum, 2000). Such circumstances, previous trauma, and even the perception that there is a lack of social support can increase the distress responses of individuals affected by a disaster (Kaniasty & Norris, 1995). Many immigrants, especially those who are undocumented fall into this high-risk category. In the early days following 9/11, much of the diversity of the American citizenship dissipated and communities across the country were suddenly one against the terrorists. At the same time the search for the terrorists brought fear as many individuals were held for questioning. Such activities can exacerbate the group paranoia and create more fear and trauma in an already traumatized group, population, or community.

The Asian / Pacific Islander Community

At the time of the World Trade Center attacks, the Asian/Pacific Islander community closest to Ground Zero, Chinatown, encompassed many subcultures speaking various dialects of Chinese, Mandarin, and Cantonese. People were remaining indoors to insulate themselves from the stark physical reminders of the attacks, the lights and grinding sounds of the recovery effort, and the pervasive odor of continuous fires and burned remains that assailed their senses 24 hours a day. A large community center near Ground Zero became a rest area for rescue and recovery workers in addition to having its "front yard" used to store vehicles destroyed in the collapse of the towers. This made their exposure level high over a long period of time. It was clear that outreach efforts would have to be made by multilingual, culturally sensitive staff hired from within the area.

Once it was discovered that the community held a deep fear that the outreach workers were not who they appeared to be, the outreach staff began to wear clearly identifying hats and shirts with imprinted messages in native tongues. The staff avoided the stigmatization of mental health services simply by referencing the local community center and the "branded" project, which was being advertised on the local Chinese television and radio.

Outreach was also very active at the local health care clinic where physicians were reporting some of the most typical disaster distress symptoms, such as sleeplessness and stomachaches. Staff at the clinic and the community center taught the outreach workers that most Asian/Pacific Islander cultures have no word for "trauma"—that the concept does not even exist, as we understand it in English. In this culture, adaptation is expected to occur immediately and individuals who are unable to cope with "life" are seen as weak and an embarrassment to their families. One individual receiving crisis counseling spent long periods of time in the meetings crying with grief over the loss of a loved one. After several meetings the individual reported to the outreach worker the need to stop the meeting for fear of being shunned if this was discovered by family.

The disaster mental health hotline had an Asian line that was answered by a multilingual staff. All the disaster brochures were translated with the main message normalizing the individual's disaster distress responses, highlighting the physical symptoms, and referring to "stress" as a generally accepted term for the problems.

Outreach to the Asian/Pacific Islander community was also provided through services to school-age children as parents more readily supported the disaster relief efforts after the association between distress relief and achievement was introduced. Over time, open conversations about the effects of the attack on this community in particular were led in the faith-based temples, where many were gathering.

The Hispanic American Population

In contrast to the Asian/Pacific Islander culture, many Latino communities came together immediately after the World Trade Center attacks and the American Airlines plane crash that occurred 2 months later, to support each other. The Dominican community in particular suffered significant losses in both these disasters. Families of victims needed to grieve and to retell their stories often. Disaster relief staff were invited to be with the family groups, and several staff members were overcome with emotion in a number of the groups. After verbalizing the staff's concern about being intrusive and disturbing the privacy of individuals who were visibly overwrought with emotion throughout the visits, one of the leaders explained that the staff's presence was vitally important. He indicated that if we did not listen, emote, and share a meal with the group, we would not be seen as sincere in our concern and support. Being together encouraged both the processing of pain and the movement toward recovery.

The outreach staff who were bilingual and from local neighborhoods of the community centers recognized that they needed mental health professionals to assist with the grieving families. They reached out to the local academic and hospital staffs with whom they had preexisting relationships and received training in running trauma-focused, family psychoeducation groups.

All the media around the disaster mental health response programs in the Latino communities included Spanish-language print ads and brochures as well as radio and television commercials. Both male and female figures and voices were used in an attempt to address the gender-related issues so strongly ingrained in the culture. Many comments from this community referenced the identification with the female, mother-like voice or the male's gentle, apparent strength. These layered supports helped create stronger bonds among community members who seemed to know they would need to stay close to each other to get through pain of their overwhelming grief.

The African American Population

In working with many communities of African Americans throughout New York, the most successful outreach strategies centered on activities with the faith-based organizations. Leaders of local churches and faith-based groups were able to gather large neighborhood groups together where outreach workers joined with them to provide crisis counseling services. In many areas, the faith-based leaders themselves became the outreach staff and delivered public education and counseling within their respective areas. These leaders were also influential in paving the way for family members to be receptive to disaster response services that were being delivered to children in schools. The outreach staff and school staff encouraged the children to have a voice, to gain positive recognition, and to take advantage of outlets that taught channeling of emotion in constructive ways like participating in music, art and drama projects.

Leaders in certain boroughs such as the Bronx taught outreach staffs that the World Trade Center attacks were seen as just another event for many in their communities, as their children were growing up in a culture dominated by violence; and they described lying awake at night listening to shooting. The staff were taught the reality that simple coping techniques were not appropriate in groups in which people were dealing with these survival skills. The outreach staff elicited ideas from the leadership in the community as to the most appropriate ways to engage the members of various neighborhoods and schools. Together they developed public education groups for families, in which they discussed the need to learn coping and self-care in the form of negotiation skills, conciliation skills, anger management, and the importance of modeling and boundaries.

One of the largest providers of disaster response services in New York City had their outreach staff use the "person on the street" methodology. They approached passers-by in an effort to engage them in brief psychoeducational contacts or crisis counseling and referral where appropriate. Staff wore identifying tags and made themselves very public to attract attention to the well-publicized mental health response program while they asked questions and distributed educational brochures. This modality was very well received in many areas and allowed the outreach to this population to soar.

The Native American Community

Disaster relief staff need to allow various groups to be heard in their own voices. This is particularly true of populations that bring a history of having their concerns ignored or invalidated. Staff must remain open and ensure that the issues to be addressed will come from the community itself rather than from a prescribed approach. One way of doing this is for the outreach staff to participate in ritual group activities and discuss with the leaders which rituals can be used in what situations. Based on the particular incident, determinations can be made regarding which rituals could be altered and which should be replaced with new ones developed by the group.

The prior traumatic experiences of this community was of major consideration in working with many members after the 9/11 attacks in New York City. Because the disaster was a terrorist attack as opposed to a naturally occurring incident, many similarities were identified between this and events in the Native American community's past. Common themes were the intrusion of foreigners into one's homeland, destruction of property, mass killings of innocents, pervasive fear, and a general mistrust of authority. It was an eye-opener for many staff to hear that the symbol of the Statue of Liberty was offensive and perceived as oppressive. Staff had to reframe their own preconceptions about the distress in this population.

A preexisting relationship between community leaders and local academic staff provided a link allowing several outreach staff to begin working within the community. They began hearing of all the historical pains, ills, and assaults that had been thrust upon this population for several hundred years. The strain of attempting to address so many traumatic events, which seemed to far outweigh the World Trade Center attacks in the collective mind of this group, felt like it might not be overcome. But the acknowledgment of this population's historical experience, coupled with patient listening and confirmation of their parallel responses to this disaster, and finally the guidance about coping skills and future planning, moved the group toward a healing path.

Holocaust Survivors

Another population with the similar experience of reliving historical trauma is the Holocaust survivors. The 9/11 event sparked flashbacks and other intolerable emotional reactions, forcing many to seek out the disaster mental health staff. Differing from Native American history, the Holocaust trauma has been acknowledged internationally. Permanent memorials, historical documentaries, films, and entire museums have been dedicated to the goal of remembering the atrocities of the Holocaust. While these efforts have helped a culture to heal, some individuals who had never attended to their personal pain were retraumatized by the 9/11 disaster, requiring support to help address their distress responses. Outreach was primarily conducted through the Jewish networks of rabbinate councils, community centers, and synagogues with much of the disaster literature that was translated into Hebrew and Russian.

The pride of individuals who had survived encampment, torture, excessive losses, and attempted genocide had to be maintained while allowing grief and fear to be expressed. Outreach staff were almost exclusively from within the community, including multilingual paraprofessional and professional staff, who addressed the issues of prior trauma and immigration and the implications of terrorism having reached these survivors' safe haven.

Closed Communities: Rescue, Recovery, Emergency, and Construction Personnel

The male-dominated world of police officers, fire department personnel, emergency services staff, and construction workers may not easily accept crisis counseling as these tight-knit communities are self-protective and fiercely independent. But they are highly social and the closeness of their cultures can serve as a strength to be utilized when attempting outreach. Because of the strong boundaries that limit outside intervention, all possible demographic issues need to be considered when developing outreach strategies. Race, ethnicity, and familiarity play a large role in the ability to engage and connect with such tight social circles. Hiring outreach workers with similar ethnic backgrounds, who come from the same neighborhoods or schools or whose family members share the same professions seems to break the ice more easily than bringing in people who are unknown. Confidentiality concerns in the form of possibly knowing the outreach workers or their families were less of an issue than was the importance of working with a peer or someone with a connection to their field.

On 9/11/01, the Fire Department of New York (FDNY) suffered painfully extensive losses of personnel in all the boroughs, and especially in Staten Island. The FDNY's own psychological support services unit was mobilized rapidly and effectively, attending to those who required immediate treatment. Many other members of the department used their own mental health support services, which caused great controversy. The psychological support services unit was known to assist those personnel who were experiencing alcohol or other substance abuse problems as well as to have the ability to remove staff from duty as necessary. This caused many FDNY staff to avoid accessing mental health disaster response services from this unit. The unit's director attended to the problem by applying a multitiered structure of access to engage department personnel and their families.

The FDNY subcontracted with mental health counselors from the local private practice pool, allowing personnel to be seen by someone outside the department's counseling unit. This helped to decrease the fear of job loss, but facilitating the connections was a slow process. It was also difficult to control for the type and quality of services delivered as well as monitoring secondary stress in the counselors. The advantage to working with these counselors was their ability to provide assessments to ensure people were being seen at appropriate levels of care.

Another route to working with this population was through the provision of outreach to every firehouse in New York City. The counseling unit hired retired firemen, friends of firemen, and brothers, uncles, and nephews of firemen. Outreach workers assimilated into their assigned firehouses in whatever manner they could—by hanging around, engaging in station chores—whatever worked. Access to this community was also successfully accomplished in the New York response by offering assistance to family members. Family meetings were centered on the types of events that were routine such as family picnics, potluck dinners, work-sponsored socials, and faith-based rituals. Outreach workers participated in such events to create a consistent presence, fostering familiarity and a supporting and caring connection.

The effect of the deaths of New York Police Department (NYPD) personnel in the World Trade Center disaster was painful and put a tremendous strain on the department that was now expected to provide the physical and emotional security of the entire city. These personnel were assigned long hours in tenuous situations—checking trucks at the bridges and tunnels, examining cars going into large public parking areas, and stopping to help reorient people who were no longer able to use the Twin Towers as their compass.

Prior to 9/11 a peer support model had been widely used in the NYPD and it became highly accessed as part of the disaster response program. In addition, the Police Foundation had a long and respected history of assisting families of personnel who had been injured or killed. A significant effort was launched to provide outreach and support services to spouses, children, and other family members in various modalities through the Foundation's partnership with the disaster mental health response.

CONCLUSION

There is much to learn from our experiences as a result of the 9/11/01 attacks perpetrated on the United States. America did not expect to have to cope with such a huge disaster affecting five states and the psyche of the nation. There was no reference point outside the state of war, which many had never been exposed to. The emotional responses that many victims exhibited were similar to what has been seen in the past—sleeplessness, nightmares, flashbacks, anxiety and depressive symptoms, displaced anger, and fear. But the terrorist disaster followed by ongoing threats has created a change in the pattern of disaster recovery. Rather than the usual peaks and valleys seen in accessing supports, service utilization in New York rose steadily spiking at 6 months postincident and reached an all-time high during the weeks surrounding the first-year anniversary. What remained constant was the extraordinary community response, as is often the case in emergency situations. The best of the human spirit that emerged, allowing people to work well together, remained for a significant period.

The federal crisis counseling disaster response model seems to address the majority of the concerns of most communities. The use of outreach as a modality for delivering disaster crisis counseling services in a city that is widely diverse seemed to guide the mental health disaster response program toward success in the aftermath of 9/11. People from all over the disaster area who watched crisis counseling television commercials, read narratives on subway cars, and/or received services in community-based locations reported positive effects.

Crisis counselors with varying levels of experience and education may benefit from the use of a screening or referral tool early on in the disaster response. Such tools may assist in identifying individuals who suffer with prolonged distress responses and need attending to at an appropriate point in their own phase of recovery. An intermediate level of intervention, such as the brief intensive services implemented in the latter phase of the New York disaster response program, may need to be integrated as an overall component of future programs to ensure timely delivery. The final evaluation describing the outcomes of service delivery, coupled with the descriptions of the experiences of individuals who received assistance from the disaster response staff, will offer more information that will help drive decisions about future mental health disaster responses.

REFERENCES

American Red Cross. (n.d.). *A brief history of the American Red Cross*. Retrieved August 4, 2003, from www.redcross.org

Center for Mental Health Services. (1995). *Psychosocial issues for children and families in disaster: A guide for the primary care physician* (SMA953022). Washington, DC: U.S. Department of Health and Human Services.

Center for Mental Health Services. (2001, September 21). *An overview of the crisis counseling assistance and training program* (CCP-PG-01). Rockville, MD: Author.

Galea, S., Ahern, J., Resnick, H., Kilpatrick, D., Mucuvalas, M., & Gold, J. (2002). Psychological sequelae of the September 11 terrorist attacks in New York City. *New England Journal of Medicine, 346,* 982–987.

Gilbert, N., Specht, H., & Terrell, P. (1993). *Dimensions of social welfare policy* (3rd ed.). Englewood Cliffs, NJ: Simon & Schuster.

Green, B., & Solomon, S. (1995). The mental health impact of natural and technological disasters. In S. Freedys & S. Hobfoll (Eds.), *Traumatic stress: From theory to practice* (pp. 163–180). New York: Plenum Press.

Jankowski, K., & Hamblen, J. (2001). *The effects of disaster on people with severe mental illness.* Retrieved August 4, 2003, from www.ncptsd.org

Kaniasty, K., & Norris, F. (1995). In search of altruistic community: Patterns of social support following hurricane Hugo. *American Journal of Community Psychology, 23*(4), 447.

Lash, J. P. (1971). *Eleanor and Franklin.* New York: New American Library.

Lum, D. (2000). *Social work practice and people of color: A process-stage approach* (4th ed.). Belmont, CA: Brooks/Cole.

McFall, M., Malte, C., Fontana, A., & Rosenheck, R. A. (2000). Effects of an outreach intervention on use of mental health services by veterans with posttraumatic stress disorder. *Psychiatric Services, 51*(3), 369–374.

McFarlane, W. R., & Piveral, K. (1996). Multiple family group psychoeducation: Creating therapeutic social networks. In G. Clark & G. Vaccaro (Eds.), *Practicing psychiatry in the community: A manual* (pp. 387–406). Washington, DC: American Psychiatric Association Press.

Norris, F., Byrne, C. M., & Diaz, E. (2001, October 4). *Risk factors for adverse outcomes in natural and human caused disasters: A review of the empirical literature.* Retrieved December 5, 2001, from www.ncptsd.org

Norris, F., Phifer, F., & Kaniasty, K. (1994). Individual and community reactions to the Kentucky floods: Findings from a longitudinal study of older adults. In R. Ursano, B. Mccaughey, & C. Fullerton (Eds.), *The structure of human chaos: Individual and community responses to trauma and disaster.* Cambridge, UK: Cambridge University Press.

Solomon, S. D., & Green, B. L. (1992). Mental health effects of natural and humanmade disasters. *National Center for Post-Traumatic Stress Disorder Research Quarterly, 3*(1), 1–8.

Stamm, B. H., & Friedman, M. J. (2000). Cultural diversity in the appraisal and expression of trauma. In A. Shalev, R. Yehuda, & A. McFarlane (Eds.), *International handbook of human response to trauma* (pp. 69–85). New York: Plenum Press.

Substance Abuse and Mental Health Services Administration. (2003). *Developing cultural competence in disaster mental health programs: Guiding principles and recommendations* (SMA3828). Rockville, MD: U.S. Department of Health and Human Services.

University of Illinois at Chicago. (n.d.). *Urban experience in Chicago: Hull*

House and its neighborhoods, 1889–1963. Retrieved July 24, 2003, from www.uic.edu

Young, B. H. (2002). Emergency outreach navigational and brief screening guidelines for working in large group settings following catastrophic events. *National Center for Post-Traumatic Stress Disorder Clinical Quarterly, 11*, 1–7.

Young, B. H., Ford, J. D., Ruzek, J. I., Friedman, M. F., & Guzman, F. D. (1998). *Disaster mental health services: A guidebook for clinicians and administrators.* St. Louis, MO: Department of Veterans Affairs Employee Education System.

PART V

CREATING AN AGENDA FOR THE FUTURE

Conducting Research
on Mental Health Interventions

BRETT T. LITZ and LAURA E. GIBSON

Who is most at risk for developing chronic mental health problems as a result of exposure to mass violence? Is there a reliable and valid way of screening individuals who are at risk? Are there evidence-based methods of preventing chronic posttraumatic stress disorder (PTSD) and other mental health problems implicated from exposure to mass violence? The sobering truth is that because the field of early intervention is in its infancy, particularly in the context of mass violence, answers to these and other important questions remain unanswered. There is a dearth of sufficiently rigorous social and clinical science that policymakers, planners, first responders, and clinicians can use to shape plans and contingencies to help people who are most likely to suffer the psychological, social, and ultimately societal consequences of exposure to mass violence. Unfortunately, but understandably, at present, the policies and procedures employed to assist victims of mass violence (and other disasters) and first responders taxed by their helping roles are based on inadequate evidence and clinical lore.

This state of affairs is unacceptable. Because most people are remarkably resilient in the face of severe trauma and intensive and draining occupational demands, blindly promoting and implementing secondary preventions of any kind is a waste of precious resources. Also, if first responders and clinicians at any point in the response chain provide interventions without a sufficient evidentiary base then, at best, some victims will waste their time captive to an inert process, and, at worst, others will be exposed to something that is harmful in unappreciated and unmonitored ways (Litz, Gray, Bryant, & Adler, 2002).

We argue that promoting, conducting, and disseminating systematic and well-controlled empirical research on early intervention is the most important agenda for the future of this field. In this chapter, we provide an overview of the process of conducting research in early intervention. We also present priorities for research in early intervention, methodological considerations, common challenges, and possible solutions to some of these challenges.

WHAT IS THE CURRENT STATE OF AFFAIRS?

While researchers may take it for granted that interventions need to be based on well-controlled clinical studies, this notion is not always obvious to consumers, clinicians, or policymakers. Individuals who work in the field may have spent many years observing what seems to work and what does not seem to work and may steadfastly believe that research only serves to validate what clinicians or policymakers have long known. It is the responsibility of clinical investigators to make the case that we do not in fact know what works in terms of early interventions for trauma-exposed populations. On the other hand, this cannot be done brashly or without appreciation for the wisdom of first responders and clinicians who have been working with people who are in anguish as a result of trauma.

Unfortunately, there is a vast divide between academic researchers and front-line clinicians. What the field needs is meaningful collaboration, based on mutual respect and trust, with a shared appreciation for the fact that research on early interventions is lacking and that there is a subsequent pressing need for research in this area. Clinicians such as Red Cross mental health planners, trainers, and responders need to be partners in the process of discovery and verification. The field will not advance unless there is openness to research findings; on the other hand, for research to have any impact there needs to be a collaboration between researchers and people at all levels invested in helping victims of mass violence.

It is unacceptable that the current standard of care in treatment for survivors of mass violence/disasters is critical incident stress debriefing (CISD), given the nonsupporting evidence or lack of evidence for its efficacy (Litz et al., 2002; Rose, Bisson, & Wessely, 2001; Watson et al., 2003). Yet, it is understandable that CISD embedded in the broader framework of critical incident stress management (CISM) is the guiding conceptual framework at disaster sites. Although CISD/CISM is based on anachronistic notions of crisis intervention and grief counseling, it is a highly face-valid set of procedures that resonates with organizations, planners, administrators, and clinicians. CISD is a semistructured intervention that can be implemented in either an individual or a group format. It typically involves psychoeducation about stress and coping, normalization of stress reactions, promotion of emotional processing through discussion of the experience, and provision of information about further interventions (Bryant, 2002). The model has appeal in part because it is the only game in town; outside of CISD/CISM, at present, there is no meaningful guiding conceptual framework and there is no consensus on a set of prescriptive interventions.

Brief, multisession cognitive-behavioral treatments (CBTs) have been developed and appear to hold great promise in terms of reducing chronic PTSD (Bryant, Harvey, Dang, Sackville, & Basten, 1998; Bryant, Sackville, Dang, Moulds, & Guthrie, 1999). CBT generally contains the common elements of psychoeducation, anxiety management techniques, exposure techniques, and cognitive restructuring. However, these treatments await evaluation in the context of well-designed and well-controlled clinical trials with larger and more diverse samples before they can be routinely recommended as early interventions for mass violence or disasters. At present, the CBT approach fails to offer much for the front-line clinician at a disaster site. CISD has been put into widespread use because of the pressing and understandable desire to attempt to help people in acute distress. To replace CISD with interventions that work, we must first develop and then systematically test alternative treatments. If the current state of affairs is allowed to continue, we are concerned that it may actually increase the likelihood that victims' distress will persist. Under the current system of care, both survivors and clinicians may assume that CISD is the most effective treatment available, given its widespread implementation.

RESEARCH PRIORITIES IN EARLY-INTERVENTION RESEARCH

Because there are many diverse empirical questions in the early-intervention arena, we next prioritize a set of research agendas for the future.

1. *Well-designed and well-controlled trials of a variety of secondary prevention strategies.* Because most people get better on their own over time, studies that include randomization to conditions are critical. Because CBT shows great promise, but the existing studies suffer from external validity problems, resources should be devoted to controlled trials applying CBT to a variety of victims of disaster. Because CBT requires considerable expertise and therapist resources, it is important to examine self-help

approaches with minimal therapist contact and efficient methods of delivering care (telemedicine, Internet, etc.).

Several recent reviews of the early-intervention literature have concluded that CISD may be ineffective (at best) or may exacerbate or worsen symptoms (Litz et al., 2002; Rose et al., 2001; Watson et al., 2003). However, several of the studies on which these reviews were based contained serious methodological limitations, including lack of a uniform CISD protocol, lack of objective treatment adherence measures, and lack of clearly defined target symptoms. Well-controlled, randomized controlled trials (RCTs) approved by the CISM organization are needed to faithfully assess the possible efficacy of CISD.

While RCTs are essential to advance the field, some experimental and quasi-experimental research designs are more feasible and potentially more acceptable to consumers, policymakers, and clinicians, particularly under the rushed and chaotic conditions ubiquitous to mass violence and disasters. One such design is a balanced design, which would entail providing an intervention at Site A but not at Site B (Yule, 1992). Another research strategy that might be more acceptable to survivors, clinicians, and so on might entail block random assignment. In a randomized block design, random assignment would occur at the group level (schools, neighborhoods, classes, etc.) rather than at an individual level (Hardin et al., 2002). Again, such research strategies are likely to be most successful if they are designed ahead of time and can be transported into the disaster-stricken community.

2. *Naturalistic longitudinal studies of the trajectory of posttraumatic adaptation, especially the course of adjustment to mass violence and traumatic loss.* While cross-sectional epidemiological studies that describe the scope and impact of trauma are important, they are not sufficient. Posttraumatic responses ebb and flow and multiwave examinations of the factors that covary with symptom onset or exacerbation and symptom attenuation (or effective functioning) will generate knowledge about mechanisms of risk and resilience that will inform future secondary interventions. At present, we know a lot about factors that are correlated with chronic impairment—so-called *risk indicators* (King, Vogt, & King, 2004; Litz et al., 2002; Norris et al., 2002). However, we know very little about *risk mechanisms*. In other words, we do not know why or how a risk indicator affects adaptation to trauma (nor do we know the direction of the relationship). For example, we know that prior trauma history is highly associated with risk for PTSD after an index trauma, but we do not understand why this is the case. Another example is social support, which is a robust predictor of chronic PTSD. It remains unclear how social supports facilitate or impede recovery specifically over the life course. We also lack an informed understanding of how resilient people naturally cope with severe trauma and of whether resilience is lifelong or phasic (e.g., a period of adjustment

could be followed by a period of severe impairment). Greater knowledge of factors that promote resilience among individuals who recover from severe trauma will inform and shape the next generation of clinical interventions. For example, preliminary research suggests that beta-adrenergic receptor blocking in the immediate aftermath of trauma may speed rate of recovery from trauma (Pitman et al., 2002).

3. *Research on screening models and screening methods.* Despite theories about what places individuals at risk for developing chronic PTSD, there are few well-designed empirical studies and there are no cogent conceptual frameworks to draw from when considering practical screening programs for early trauma intervention. Serious questions remain regarding when to screen, how to screen, and what questions to ask. Should screening be based on extent of exposure, presence of risk factors, or symptoms during and/or after the disaster? Are there certain individuals who should not be screened? Are there iatrogenic or stigmatizing effects associated with screening? These remain empirical questions that should be addressed through controlled research.

We need more evidence about personal liabilities and the social and cultural factors that affect chronic posttraumatic problems. This information then needs to be shaped into different testable methods of screening people who will have difficulty recovering on their own. Because most people are capable of using their existing support systems and are resilient in the face of mass violence (Galea et al., 2002; Schlenger et al., 2002), we need to find methods of providing immediate psychological first aid and sustained secondary prevention to the people who have the greatest need.

4. *Research on the optimal timing of various interventions.* We have argued that in the immediate aftermath of trauma, formal secondary prevention interventions should not be used (Litz et al., 2002). Rather, on the scene, people are likely to require psychological first aid, which is designed to provide a supportive human presence, safety, reassurance, and information. We have argued that in the first hours and days after exposure to tragedy, people are not cognitively or emotionally prepared to undergo the hard work of secondary-prevention interventions, such as CBT procedures (Litz & Gray, 2004). Ehlers and Clark (2003) have suggested offering assessments (but not treatment) in the first 1–2 months after trauma, followed by an intensive course of treatment at 2–3 months for those survivors who continue to be symptomatic. On the other hand, it is possible that a few days after a trauma, some individuals may be emotionally and intellectually prepared to absorb CBT and do the work necessary to recover from trauma, which requires attention and sustained action over time. If there were a more reliable way of identifying which survivors were at risk of developing long-term psychopathology, it would be ideal to offer an intervention as soon as an individual might be capable of benefiting from it. Research that

examines the effects of intervention timing (e.g., 2 days vs. 1 month) is critically needed to address these knowledge gaps.

5. *Research on the critical components and necessary change agents of early interventions.* Dismantling studies of CBT are needed in order to determine the relative contributions of core techniques, such as anxiety management, cognitive restructuring, and exposure methods. It would be useful to know the relative contributions of these components to positive outcomes. In addition, it would be useful to examine whether certain techniques are better suited to certain clinical presentations. For example, it is possible that an individual with a preponderance of severe reexperiencing symptoms may benefit more from an emphasis on exposure techniques than someone with minimal reexperiencing symptoms. Similarly, an individual with PTSD and major depressive disorder may require more emphasis on cognitive restructuring to address depressive cognitions. At present, practitioners must largely rely on clinical judgment to decide where to place the emphasis in their interventions, and which interventions to implement. Dismantling studies aimed at examining the relative contributions of various therapeutic techniques would be extremely useful in terms of developing a more empirically based guide to practice.

6. *Research on the needs of victims.* Surprisingly, there are no well-designed descriptive studies of the various biopsychosocial needs of victims of disasters and terrorism. There are good conceptual models that guide our understanding of what victims might need (e.g., Hobfoll's conservation of resources theory [Hobfoll, 1989; Hobfoll, Dunahoo, & Monnier, 1995]), but there are few data regarding what victims need at various points in time.

7. *Research on the unique burden of traumatic loss.* There is little sound research on the unique psychosocial needs of individuals who suffer traumatic loss or those who suffer the dual burden of losing a loved one through trauma while experiencing their own acute trauma (Neria & Litz, 2004; Raphael, Minkov, & Dobson, 2001). Although there are some promising uncontrolled intervention trials (Shear et al., 2001; Sireling, Cohen, & Marks, 1988), there are no published randomized controlled trials of early interventions for traumatic bereavement.

8. *Broadening conceptualizations of posttraumatic adaptation.* A strong emphasis has been placed on the measurement of PTSD symptoms as the *sine qua non* indicator of posttraumatic malady. However, other problems such as depression, substance abuse, and other anxiety disorders are common (Norris et al., 2002; North, 2003). Future research should include a broader range of outcome measures, including occupational and interpersonal functioning, depression, anger, substance use, and somatic complaints, among others.

OBSTACLES AND SOLUTIONS TO CONDUCTING
SOUND EARLY-INTERVENTION RESEARCH

There are numerous significant obstacles to conducting rigorous investigations in the chaotic aftermath of a disaster or mass violence situation. These barriers present unique and difficult challenges to early-intervention researchers. However, we do not believe that these challenges are insurmountable. It will be critical for the field of early-intervention research to collectively address and overcome the challenges inherent in this type of research.

One common challenge faced by mass violence and disaster researchers is that a study design or research infrastructure has not been put into place prior to the trauma. A common example of this can be seen when a disaster strikes a given community, and a researcher from that community quickly designs a study in an attempt to assess the effectiveness of community interventions that are being implemented under chaotic conditions. Almost inevitably, a clinical outcome study undertaken under such rushed conditions will result in a methodologically flawed research design with limited conclusions and generalizability. To meet this challenge, researchers with an interest in early intervention must design studies that are portable. In essence, studies would need to be funded and designed ahead of time that could be brought into a disaster-stricken community.

Another challenge that can be faced by early-intervention researchers concerns the long-standing theoretical clashes or misunderstandings between researchers, practitioners in the field, and policymakers. Although a recent joint conference on early interventions (National Institute of Mental Health, 2002) suggested that these historically disparate groups are beginning to work more collaboratively, misunderstandings continue to arise and present further logistical challenges in terms of the implementation of RCTs as early interventions after disasters.

Anecdotally, we have heard about reluctance to recruit disaster-exposed individuals into research studies out of fear of taking advantage of vulnerable populations by using them as research participants, or "test cases." Similarly, we have heard voiced concerns about assigning individuals to control groups and therefore withholding potentially useful treatment to consumers who are suffering from high levels of distress. Incidentally, these concerns may be voiced not only by policymakers or responders in the field but also by institutional review boards or funding sources.

We cannot overstate the importance of educating policymakers, clinicians, and even consumers about the need for well-designed and well-controlled studies. While RCTs will ultimately be most informative, studies utilizing randomized block or balanced designs could also contribute substantially to our understanding of effective interventions after mass violence and disasters. If quasi-experimental designs are used, there should be multiple replications to bolster the validity of the conclusions. Concerns about research (and researchers) are rooted in an understandable desire to help clients exposed to disasters and not to be intrusive. For concerned policymakers and practitioners to be persuaded to support carefully controlled research, they need to understand that the purpose of empirical trials is ultimately to more effectively relieve human suffering by providing scientifically grounded answers to crucial clinical questions. We do not yet know what interventions work best, for whom, and at what point in time. We will not have adequate answers to these questions until further well-controlled studies have been undertaken.

Another typical barrier to conducting solid empirical research in the aftermath of mass violence or disaster revolves around recruitment of trauma survivors as participants. Researchers may encounter challenges in gaining access to survivors in the first place and then must contend with whether those survivors who are willing to participate in a research study are actually representative of other traumatized individuals. Understandably, many survivors will leave an area exposed to disaster or mass violence as soon as possible, in an attempt to seek refuge, comfort, or safety. This presents another practical challenge. Also, after a massive disaster or violence situation, many individuals may be forced to leave their homes for extended periods of time and it may be logistically impossible to reach and follow-up with a representative sample of exposed individuals. In addition, survivors of trauma may be unwilling or unable to discuss their emotional reactions due to high levels of emotional suffering or fear of overwhelming distress. At this point, there is minimal research to draw from regarding the impact of participation in research—whether it is the ability to give informed consent or to participate in screening, more in-depth assessment, or clinical trial. Again, further research is needed before informed recommendations can be made regarding these issues.

Ethical issues also complicate the implementation of solid empirical research after disaster or mass violence. One key ethical debate, about which there is ongoing disagreement among traumatologists, concerns the issue of obtaining informed consent from acutely traumatized individuals. While researchers are clearly in agreement that informed consent is a necessary prerequisite to participation in a clinical trial, they differ in their opinions regarding the capability of acutely traumatized survivors to actually give informed consent.

There should be caution and concern about the ability of acutely traumatized survivors to consent to research. For example, consider the fact that the diagnosis of acute stress disorder (ASD) cannot be given within the first 2 days of trauma exposure due to the expectation that most severely traumatized individuals will endure an initial period of shock and extreme emotional distress. It would seem reasonable to expect that individuals could have trouble fully understanding the implications of participation in a study during this initial period after a severe trauma. Also, after severe trauma, the stress reaction involves higher circulating levels of epinephrine and cortisol. When combined with emotional distress, these physiological responses may impair coping, attention, and information-processing capacities (Christianson, 1992; Eysenck & Calvo, 1992). Theoretically, survivors would be better equipped to make decisions regarding participation in research after at least some minimal period of time has elapsed. Until these issues are better understood, it seems wise to avoid the implementation of emotionally and cognitively complex and demanding treatments or obtaining informed consent for such treatments within the first few days following a trauma. However, we would add that this time frame could ultimately be modified forward or backward, pending further empirical work on emotional and cognitive processing in the early stages posttrauma.

Another ethical concern that arises in regard to early intervention research revolves around the issue of random assignment, when one condition is considered more likely to lead to clinical improvement. A related question concerns whether it is ethical to randomly assign recent trauma victims to no-treatment or nonspecific factors/placebo control conditions. As discussed by Gray, Litz, and Olson (2004), it is instructive to consider both of these issues with reference to the concept of "clinical equipoise." (Freedman, 1987). Ethical clinical research demands a state of equipoise, which refers to true uncertainty concerning the relative merits of the interventions under study. A violation of equipoise (and of ethics) occurs when participants are randomly assigned to an intervention that is scientifically known to be inferior to another intervention. A violation would also occur if it became convincingly clear during the course of a clinical trial that one of the treatments far outweighed another in terms of positive or negative outcome. In such a case, it would be incumbent upon investigators to stop the investigation and recommend the more effective treatment to all participants involved in the study (Freedman, 1987). In most cases, the scientific superiority of one intervention relative to others would not be established until the conclusion of a study.

Confusion arises in regard to the ethics of RCTs when investigators misapply the concept of clinical equipoise at the level of the individual scientist rather than at the level of the scientific community as a whole. In other words, some investigators may believe (in the absence of clear scientific evidence) that one treatment is likely to be superior to another and they may erroneously conclude that equipoise is therefore disturbed and that the trial cannot ethically continue (Weijer, Shapiro, Glass, & Enkin,

2000). Freedman (1987) refers to this situation as "theoretical equipoise" as opposed to clinical equipoise and notes that it is "conceptually odd and ethically irrelevant" (p. 143). Freedman's (1987) critique is based on the fact that theoretical equipoise would be subject to the idiosyncrasies of the individual scientist and would require that a study be terminated each time an investigator were to perceive a slight superiority of one treatment over another, without regard to actual objective or scientific data. In other words, in a theoretical equipoise situation, any bias or hunch would be grounds for discontinuing an investigation. In a situation of theoretical equipoise, the basis for a clinical trial—informed disagreement among a community of clinicians and scholars—is given less weight than the subjective intuition of a single individual. As stated by Gray and colleagues (2004), a controlled clinical trial is ultimately the only way to resolve legitimate disagreement within the clinical community. It is both appropriate and necessary for a controlled clinical trial to be undertaken to resolve substantive disagreement in the field, even if the experimenter believes in the superiority of one of the interventions relative to the alternatives (Weijer et al., 2000).

A state of clinical equipoise exists in regard to appropriate early intervention for trauma survivors. Disagreement exists among members of the scientific and professional communities regarding whether to provide early-intervention services to survivors, when to provide them, and which treatments to offer. It is arguably the failure to conduct RCTs, rather than to implement them, that represents an ethical problem.

It is also unclear why ethical concerns would be raised regarding the use of nonspecific factors/placebo control conditions in early-intervention research. Psychological debriefing, which is currently widely used, appears to be inert (at best)—and some have suggested that it may even be harmful (Bisson, Jenkins, Alexander, & Bannister, 1997). The principle of clinical equipoise suggests that placebos are unacceptable in any treatment situation for which a validated and effective treatment has been established (Young, Annable, & Stat, 2002). This situation simply does not apply to the case of early intervention for traumatized individuals, because there are no established, effective, validated early interventions for this population. There is growing consensus on this issue among the research community. For example, the Declaration of Helsinki, the World Medical Association Council, the Canadian Institutes of Health Research, the Natural Sciences and Engineering Research Council of Canada, the Social Sciences and Humanities Research Council, and the U.S. Food and Drug Administration all condone the use of placebos in instances in which no standard treatment exists that has been shown to be more effective than no treatment (Young et al., 2002). As we have argued elsewhere (Gray et al., 2004), given the paucity of the evidence base regarding early trauma interventions, it is unquestionably permissible to utilize RCTs to test promising new interventions for trauma survivors and to employ placebo/nonspecific factors control conditions. In addition, we would argue that it is actually unethical to fail to conduct RCTs, as this failure would likely perpetuate the current state of affairs in which acutely traumatized individuals are generally offered useless interventions that we know will not help to alleviate their suffering.

METHODOLOGICAL CONSIDERATIONS IN EARLY-INTERVENTION RESEARCH

One of the criticisms of the extant research literature concerning early interventions is that there are multiple threats to internal and external validity. Much of this research has been undertaken quickly, and under the rushed conditions that are inevitable in the aftermath of a disaster. Foa and Meadows (1997) have described seven criteria or "gold standards" that should be met to increase the validity of clinical research. A recent review of the research on early intervention found only a handful of studies that met all seven criteria (National Institute of Mental Health, 2002). When these standards are not met, it makes it difficult (and oftentimes impossible) to draw conclusions from the results. Not only is this situation frustrating for consumers of research, but it is a waste of time and money for researchers, participants, and funding agencies when expensive and time-consuming clinical trials are undertaken that lead to little to no meaningful conclusions. It needs to be emphasized that the chaotic conditions involved in a mass violence or disaster situation present real difficulties for researchers that can render research extremely challenging. However, we would hope that clinical researchers would strive to meet as many of these conditions as is feasible. The scientific community can address the limitations of prior studies by actively correcting for methodological weaknesses in existing studies. Furthermore, if multiple studies are conducted, this can help to correct the limitations that will inevitably be present in individual trials.

Foa and Meadows's (1997) suggested standards for clinical research include (1) clearly defined target symptoms; (2) unbiased (random) assignment to treatment; (3) reliable and valid measures; (4) blind evaluators; (5) assessor training; (6) manualized, replicable, specific treatment programs; and (7) objective treatment adherence measures. In addition to these standards, we discuss the importance of assessing multiple outcomes, by multiple informants, in the context of early-intervention research.

Clearly Defined Target Symptoms

Given that the vast majority of individuals recover from the experience of trauma without developing psychiatric illnesses, it is unacceptable to merely use the experience of trauma itself as a basis for providing treatment. Foa and Meadows (1997) also suggest that researchers develop a threshold of symptom severity to use for inclusion in clinical trials, in addition to diagnostic status alone.

In addition to these factors, Foa and Meadows (1997) discuss the importance of establishing inclusion and exclusion criteria for treatment studies. Researchers should clearly demarcate what populations are and are not included in any given clinical trial in order to best assess which problems a given treatment can effectively address and which it cannot. In addition, researchers should expect that findings between studies will probably differ, based on the severity of participants' symptoms and the presence of comorbid diagnoses.

Random Assignment to Treatment

We have already made mention of the importance of RCTs for the assessment of treatment efficacy. Randomization allows the clinical researcher to compare the efficacy of treatments under highly controlled conditions. It is the only way to control for the multitude of other factors that may affect symptom change, such as regression to the mean, passage of time, and individual therapist or client factors. Foa and Meadows (1997) also suggest that in order to separate the effects of the experimental treatments from therapist effects, each treatment should be delivered by at least two therapists who are randomly assigned within that treatment condition. When random assignment to condition is simply not possible, randomization by neighborhood, school, and so on, would be indicated.

Reliable and Valid Measures

Once target symptoms are identified, appropriate measures need to be selected that can reliably measure change in those specific symptoms. Without reliable and valid measures, it is impossible to know how to interpret the results of any given clinical trial. Poor measures could lead researchers to falsely conclude that there has been symptom change when indeed there has been none (Type II error), or, conversely, to erroneously conclude that an effective treatment has had no impact on symptoms (Type I error). Researchers must ensure that the measures they select can reliably measure the symptoms that they are targeting, and that they are capable of capturing the degree of change that would be reasonably expected to occur within the parameters of a clinical trial.

In addition to self-report measures (which are the most typical means of evaluating treatment response), investigators should consider using structured clinical interviews to gain more detailed information about symptom frequency, severity, and level of impairment. Investigators should, to the extent possible, utilize multiple informants in assessing treatment response. The inclusion of multiple informants may provide a more objective measure of treatment outcome.

Blind Evaluators

Evaluators should be kept blind to treatment condition in order to provide an objective assessment of symptoms, without being biased by their individual beliefs about which treatment condition is most likely to be effective. Investigators should take measures to ensure that assessors remain blind to treatment group. This might include instructing participants to refrain from discussions of the particularities of their experimental treatment with their assessors and/or ensuring that therapists in the study and assessors are not housed in close proximity if this would likely result in assessors observing which participants are seeing which therapists. It should go without saying that assessments should not be conducted by therapists who are implementing the experimental treatments, given that they would not be blind to treatment condition and would be unable to provide unbiased assessments.

Assessor Training

Assessors/evaluators should be given specialized training in administering and scoring standardized clinical interviews and other standardized assessment measures and should reach some specified minimum criterion before they provide ratings within a research study. Given the pivotal role of a thorough and objective assessment of symptoms, it is crucial that the assessment itself is conducted reliably. Foa and Meadows (1997) also cite the importance of establishing interrater reliability and calibrating assessment procedures during the study in order to prevent evaluators from drifting in their ratings.

Manualized, Replicable Specific Treatment Programs

For treatments to be objectively evaluated, it is critical that they are manualized and replicable. Without detailed documentation of the experimental treatment being provided, there is no way of examining which component parts of the treatment are effective and which are not. In addition, it is critical that these component parts are explicitly defined. It is not enough to state that a treatment contains "cognitive restructuring" or "exposure," for example, without explicit descriptions of these complex interventions. In addition, detailed descriptions of an intervention, rather than a brief listing of treatment components, would permit early-intervention researchers to revise potentially helpful interventions rather than summarily concluding that a treatment does not work. Detailed manuals can also aid in the routine assessment of treatment adherence, by providing raters with explicit guidelines.

Objective Treatment Adherence Measures

Objective treatment adherence or fidelity ratings allow researchers to determine whether the experimental treatments were administered as they were designed. They also allow investigators to determine whether the treatment conditions overlapped substantially, which would obscure interpretation of the results. In addition, objective assessments of treatment fidelity will aid researchers in determining whether apparently ineffectual treatments are indeed lacking in efficacy—or whether apparent treatment failures are due to poor implementation or administration of theoretically sound interventions. Likewise, evidence of high treatment fidelity in clinical trials can lead to increased confidence in the trial outcomes.

Consider the following theoretical example that demonstrates the importance of treatment adherence measures. In a theoretical study, trauma survivors with ASD are randomly assigned to an early intervention that is anticipated to be quite beneficial (e.g., five sessions of cognitive-behavioral therapy), to a placebo/non-specific factors control condition (also five sessions), or to a no-treatment control condition. At the end of the clinical trial, the CBT condition results in a 50% reduction in symptom severity relative to no-treatment control participants and the nonspecific factors condition. In this situation, it would be tempting to immediately conclude that the five sessions of CBT (hypothesized to be especially helpful) promoted positive posttraumatic adjustment to a greater extent than nonspecific therapeutic factors such as basic empathy and support. That is, one might readily conclude that the unique components of the CBT intervention such as imaginal and *in vivo* exposure were associated with incremental treatment gains above and beyond nonspecific therapeutic factors. To increase confidence in these results, it would be helpful to ensure that the "nonspecific factors" condition did not include any unintended exposure component, and that the two conditions were indeed distinct in terms of potential therapeutic components. An evaluation of the integrity of the nonspecific factors condition would allow investigators to ensure that the conditions were in fact distinct. For example, the researchers could ensure that clients in the nonspecific factors control group did not spontaneously discuss their trauma and that clients in the exposure condition had indeed received systematic exposure. Likewise, had this theoretical study failed to demonstrate differences between the conditions, it would be useful to make sure that the conditions had indeed been distinct, before concluding that the additional components of the CBT condition did not add benefit beyond the nonspecific factors control condition. We would argue that the scientific community must provide more detailed accounts of early interventions, as well as attend to and document the fidelity with which our interventions are delivered.

Evaluation of Multiple Outcomes

Although most of the research to date on the psychological aftermath of trauma focuses on PTSD, it is clear that mass violence and disaster are associated with a wide range of emotional and behavioral difficulties. A recent review indicated that specific psychological problems (PTSD, major depressive disorder, panic disorder, and generalized anxiety disorder), nonspecific emotional distress, health problems, substance abuse and dependency, occupational and financial stress, impairments in social supports and interpersonal relationships, and age-specific problems (e.g., temper tantrums, incontinence, and hyperactivity in children) are all common in the aftermath of mass violence or disaster situations (Norris et al., 2002).

It is necessary to study a broad range of outcomes in order to determine whether standard psychological interventions are having an impact on the range of symptoms commonly seen after mass violence or disaster. It is possible that some treatments may be useful for a broad range of symptoms (e.g., anger, substance abuse, and social withdrawal) that are common in the aftermath of mass violence. For example, a treatment that included a module on healthy coping skills might prove useful for a variety of psychological difficulties. In addition, treatments could be designed that included modules based on the psychological difficulties found to be most prevalent in mass violence situations. For example, it seems likely that all treatments for survivors of a mass violence situation might include some basic psychoeducation about common reactions to mass violence (e.g., PTSD, depression, and survivor guilt) and might include some basic anxiety management skills. Researchers must examine the extent to which similar treatments might prove useful in meeting the diverse needs of survivors.

We would also argue that greater attention needs to be paid to differential rates of recovery between experimental treatments. For example, if two treatments appear to have comparable effect sizes yet one of them leads to a faster reduction of symptoms (Kenardy et al., 1996), this should be examined carefully, given the important clinical implications. However, the rate of recovery is not a variable that has traditionally received much research attention.

CONCLUSION

A state of clinical equipoise exists with respect to how best to prevent chronic PTSD and other mental health problems that stem from exposure to mass violence and traumatic loss. This has motivated researchers and policymakers to attend to the need for systematic research. In this chapter, we offered some research priorities. In addition, we reviewed obstacles to and suggestions for conducting research on early interventions, as well as methodological standards that researchers should strive to meet whenever feasible. Although the challenges to conducting methodologically sound research on early interventions are great, they can be overcome.

REFERENCES

Bisson, J. I., Jenkins, P. L., Alexander, J., & Bannister, C. (1997). Randomized controlled trial of psychological debriefing for victims of acute burn trauma. *British Journal of Psychiatry, 171,* 78–81.

Bryant, R. A. (2002). Early interventions following psychological trauma. *CNS Spectrums, 9,* 650–654.

Bryant, R. A., Harvey, A. G., Dang, S. T., Sackville, T., & Basten, C. (1998). Treatment of acute stress disorder: A comparison of cognitive-behavioral therapy and supportive counseling. *Journal of Consulting and Clinical Psychology, 66,* 862–866.

Bryant, R. A., Sackville, T., Dang, S. T., Moulds, M., & Guthrie, R. (1999). Treating acute stress disorder: An evaluation of cognitive behavioral therapy and supportive counseling techniques. *American Journal of Psychiatry, 156,* 1780–1786.

Christianson, S. A. (1992). *The handbook of emotion and memory: Research and theory.* Mahwah, NJ: Erlbaum.

Ehlers, A., & Clark, D. M. (2003). Early psychological interventions for adult survivors of trauma: A review. *Biological Psychiatry, 53,* 817–826.

Eysenck, M., & Calvo, M. (1992). Anxiety and performance: The processing efficiency theory. *Cognition and Emotion, 6,* 409–434.

Foa, E. B., & Meadows, E. A. (1997). Psychosocial treatments for post-traumatic stress disorder: A critical review. In J. Spence, J. M. Darley, & D. J. Foss (Eds.), *Annual review of psychology* (pp. 449–480). Palo Alto, CA: Annual Reviews.

Freedman, B. (1987). Equipoise and the ethics of clinical research. *New England Journal of Medicine, 317,* 141–145.

Galea, S., Ahern, J., Resnick, H. S., Kilpatrick, D., Bucuvalas, M., & Gold, J. (2002). Psychological sequelae of the September 11 terrorist attacks in New York City. *New England Journal of Medicine, 346,* 982–987.

Gray, M. J., Litz, B. T., & Olson, A. R. (2004). Methodological and ethical issues in early intervention research. In B. T. Litz (Ed.), *Early intervention for trauma and traumatic loss* (pp. 179–198). New York: Guilford Press.

Hardin, S. B., Weinrich, S., Weinrich, M., Garrison, C., Addy, C., & Hardin, T. L. (2002). Effects of a long-term psychosocial nursing intervention on adolescents exposed to catastrophic stress. *Issues in Mental Health Nursing, 23,* 537–551.

Hobfoll, S. E. (1989). Conservation of resources: A new attempt at conceptualizing stress. *American Psychologist, 44,* 513–524.

Hobfoll, S. E., Dunahoo, C. A., & Monnier, J. (1995). Conservation of resources and traumatic stress. In J. R. Freedy & S. E. Hobfoll (Eds.), *Traumatic stress: From theory to practice* (pp. 29–47). New York: Plenum Press.

Kenardy, J., Webster, R., Lewin, T., Carr, V., Hazell, P., & Carter, G. (1996). Stress debriefing and patterns of recovery following a natural disaster. *Journal of Traumatic Stress, 9,* 37–49.

King, D. W., Vogt, D. S., & King, L. A. (2004). Risk and resilience factors in the etiology of chronic posttraumatic stress disorder. In B. T. Litz (Ed.), *Early intervention for trauma and traumatic loss* (pp. 34–64). New York: Guilford Press.

Litz, B. T., & Gray, M. J. (2004). Early intervention for trauma in adults. In B. T. Litz (Ed.), *Early intervention for trauma and traumatic loss* (pp. 87–111). New York: Guilford Press.

Litz, B. T., Gray, M. J., Bryant, R. A., & Adler, A. B. (2002). Early intervention for trauma: Current status and future directions. *Clinical Psychology: Science and Practice, 9,* 112–134.

National Institute of Mental Health. (2002). *Mental health and mass violence: Evidence-based early psychological intervention for victims/survivors of mass violence: A workshop to reach consensus on best practices* (NIH Publication No. 02-5138). Washington, DC: U.S. Government Printing Office.

Neria, Y., & Litz, B. (2004). Bereavement by traumatic means: The complex synergy of trauma and grief. *Journal of Loss and Trauma, 9,* 73–87.

Norris, F. H., Friedman, M. J., Watson, P. J., Byrne, C. M., Diaz, E., & Kaniasty, K. Z. (2002). 60,000 disaster victims speak: Part I, an empirical review of the empirical literature, 1981–2001. *Psychiatry, 65,* 207–239.

North, C. S. (2003). Psychiatric epidemiology of disaster responses. *Review of Psychiatry, 22,* 37–62.

Pitman, R. K., Sanders, K. M., Zusman, R. M., Healy, A. R., Cheema, F., Lasko, N. B., et al. (2002). Pilot study of secondary prevention of post-traumatic stress disorder with Propranolol. *Biological Psychiatry, 51,* 189–192.

Raphael, B., Minkov, C., & Dobson, M. (2001). Psychotherapeutic and pharmacological interventions for bereaved people. In M. S. Stroebe, R. O. Hansson, W. Stroebe, & H. Schut (Eds), *Handbook of bereavement research: Consequences, coping, and care* (pp. 587–612). Washington, DC: American Psychological Association.

Rose, S., Bisson, J., & Wessely, S. (2001). *Psychological debriefing for preventing posttraumatic stress disorder (PTSD)* (The Cochrane Library, Issue 3). Oxford, UK: Update Software.

Schlenger, W. E., Caddell, J. M., Ebert, L., Jordan, B. K., Rourke, K. M., Wilson, D., et al. (2002). Psychological reactions to terrorist attacks: Findings from the national study of Americans' reactions to September 11. *Journal of the American Medical Association, 288,* 581–588.

Shear, M. K., Frank, E., Foa, E., Cherry, C., Reynolds, C. F. III, Vander Bilt, J., et al. (2001). Traumatic grief treatment: A pilot study. *American Journal of Psychiatry, 158,* 1506–1508.

Sireling, L., Cohen, D., & Marks, I. (1988). Guided mourning for morbid grief: A controlled replication. *Behavior Therapy, 19,* 121–132.

Watson, P. J., Friedman, M. J., Gibson, L. E., Ruzek, J. I., Norris, F. H., & Ritchie, E. C. (2003). Early intervention for trauma-related problems. *Review of Psychiatry, 22,* 97–124.

Weijer, C., Shapiro, S. H., Glass, K. C., & Enkin, M. W. (2000). Clinical equipoise and not the uncertainty principle is the moral underpinning of the randomised controlled trial. *British Medical Journal, 321,* 756–758.

Young, S., Annable, L., & Stat, D. (2002). The ethics of placebo in clinical psychopharmacology: The urgent need for consistent regulation. *Journal of Psychiatry and Neuroscience, 27,* 319–321.

Yule, W. (1992). Post-traumatic stress disorder in child survivors of shipping disasters: The sinking of the "Jupiter." *Psychotherapy and Psychosomatics, 57,* 200–205.

CHAPTER 21

Mental Health and Behavioral Interventions for Victims of Disasters and Mass Violence

Systems, Caring, Planning, and Needs

ROBERT J. URSANO and MATTHEW J. FRIEDMAN

Disasters and mass violence are an all too common part of life. They affect all strata of life—the rich and the poor, at work and at home, children and adults, and across all ethnic and religious backgrounds. Disasters may range from the typhoon, tornado, or tsunami to transportation accidents and epidemic outbreaks of severe acute respiratory syndrome (SARS), influenza, or avian flu. Across the world those who are disadvantaged are at greatest risk of disasters because of where they live, work, and play—often where land is less expensive, in homes and work sites that are less protected and near dangerous industrial areas. Mass violence is also a result of human-made or intentional events—industrial and transportation accidents as well as terrorism and war. These may carry more behavioral and mental health consequences. Terrorism raises particular challenges for mental health and behavioral consequence management. The mental health and behavioral consequences of terrorism will be the most significant, long term, and most costly effects of a terrorist attack. The primary goal of terrorism's is to alter one's trust in public institutions and change people's beliefs, sense of safety, and behaviors (Holloway, Norwood, Fullerton, Engel, & Ursano, 1997). For this reason mental health experts are an essential part of planning for and responding to terrorism.

Discussions of early intervention following mass violence and large-scale disasters generally address two major areas: public health concerns and clinical treatment for distressed individuals. Although these two levels of concern are obviously interrelated in many important ways, they can also be addressed separately from both a conceptual and a practical perspective. Public mental health considerations focus on the capacity of current systems to provide adequate protection at the societal or community level. The orientation is "wellness." Interventions are designed either to promote resilience or to detect those in need, and the expectation is recovery for the vast majority of people with provision of services for those who remain symptomatic. Discussions of interventions for individuals, in contrast, generally have an "illness" perspective. Interventions are designed to reduce pathological symptoms or maladaptive behavior. Such discussions are usually embedded within a more traditional clinical mental health context.

This book reflects these two different orientations, with some chapters focusing on public health initiatives while others address the clinical challenge of intervention to ameliorate individual posttraumatic distress. There are other topics that do not fit neatly into this dichotomy such as the training and credentialing of disaster mental health professionals, which has both public health and traditional clinical components. Likewise chapters on theory, research, cultural sensitivity, and, possibly, outreach need to be considered from both perspectives.

PUBLIC HEALTH PERSPECTIVE

Disasters and mass violence overwhelm local resources and can threaten the function and safety of a community. Instantaneous communication and media coverage disseminate the events in real time and the world becomes a witness as relatives and friends begin to grieve even before complete information is available. The disaster community is often flooded with outsiders: those who offer assistance, curiosity seekers, and the media. This sudden influx of strangers can be experienced as intrusive and insensitive. Hotel rooms fill up, restaurants become crowded with unfamiliar faces, the community's normal routine is lost, and social supports as well as social services are strained and disrupted.

Cohesion of communities is common early after a disaster. Most communities respond well and adaptively to all types of disasters. The period of cohesion is also an opportunity to mobilize communities and natural support groups to contribute to the recovery of the community. During this phase, the media serve as a vector for both knowledge and, potentially, for distress in how they transmit pictures of injury and fear or information and aid. Inevitably, after any major trauma, there are rumors circulated within the community about the circumstances leading up to the traumatic event and the government response. Sometimes there is a heightened state of fear as additional disaster or violent events are anticipated or feared. In this potentially chaotic setting mental health care targets the relief of suffering and distress, treatment of psychiatric illness, and the prevention of behavioral breakdown, especially among first responders

We have not developed a systematic approach to the provision of mental health care after disasters and mass violence. Worker support, rape counseling, treatment of combat veterans, and even traditional mental health services models fail to address the breadth of needs for care across populations and time (Ruzek, Chapter 2). Health care delivery plans must recognize that most people will recover, that we do not know the optimum time for interventions for direct survivors (as well as for friends and relatives), that our understanding of effective educational interventions (including those utilizing the media) is in its infancy, and that social supports appear to be important to natural recovery and adaptive coping. Active outreach, in particular to high risk and or forgotten groups (e.g., elderly and children) is important for service delivery, while triage may be important in the early stages of health care delivery. In addition, the economics of disasters generally require that early interventions be brief and highly cost-effective if they are to be able to be delivered widely.

There is little public medical care for mental health problems across the entire range of primary, secondary, and tertiary prevention, including health behaviors and traditional mental health—from community-based prevention programs to outpatient clinics, inpatient hospital care, and care in the primary care setting where most mental health problems present. With rare exceptions, the public health component of our mental health system refers to community-based services for people with serious and persistent mental illness, not to a comprehensive public health approach to the entire mental health and behavioral needs of the community including for disasters and mass violence (Institute of Medicine, 2002).

Care for the mental health and behavioral health needs of disaster and mass violence requires a systematic approach to the provision of public medical care for mental health problems across the entire range of primary, secondary, and tertiary prevention. This includes care for health behaviors that may increase distress and morbidity as well as traditional mental health care. Such health care is needed from community-based prevention programs to outpatient clinics and to inpatient hospital care, including those who are injured and the health care providers themselves when true disaster strikes and resources are overwhelmed. The private health care system and the primary care setting where most mental health problems present are part of the mental health care response network.

Traditional natural disaster or transportation accident models of providing health services after a disaster have limited applicability in terrorism.

Effective, consistent health responses to the psychological, behavioral and mental health needs after disasters and mass violence require preparedness and response activities within the framework of all-hazards disaster planning (Flynn, 2003).

The mental health care system, as part of the medical care system for disasters and mass violence, must join with the public health and emergency response systems to address needs for triage, surge capacity, and health surveillance in order to best provide care for disaster communities. This requires coordination across public health, health and mental health authorities, state and local emergency planners, disaster relief organizations, health care institutions and providers and representatives of critical infrastructure entities (Ursano, Fullerton, & Norwood, 2003a).

Speier (Chapter 5) insists that such planning must be based on useful and accurate data; he illustrates how the current methodology for postdisaster needs assessment is inadequate. Ørner, Kent, Pfefferbaum, Raphael, and Watson (Chapter 7) emphasize that any systemic approach to planning must consider basic contextual factors that will affect success; they insist that the most effective early interventions are those that recognize and promote individual and group competencies among survivors. Pastel and Ritchie (Chapter 16), when discussing how to mitigate psychological reactions following chemical, biological, radiological, and nuclear events, emphasize public health approaches that include preparation, risk communication, and the importance of establishing separate stress centers at hospitals to triage and diagnose the surge of people reporting posttraumatic distress and somatic complaints. Leskin, Huleatt, Herrmann, LaDue, and Gusman (Chapter 14), recounting the establishment of post-9/11 family assistance centers in New York City and near the Pentagon, emphasize the necessity for community planning, coordination, training, collaboration, cooperation, and working with the media. Norris and Alegría (Chapter 17) admonish us to ensure that cultural competence among caregivers be optimized and that cultural sensitivity inform the design and implementation of postdisaster interventions. And Norris and colleagues (Chapter 18), drawing on their post-9/11 New York case study, provide a systems perspective on a public mental health response that focuses on preparation, systemic response, coordination, training, caring for providers, and serving the consumer.

INDIVIDUAL CARE

The psychological and behavioral consequences of disasters and mass violence include behavior change, distress symptoms, and, for some, psychiatric illness (for review, see Norris et al., 1999, 2002). In the immediate aftermath of a disaster or mass violence, individuals, whether as part of a community or a workplace site, may respond in adaptive, effective ways or they may make fear-based decisions, resulting in unhelpful behaviors. The adaptive capacities of individuals and groups within a community are variable and need to be understood before a crisis in order to effectively identify postevent needs (Ursano & Norwood, 2003). Acute posttraumatic reactions such as hypervigilance and difficulty sleeping are prominent early on. Recovery is rapid for most, slower for others, and may not occur for some people who develop chronic problems lasting 6 months or more. Individuals exposed to terrorism and other disasters have been found to increase their use of alcohol, tobacco, and other drugs, especially those with preexisting alcohol abuse or other psychiatric difficulties (Galea et al., 2002; North et al., 1999; Pfefferbaum & Doughty, 2001; Ursano et al., 2003b; Vlahov et al., 2002).

We do not know the course of these behavioral changes. In Manhattan, 1–2 months after 9/11, residents south of 110th Street reported increased substance use (alcohol, cigarettes, or marijuana) that remained the same 6 months later: 24.6% reported increased alcohol use; 9.7% showed increased cigarette smoking; 3.2% increased use of marijuana (Vlahov et al., 2002).

Interventions are dependent on the rapid, effective, and sustained mobilization of resources. Knowledge of a community's resilience and vulnerability factors before a disaster or terrorist event, as well as understanding the psychological responses to such an event, enables leaders and medical experts to talk to the public, promoting resilient healthy behaviors, sustaining the social fabric of the community, and facilitating recovery (Institute of Medicine, 2003).

After a disaster or mass violence event those who are injured are in need of mental health care (Wain, Grammer, Stasinos, & DeBoer, Chapter 15). In addition, traditional mental health problems may appear as physical health problems (Rundell, 2003). In a new infectious outbreak by a new agent, the only available interventions will be behavioral interventions, such as quarantine and protective behaviors, until new vaccination and treatments can be developed. In the face of fears of contamination, multiple unexplained physical symptoms may be the presentation of distress in the outpatient and emergency setting. Belief in exposure, rather than actual exposure, leads to health care seeking (Stuart, Ursano, Fullerton, Norwood, & Murray, 2003). Health education and risk communication can minimize the numbers seeking health care and strengthen the public health response in both the medical and mental health arena (Tucker, 1997).

Behavior changes (e.g. altered smoking behaviors, travel behaviors, and willingness to leave home), distress symptoms, and illness vary after disasters and mass violence, depending on many factors including the characteristics of the event and the degree of exposure. Bereavement is an inevitable component of disasters (Prigerson et al., 1999). Bereavement begins early after a loss both as an individual and as a community event, but often the community moves onward before the individuals themselves are recovered. Bereavement is complicated by ongoing identification of remains, the complexity of possible financial remuneration for victims, and the criminal justice system, often experienced by victims as circuitous and puzzling.

We have focused on the alleviation of posttraumatic distress among individuals as immediate, intermediate, and long-term interventions. There has actually been more progress in this conceptual thinking rather than in the public mental health arena. We now understand the advisability of psychological first aid rather than psychological debriefing during the immediate aftermath. (Young, Chapter 8). The efficacy of brief CBT interventions during the intermediate phase has good empirical support (Bryant & Litz, Chapter 9). A variety of CBT and pharmacological treatments for PTSD, bereavement, and traumatic grief have been successfully tested (Raphael & Wooding, Chapter 10). As usual progress on evidence-based treatments for children and adolescents has lagged far behind although there have also been promising developments in that area (Cohen, Mannarino, Gibson, Cozza, & Murray, Chapter 13). This is only a beginning, however, because as Shalev (Chapter 6) cautions, we must do a better job developing a theoretical context within which to conceptualize acute posttraumatic reactions and early interventions designed to foster recovery and ameliorate distress. He believes that the key to such a process is to distinguish stress theory from a theory of psychological trauma. Finally, Litz and Gibson (Chapter 20) identify key challenges to research in this field.

FORGOTTEN CARE NEEDS

First responders following a terrorist attack include not only the traditional firefighters, police, and military but also health care providers. Because the medical community is a "first responder" particularly in a bioterrorist attack, a broad-based educational plan for health care providers and organizations is essential. Hospital response plans must incorporate mental health and behavioral interventions at all levels. Medical care for infected/injured people as well as for those people who fear they were infected must be based on proven psychological and behavioral principles (Joint Commission on Accreditation of Health Care Organizations, 2003).

Children are at risk both from their own exposure and that of their caregivers. Perhaps the most common response in Western cultures to a disaster is to pull the family in closer and keep children home. Although this offers increased family support, it may also decrease the availability of an important part of children's recovery process, the school system, and interaction with friends. The effect of depression and PTSD in caregivers on their children is only beginning to be examined but certainly includes less awareness of the child's needs and therefore altered parenting. Children with direct exposures or who have had a caregiver killed or injured have special needs. School health care programs and teacher training for identifying children in need are important parts of the public health care of children of all ages. Teaching psychological first aid, ("buddy care") to "friends" can also facilitate identification of those children, particularly adolescents, who may be less likely to let adults know of their or their family's distress.

The elderly may have substantial practical needs that go unaddressed when social services disappear. From finding a new grocery store to obtaining medication or transportation for renal dialysis, social service outreach is critical for this group. Similarly, for all chronic medical illnesses, including chronic mental illness, loss of critically important medications and loss of the care provider availability can greatly increase morbidity and mortality.

FUTURE DIRECTIONS

An enhanced public health infrastructure for disaster mental health requires the means to quickly detect, track, and monitor disaster-related psychological and behavioral casualties. This entails enhancing the medical incident management infrastructure through standardizing and expanding the manner in which certain illnesses and symptoms are described, recorded, and tracked. In addition, the system requires improved ability to share this information quickly and efficiently both locally and across the nation. Knowledge of a community's resilience and vulnerability factors before a disaster or terrorist event, as well as understanding the psychological responses to such an event, enables leaders and medical experts to talk to the public, promoting resilient healthy behaviors, sustaining the social fabric of the community, and facilitating recovery (Institute of Medicine, 2003).

The knowledge base for interventions to alleviate distress, behavioral changes, and illness draws from a variety of disciplines, including sociology, risk communication, education, and disaster mental health to provide guidance to community leaders, local emergency planners, health and mental health planners, and health care providers to develop integrated plans and linked preparations for psychological and behavioral consequences of a disaster or mass violence event (Litz, Gray, Bryant, & Adler, 2002; National Institute of Mental Health, 2002).

The development of specific recommendations for the integration of mental health and public health in responding to a terrorist event is critical (Institute of Medicine, 2003; Joint Commission on Accreditation of Health Care Organizations, 2003; Ursano, Fullerton, & Norwood, 2001, 2002). Preparedness planning is the first of the mental health and behavioral planning needs.

Evidence-based interventions are needed. This includes the need for studies of psychological first aid, early education and support, and leadership behaviors. In addition, critical components of our treatment armamentarium require further knowledge: treatment of acute stress disorder and PTSD and disaster-related depression and increased alcohol use and smoking behaviors. We know little about the course of these disorders in the multiple populations that may be exposed to a disaster. Clinician training to provide appropriate evidence-based care is also needed to ensure the availability of services.

Because we see this book as a stepping-stone between work accomplished to date and future advancement of the field, it is, useful to reconsider our previous report card (Friedman, Ritchie, & Watson, Chapter 1), to see what progress, if any, we have made in recent years.

A number of federal initiatives are underway to develop epidemiological predictive models, population-based surveillance methodologies, and reliable instrumentation procedures to characterize the full range of acute phase reactions and to predict chronicity. The mental health and behavioral consequences of terrorism will be the most significant, long-term, and most costly effects of a terrorist attack. As for theory, conceptual advances in our understanding of both psychological processes and psychobiological mechanisms that mediate acute posttraumatic reactions have begun to inform current research protocols. Intervention research, especially with children, is moving forward to develop and test a variety of treatment approaches that might reduce acute posttraumatic distress and prevent the later development of PTSD, depression, alcohol/drug misuse, and other posttraumatic psychiatric sequelae. Such progress is essential to the development of an evidence-based approach to early intervention that will guide prevention, policy, and practice in the future.

Much of what is spoken of here and needed is still on the drawing board—but it is a start in the right direction. Therefore, we end this book, as it began, with a realistic assessment of the current state-of-the-art determination to close identified gaps in knowledge as soon as possible and hope for the future.

REFERENCES

Flynn, B. W. (2003). *Promoting psychosocial resilience in the face of terrorism.* Briefing for members of the U.S. House of Representatives and their staffs.

Galea, S., Ahern, J., Resnick, H., Kilpatrick, D., Bucuvalas, M., Gold, J., & Vlahov, D. (2002). Psychological sequelae of the September 11 terrorist attacks in New York City. *New England Journal of Medicine, 346,* 982–987.

Holloway, H. C., Norwood, A. E., Fullerton, C. S., Engel, C. C., & Ursano, R. J. (1997). The threat of biological weapons: Prophylaxis and mitigation of psychological and social consequences. *Journal of the American Medical Association, 278,* 425–427.

Institute of Medicine. (2003). *Preparing for the psychological consequences of terrorism: A public health strategy.* Washington DC: National Academies Press.

Joint Commission on Accreditation of Health Care Organizations. (2003). *Health care at the crossroads. Strategies for creating and sustaining community-wide emergency preparedness systems.* Washington, DC: Author.

Litz, B. T., Gray M. J., Bryant, R. A., & Adler, A. B. (2002). Early intervention for trauma: current status and future directions. *Clinical Psychology: Science and Practice, 9,* 112–134.

National Institute of Mental Health. (2002). *Mental health and mass violence: Evidence-based early psychological intervention for victims/survivors of mass violence. A workshop to reach consensus on best practices* (NIH Publication No. 02-5138). Washington, DC: U.S. Government Printing Office. Available online at www.nimh.nih.gov/research/massviolence.pdf

Norris, F. H., Friedman, M. J., Watson, P. J., Byrne, C. M., Diaz, E., & Kaniasty, K. Z. (2002). 60,000 disaster victims speak, Part I. and Part II. An empirical review of the empirical literature: 1981–2001. *Psychiatry, 65,* 207–239.

North, C. S., Nixon, S. J., Shariat, S., Mallonee, S., McMillen, J. C., Spitznagel, E. L., & Smith, E. M. (1999). Psychiatric disorders among survivors of the Oklahoma City bombing. *Journal of the American Medical Association, 282,* 755–762.

Pfefferbaum, B., & Doughty, D. E. (2001). Increased alcohol use in a treatment sample of Oklahoma City bombing victims. *Psychiatry, 64,* 296–303.

Prigerson, H. G., Shear, M. K., Jacobs, S. C., Reynolds, C. F., Maciejewski, P. K., Davidson, J. R., et al. (1999). Consensus criteria for traumatic grief: a preliminary empirical test. *British Journal of Psychiatry, 174,* 67–73.

Rundell, J. R. (2003). A consultation–liaison psychiatry approach to disaster/terrorism victim assessment and management. In R. J. Ursano, C. F. Fullerton, & A. E. Norwood (Eds.), *Terrorism and disaster: Individual and community mental health interventions* (pp. 107–120). Cambridge, UK: Cambridge University Press.

Stuart, J., Ursano, R. J., Fullerton, C. S., Norwood, A. E., & Murray, K. (2003). Belief in exposure to terrorist agents: Reported exposure to nerve/mustard gas by Gulf War Veterans. *Journal of Nervous and Mental Disease, 191*(7), 431–436.

Tucker, J. B. (1997). National health and medical services response to incidents of chemical and biological terrorism. *Journal of the American Medical Association*, *278*, 362–368.

Ursano, R. J., Fullerton, C. S., & Norwood, A. E. (2001). Planning for terrorism: behavioral and mental health responses to weapons of mass destruction and mass disruption. Bethesda, MD: Uniformed Services University of the Health Sciences.

Ursano, R. J., Fullerton, C. S., & Norwood, A. E. (2002). *Responding to terrorism: Individuals and community needs*. Bethesda, MD: Uniformed Services University of the Health Sciences.

Ursano, R. J., Fullerton, C. S., & Norwood, A. E. (2003a). *Terrorism and disaster: Individual and community mental health interventions*. Cambridge, UK: Cambridge University Press.

Ursano, R. J., Fullerton, C. S., & Norwood, A. E. (2003b). Traumatic death in terrorism and disasters: The effects on posttraumatic stress and behavior. In R. J. Ursano, C. F. Fullerton, & A. E. Norwood (Eds.), *Terrorism and disaster: Individual and community mental health interventions* (pp. 308–332). Cambridge, UK: Cambridge University Press.

Ursano, R. J., & Norwood, A. E. (Eds.). (2003). *Trauma and disaster: Responses and management*. Washington, DC: American Psychiatric Association Press.

Vlahov, D., Galea, S., Resnick, H., Boscarino, J. A., Bucuvalas, M., Gold, J., et al. (2002). Increased use of cigarettes, alcohol, and marijuana among Manhattan, New York, residents after the September 11th terrorist attacks. *American Journal of Epidemiology, 155*, 988–996.

Index

Page numbers followed by *f* indicate figure; *t* indicate table.